Malocclusion: Clinical Dentistry

Edited by Philip Chiders

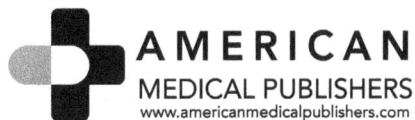

AMERICAN
MEDICAL PUBLISHERS
www.americanmedicalpublishers.com

American Medical Publishers,
41 Flatbush Avenue,
1st Floor, New York,
NY 11217, USA

Visit us on the World Wide Web at:
www.americanmedicalpublishers.com

ISBN: 978-1-63927-055-2

Cataloging-in-Publication Data

Malocclusion : clinical dentistry / edited by Philip Chiders.
    p. cm.
Includes bibliographical references and index.
ISBN 978-1-63927-055-2
1. Malocclusion. 2. Malocclusion--Treatment. 3. Orthodontics. I. Chiders, Philip.
RK523 .M35 2022
617.643--dc23

Table of Contents

Preface

This book was inspired by the evolution of our times; to answer the curiosity of inquisitive minds. Many developments have occurred across the globe in the recent past which has transformed the progress in the field.

Malocclusion refers to the condition when there is misalignment between the teeth of the two dental arches when they come closer to each other as the upper jaw and lower jaw closes. Malocclusions usually don't require treatment until and unless it's very severe. Severe malocclusion is treated with orthodontic treatment. It reduces the risk of tooth decay and helps in relieving excessive pressure on the temporomandibular joint. As per the sagittal relations of teeth and jaws, malocclusions can be classified into three types - class I: neutrocclusion, class II: distocclusion and class III: mesiocclusion. Malocclusion can be caused due to lost teeth, extra teeth, abnormally shaped teeth and impacted teeth. Ill-fitting dental fillings, crowns, appliances, retainers, or braces and misalignment of jaw fractures after a severe injury are some other causes. This book unravels the recent studies in the field of malocclusion. It provides significant information of this discipline to help develop a good understanding of this domain. This book is a resource guide for experts as well as students.

This book was developed from a mere concept to drafts to chapters and finally compiled together as a complete text to benefit the readers across all nations. To ensure the quality of the content we instilled two significant steps in our procedure. The first was to appoint an editorial team that would verify the data and statistics provided in the book and also select the most appropriate and valuable contributions from the plentiful contributions we received from authors worldwide. The next step was to appoint an expert of the topic as the Editor-in-Chief, who would head the project and finally make the necessary amendments and modifications to make the text reader-friendly. I was then commissioned to examine all the material to present the topics in the most comprehensible and productive format.

I would like to take this opportunity to thank all the contributing authors who were supportive enough to contribute their time and knowledge to this project. I also wish to convey my regards to my family who have been extremely supportive during the entire project.

Editor

Cephalometric changes in Class II division 1 patients treated with two maxillary premolars extraction

Marisana Piano Seben[1], Fabricio Pinelli Valarelli[2], Karina Maria Salvatore de Freitas[3],
Rodrigo Hermont Cançado[3], Aristeu Correa Bittencourt Neto[1]

Objective: The purpose of this study was to evaluate the cephalometric alterations in patients with Angle Class II division 1 malocclusion, orthodontically treated with extraction of two maxillary premolars. **Methods:** The sample comprised 68 initial and final lateral cephalograms of 34 patients of both gender (mean initial age of 14.03 years and mean final age of 17.25 years), treated with full fixed appliances and extraction of the first maxillary premolars. In order to evaluate the alterations due the treatment between initial and final phases, the dependent t test was applied to the studied cephalometric variables. **Results:** The dentoskeletal alterations due to extraction of two maxillary premolars in the Class II division 1 malocclusion were: maxillary retrusion, improvement of the maxillomandibular relation, increase of lower anterior face height, retrusion of the maxillary incisors, buccal inclination, protrusion and extrusion of the mandibular incisors, besides the reduction of overjet and overbite. The tissue alterations showed decrease of the facial convexity and retrusion of the upper lip. **Conclusions:** The extraction of two maxillary premolars in Class II division 1 malocclusion promotes dentoskeletal and tissue alterations that contribute to an improvement of the relation between the bone bases and the soft tissue profile.

Keywords: Corrective Orthodontics. Cephalometry. Retrospective studies. Tooth extraction.

[1] MSc in Orthodontics, Inga Dental School, Maringá/PR, Brazil.
[2] Assistant Professor, MSc Program at Inga Dental School, Maringá/PR, Brazil.
[3] Post-doc in Orthodontics, University of Toronto. Assistant Professor, Inga Dental School, Maringá/PR, Brazil.

» The authors report no commercial, proprietary or financial interest in the products or companies described in this article.

Fabrício Pinelli Valarelli
Rua Manoel Pereira Rolla, 12-75 – Apto 503 – Bauru/SP – Brazil
CEP: 17012-190 – E-mail: fabriciovalarelli@uol.com.br

INTRODUCTION

Nowadays, the protocol for Class II treatment with extraction of two maxillary premolars is the second most used protocol of extraction in orthodontic treatments (20.2%), being only inferior to the protocol of extraction of the four first premolars (42.9%). It is especially recommended when there is no cephalometric discrepancy and severe crowding on the lower arch. This treatment protocol favors the patient regarding to collaboration on the use of anchorage reinforcement, once it will be required a shorter period of use of such appliances.[12]

Some authors speculate that dental extractions may cause some problems to the patient such as: Temporomandibular disorder,[2,6] lack of treatment stability,[10,17] and unwanted profile flattening, which would compromise the patient's esthetics by the end of the treatment.[22,23] However, other authors point the numerous favorable results obtained on treatment with extraction of two upper premolars with good occlusal stability in the long term[13,14] and without direct influence on the flattening of the patient's profile.[11,12,15]

The cephalometric alterations promoted by this treatment protocol and often mentioned in literature are: Increase of nasolabial angle, retraction of upper lip, reduction of profile convexity and retraction with verticalization of upper incisors,[24-27] i.e., the orthodontic treatment with extractions of maxillary premolars has little influence in relation to skeletal changes and provides greater dental and profile alterations.

Nevertheless, some doubts and questioning still persist about the real impact of extraction of upper premolars on skeletal, dentoalveolar and tissue components of patients with Class II malocclusion. Before that, this work aims to assess the cephalometric, dentoalveolar and tissue alterations in patients with Angle Class II malocclusion, division 1, orthodontically treated with extraction of two maxillary premolars.

MATERIAL AND METHODS
Material

The sample used in this retrospective study consisted of 68 initial and final teleradiographs of 34 patients (15 females, 19 males, mean age of 14.03 years ± 2.65, with amplitude of 10.83 to 25.83) treated on the course of specialization in Orthodontics at Uningá, Bauru, for a mean period of 3.21 ± 1.43 years, with amplitude of 1.25 to 7.83 and finished the orthodontic treatment with a final mean age of 17.25 ± 2.59 years, with amplitude of 13.49 to 28.24.

The criteria for inclusion of patients in the selected sample was based on presence of the following characteristics: Angle Class II malocclusion division 1 with molar relation of at least ½ Class II (cusp-to-cusp relation), absence of crowding or with mild crowding, presence of all permanent teeth erupted until the first premolars, overjet of at least 5 mm[4,25] and orthodontically treated with extractions of upper first premolars. Patients with Class II malocclusion subdivision were excluded from the sample.

Patients in the sample were treated with Edgewise technique braces, slot 0.022 x 0.028-in. The most used sequence of alignment and leveling was 0.015-in twist-flex or 0.014-in NiTi at the beginning of treatment, followed by arches 0.016, 0.018 and 0.020-in of stainless steel. For the anterior superior retraction phase it was used the arch 0.019 x 0.025-in of stainless steel and some patients used during this phase intermaxillary elastics of Class II and/or headgear for anchorage reinforcement. By the end of active treatment, the patients used a Hawley plate on the upper arch and a retainer 3 x 3 attached on the lower arch.

Methods

Lateral teleradiographs were obtained from all patients at the beginning (T_1) and end (T_2) of the orthodontic treatment. These teleradiographies were obtained in 4 different radiographic units that presented magnification factors ranging from 6 to 9.8%.

The teleradiographies were scanned with flatbed scanner *Microtek ScanMaker i800* (9600 x 4800 dpi, from *Microtek International, Inc., Carson, CA, USA*) and attached to a microcomputer Pentium. The images were transferred to *Dolphin Imaging Premium* 10.5 (*Dolphin Imaging & Management Solutions, Chatsworth, CA, USA*) through which it were unmarked the points by the same examiner and it were performed the measurements of skeletal, dental and tissue measures (Figs 1, 2, and 3).

Skeletal cephalometric measures

» SNA (°): Angle formed by lines SN and NA. It indicates the sagittal relation of the maxilla in relation to the skull base.

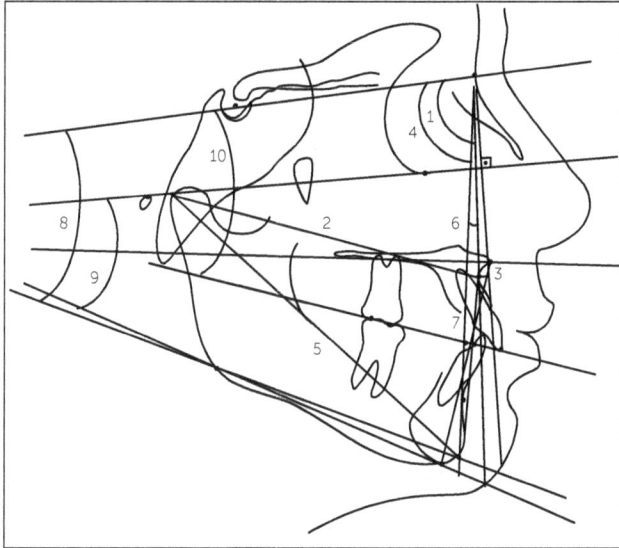

Figure 1 - Skeletal cephalometric measures: 1) SNA (°); 2) Co-A (mm); 3) A-Nperp (mm); 4) SNB (°); 5) Co-Gn (mm); 6) ANB (°); 7) AIFH (mm); 8) SN-GoGn (°); 9) FMA (°); 10) SN.Ocl (°).

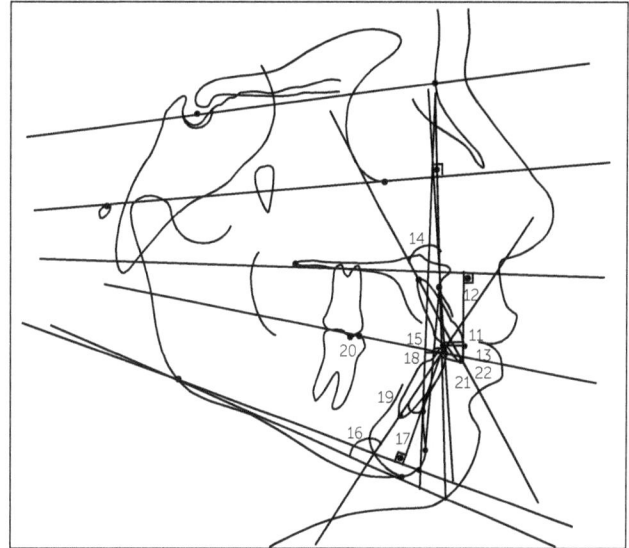

Figure 2 - Dental cephalometric measures: 11) 1-Aperp (mm); 12) 1-PP (mm); 13) 1-NA (mm); 14) 1.NA (°); 15) 1-AP (mm); 16) IMPA (°); 17) 1-GoGn (mm); 18) 1-NB (mm); 19) 1.NB (°); 20) Molar relation (mm); 21) Overbite (mm); 22) Overjet (mm).

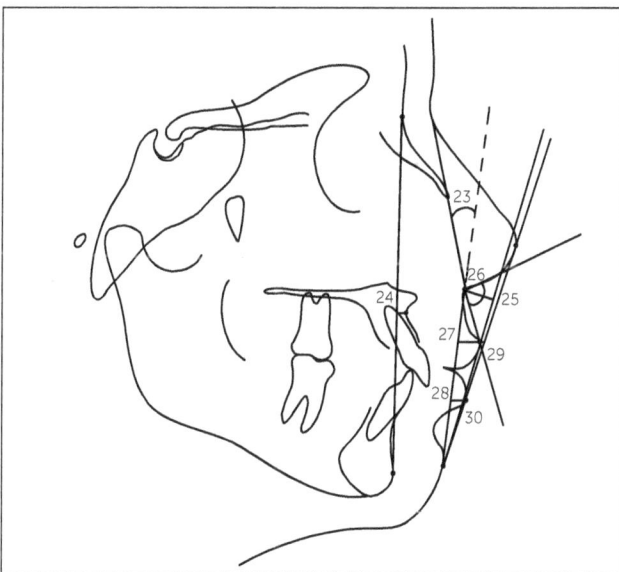

Figure 3 - Tissue cephalometric measures: 23) G'.Sn.Pog' (°); 24) A-NPog (mm); 25) Sn-H (mm); 26) ANL (°); 27) UL-SnPog (mm); 28) LL-SnPog (mm); 29) UL-E (mm); 30) LL-E (mm).

» Co-A (mm): Distance between the points Condyle and A. It represents the effective length of the mean face (maxilla).

» A-Nperp (mm): Distance between the point A and the line N perpendicular to Frankfurt's plane. It defines the sagittal position of the maxilla.

» SNB (°): Angle formed by lines SN and NB. It indicates the sagittal relation of the mandible in relation to the skull base.

» Co-Gn (mm): Distance between the points Condyle and Gnathion. It defines the effective mandibular length.

» ANB (°): Angle between the lines NA and NB. It represents the degree of sagittal discrepancy between maxilla and mandible.

» SN.GoGN (°): Defines the orientation of facial growth pattern.

» FMA (°): Angle formed by Frankfurt's and mandibular planes.

» OP.SN (°): Angle formed between the line SN and the occlusal plane. It relates the occlusal plane inclination to the skull base.

» AIFH (mm): Distance between the points anterior nasal spine and mentalis. It indicates the height of the lower third of the face.

Dental cephalometric measures

» 1-Aperp (mm): Distance from the vestibular portion of the upper central incisor to the line A-perp.

» 1-PP (mm): Distance between the incisal edge of the upper central incisor and the palatal plane perpendicularly measured. It relates the vertical positioning of the upper incisor to the maxilla.

» 1-NA (mm): Distance between the anterior point of the crown of upper central incisor and the line NA. It relates the sagittal position of upper incisor in relation to maxilla and to Nasion.

» 1.NA (°): Angle between the long axis of upper central incisor and line NA. It defines the degree of inclination of the central incisor in relation to maxilla and Nasion.

» 1-APog (mm): Distance from the incisal edge of lower incisor to line Apog.

» IMPA (°): Angle between the long axis of lower central incisor and the mandibular plane GoMe. It indicates the inclination of this tooth in relation to the mandible.

» 1-GoGn (mm): Distance from incisal edge of lower incisor to mandibular plane GoGn, measured perpendicularly to this plane.

» 1-NB (mm): Distance between the anterior point of the crown of lower central incisor and line NB. It relates the sagittal position of lower incisor in relation to mandible and Nasion.

» 1.NB (°): Angle between the long axis of lower incisor and line NB. It relates the inclination of this tooth to the mandible and Nasion.

» Molar relation (mm): Distance between the mesial cusp of upper and lower first premolars perpendicularly projected on the occlusal plane.

» Overbite (mm): Distance between the incisal edges of upper and lower central incisors measured perpendicularly to the occlusal plane.

» Overjet (mm): Distance between the incisal edges of upper and lower central incisors perpendicularly projected to the occlusal plane.

Tissue profile

» UL-SnPog (mm): Distance from the upper lip to line Subnasal Pogonion.

» LL-SnPog (mm): Distance from the lower lip to line Subnasal Pogonion.

» UL-E (mm): Distance from the upper lip to line Pronasal Pogonion.

» LL-E (mm): Distance from the lower lip to line Pronasal Pogonion.

» ANL - nasolabial angle: Formed by lines columella to Subnasal and from Subnasal to upper lip.

» G'.Sn.Pog' (°): Facial convexity angle. It's formed by lines tissue glabella to Subnasal and from Subnasal to tissue Pogonion.

» A-NPog (mm): Distance from point A to line Nasion to the Pogonion.

» Sn-H (mm): Shortest distance from point Subnasal to line H of Holdaway (Pogonion to upper lip).

For evaluation of intraexaminer error, 20 teleradiographs randomly selected were scanned and measured again after a minimum interval of 4 weeks. For evaluation of systematic error, it was applied the dependent t test and the magnitude of random error was calculated by Dahlberg's formula.

It was performed the evaluation of data normality through Kolmogorov-Smirnov test. The results showed that all variables presented normal distribution. This way, it was applied the dependent t test on the studied cephalometric variables to verify alterations due treatment between initial (T_1) and final (T_2) phases. The statistical analysis was performed with Statistica for Windows (Statistica for Windows - Release 7.0 - Copyright Statsoft, Inc. 2005). It were considered statistically significant the results with p value of $p < 0.05$.

RESULTS

Among the 30 studied cephalometric variables, only 3 presented significant systematic error (FMA, 1-PP and IMPA). The magnitude of random errors ranged from 0.22 (overjet) to 2.12 (IMPA). The results are displayed on Table 1.

Patients with Class II malocclusion, division 1, treated with extraction of two upper premolars presented the following cephalometric alterations: maxillary retrusion in relation to the skull base, increase on the mandibular length and anterior inferior facial height (AIFH), improvement on the maxillomandibular relation, upper incisors retrusion, vestibularization and protrusion of the lower dentoalveolar component, improvement on molar relation, reduction of overbite and overjet, reduction of facial convexity and upper lip retrusion.

DISCUSSION

Evaluating the results found in this work it is possible to establish and assess the alterations caused on dentoskeletal and tissue components due the extraction of upper first premolars, in Class II division 1 patients.

Regarding the maxillary component, the maxilla experienced a significant retrusion noticed by the statistically significant reduction of variables SNA and A-NPerp (Table 1). The reduction of these variables occurred due the necessity of correction of Class II relation of canines and overjet normalization, due the use of intermaxillary elastic and EOA as anchorage reinforcement.

Table 1 - Results of dependent t test comparing initial phase (T₁) and final phase (T₂) of treatment.

Variables	Initial (T₁) Mean ± SD	Final (T₂) Mean ± SD	Difference (T₂-T₁)	p
Maxillary component				
SNA (degrees)	75.66 ± 4.73	74.15 ± 3.96	-1.51	**0.017***
Co-A (mm)	84.21 ± 5.12	85.00 ± 5.00	0.78	0.084
A-Nperp (mm)	0.19 ± 3.46	-1.06 ± 3.60	-1.26	**0.024***
Mandibular component				
SNB (degrees)	70.79 ± 3.99	70.55 ± 3.57	-0.24	0.569
Co-Gn (mm)	107.50 ± 6.39	111.55 ± 5.95	4.05	**0.000***
Maxillomandibular relation				
ANB (degrees)	4.87 ± 2.58	3.61 ± 2.20	-1.27	**0.001***
Vertical component				
SN.GoGn (degrees)	30.55 ± 5.59	30.90 ± 5.61	0.35	0.338
FMA (degrees)	24.44 ± 4.21	24.54 ± 4.49	0.10	0.777
OP.SN (degrees)	11.41 ± 4.12	12.49 ± 4.21	1.08	0.016
AIFH (mm)	62.60 ± 4.39	64.93 ± 4.56	2.33	**0.000***
Upper dentoalveolar component				
1-Aperp (mm)	7.68 ± 2.23	5.22 ± 2.18	-2.45	**0.000***
1-PP (mm)	26.65 ± 2.37	26.98 ± 2.60	0.33	0.373
1-NA (mm)	6.49 ± 3.17	4.48 ± 2.67	-2.02	**0.001***
1.NA (degrees)	25.23 ± 6.76	22.76 ± 5.19	-2.47	0.080
Lower dentoalveolar component				
1-APog (mm)	1.91 ± 1.81	3.81 ± 1.76	1.89	**0.000***
IMPA (degrees)	86.21 ± 5.36	89.65 ± 6.38	3.43	**0.001***
1-GoGn (mm)	36.40 ± 2.74	37.36 ± 2.30	0.96	**0.016***
1-NB (mm)	5.93 ± 1.79	7.22 ± 1.57	1.28	**0.000***
1.NB (degrees)	24.60 ± 4.16	28.13 ± 5.04	3.52	**0.000***
Dental relations				
Molar relation	2.89 ± 1.32	4.45 ± 0.83	1.56	**0.000***
Overbite	2.90 ± 2.92	1.78 ± 1.12	-1.13	**0.011***
Overjet	7.63 ± 1.59	2.32 ± 0.84	-5.31	**0.000***
Tissue profile				
UL-SnPog (mm)	5.60 ± 1.55	4.35 ± 1.45	-1.25	**0.000***
LL-SnPog (mm)	3.81 ± 1.80	3.62 ± 1.83	-0.19	0.468
UL-E (mm)	-0.37 ± 2.20	-2.65 ± 2.12	-2.28	**0.000***
LL-E (mm)	0.77 ± 2.09	-0.07 ± 2.24	-0.85	**0.004***
ANL (degrees)	97.57 ± 7.06	99.64 ± 7.51	2.07	0.072
G'.Sn.Pog' (degrees)	18.48 ± 4.73	16.96 ± 4.80	-1.52	**0.000***
A-NPog (mm)	0.19 ± 3.46	-1.06 ± 3.60	-1.26	**0.024***
Sn-H (mm)	7.33 ± 2.01	5.74 ± 1.83	-1.59	**0.000***

*Statistically significant difference for p < 0.05.

It is notable that the antero-superior teeth retraction may affect the positioning of point A in relation to the skull base.[4,25]

Scott Conley and Jernigan[25] also observed a statistically significant reduction of the variable A-Nperp in cases treated with extraction of two upper premolars. However, Rains and Nanda[24] did not find significant alterations on point A. But in this study the variable Co-A did not present statistically significant alteration. It is speculated that there was no alteration due the fact that most patients were in growth stage, which disguised the retraction experienced by point A.

On the mandibular component, it was evidenced a significant increase of the mandible effective length (Co-Gn)

(Table 1). This was expected since the evaluated patients in this research were in growth stage, as explained above. In this study, this increase was greater than the expected being corroborated by some authors that reported similar results in literature. [4,7,23]

On the maxillomandibular relation, there was a significant alteration of the anteroposterior skeletal discrepancy, shown by the reduction of angle ANB (Table 1). This alteration was expected because the orthodontic treatment aimed the correction of Class II malocclusion and of the overjet initially increased by upper incisors retraction. Besides, the potential of mandibular growth on this age group helps the reduction of angle ANB. [25,26] Tadic and Woods[26] observed that the greater the overjet at the beginning of treatment, greater the probability of reduction of angle ANB, in cases treated with extraction of two upper premolars. Oliveira et al[20] observed that there was improvement on the anteroposterior maxillomandibular relation, shown by the reduction of ANB. Scott Conley and Jernigan[25] also observed a statistically significant reduction of the angle ANB contributing for an improvement of the existent relation between dental arches, and a significant increase of AIFH as occurred in the present study.

In the work by Chua, Lim and Lubit[5] it was found an increase of AIFH associated to a clockwise rotation of the mandible only in cases treated without dental extractions, while in treatments with extractions it was not observed any significant alteration on AIFH. Differently from the findings of these authors, most works found in literature are in agreement with the present study, in which AIFH presented a statistically significant increase during treatment. It is believed that the responsible for this alteration was the potential growth still present in patients and the orthodontic mechanics that used intermaxillary elastics during closing of spaces after extractions. Some authors observed that the increase of the lower third of the face is related to age and growth potential of the patients, besides the use of intermaxillary elastics.[19] On the work by Oliveira et al[20] the AIFH increased due the compensatory extrusion of molars during anterior retraction phase. Now Merrifield and Cross[19] emphasized that any mechanics that promote dental extrusion causes the increase of AIFH.

On the variables related to growth pattern, both SN.GoGn and FMA did not present statistically significant alterations between initial and final phases of treatment (Table 1). Scott Conley and Jernigan[25] also did not find significant alterations in relation to the change on growth pattern in cases treated with extraction of two premolars. The variable OP.SN presented a statistically significant increase during treatment. This increase does not mean in alteration of growth pattern impressing a vertical characteristic for the patients, because the other variables of this component did not present significant alteration. It is believed that the alterations observed on the variable OP.SN are related to dentoalveolar changes, for instance, the curve of Spee flattening, occurred during the treatment of patients. At the beginning of treatment, it is frequently observed an accented extrusion of lower incisors due to increased overjet.[18,28] During treatment there was flattening of curve of Spee, which led to a clockwise rotation of the occlusal plane. This effect was enough to promote statistically significant change of variable OP.SN being only a reflex of dental alterations and not skeletal since the other variables, SN.GoGn and FMA, that characterize the component, did not present statistically significant changes.

The study by Oliveira et al[20] showed compensatory extrusion of molars during retraction phase in cases with extraction of four premolars, and also did not report statistically significant differences on variables SN.GoGn and SN.GoMe that characterized the growth pattern.

On the upper alveolar component, the upper incisors presented a statistically significant retrusion (1-Aperp, 1-NA). There was no significant alteration of upper incisors on the vertical direction or in relation to inclination (1-PP and 1.NA, respectively) (Table 1). According to several authors, the skeletal effects of the treatment were more evident on the maxilla and on the superior teeth than in the mandible or lower teeth, in cases treated with extraction of two upper premolars.[25,27]

Tadic and Woods[26] verified a significant increase on the inclination of upper incisors related to line N-A also in cases with extraction of two upper premolars and observed that the greater the overjet at the beginning of treatment, greater the probability of reduction of upper incisors inclination, and that the greater the reduction on angle ANB, smaller the necessity of reduction of upper incisors inclination. In this work there was no significant difference between the inclination of upper incisors at the beginning and end of treatment, which differs from most works with extraction of two premolars. It can be asserted that there is a tendency of these teeth to obtain a more palatine inclination after the anterior retraction because the numeric value was reduced, but with no statistical significance.

Paiva et al[21] also in cases treated with extraction of 4 premolars reported a statistically significant reduction of linear values (1-NA), however the reduction on angular values (1.NA), was not statistically significant, which is in agreement with the findings in this study.

On the lower dentoalveolar component, all variables related to lower incisors experienced statistically significant alteration (Table 1). It was verified a protrusion, vestibularization and extrusion of lower incisors (1-APog, IMPA, 1-GoGn, 1-NB, 1.NB). This can be explained by the use of intermaxillary elastics of Class II that were necessary in most patients at final stage. Side effects on the inclination of incisors in patients treated with intermaxillary elastics are widely reported in literature, confirming this supposition.[19] On the other hand, Scott Conley and Jernigan[25] did not find statistically significant alterations on IMPA.

By evaluating the dental relations, it was observed a reduction of the value of molar relation, pointing the increase of Class II molar relation, which was expected, for only two upper premolars were extracted, and the cases would be finished with a full Class II molar relation in both sides (Table 1). It was observed a significant improvement on the overbite which was also already expected, for the deep overbite was corrected during treatment with the use of reverse curve wires on the lower arch and accentuated on the upper arch, including during the anterior retraction (Table 1). The overjet reduced significantly with the treatment, which was also expected, because it was taken as criteria for inclusion on the sample that the patients presented an overjet of at least 5 mm and finished the treatment with the malocclusion corrected with canines in Class I relation and normalized overjet (Table 1).

Also on the evaluation of tissue profile results, the data presented an upper lip retrusion, verified on measures UL-SnPog, A-NPog, UL-E, and a lower lip retrusion on measure LL-E, however the variable LL-SnPog did not present statistically significant difference despite presenting a tendency to reduction in its value which shows a tendency to lower lip retrusion,

contradicting the expected lower lip protrusion due to vestibularization and protrusion verified on lower incisors (Table 1). These results are in agreement with the works presented in literature.[25,27] Scott Conley and Jernigan[25] also found an unexpected result. They assigned this reduction on the lower lip projection to the presence of an everted lower lip, because with a deep overbite, an accentuated overjet and a Class II dental relation, the lower lip may be artificially kept in a more protruded position trapped in the space between lower and upper incisors and after the upper incisors retraction, returns to its normal position.

Some authors that evaluated cases with extraction of two upper premolars, realized that according to the treatment protocol used, the lip thickness at the beginning of treatment, the vertical control and variety of facial patterns, the lips may be affected by dental moves on the anteroposterior direction, however the magnitude of this alterations is of difficult predictability.[26,27]

Several authors did not find significant differences on the alterations of soft tissue between groups treated with extraction of four premolars and without extractions[7,30] while other authors observed a tissue profile retrusion.[1,3,4]

Considering that a retraction of upper incisors necessarily imply in a retrusion of the upper lip,[30] it is known that the muscle-skeletal-functional complex of the upper lip contributes for the variability observed on alterations of upper lip with the treatment protocol with premolars extractions.[29]

In this work the nasolabial angle did not present statistically significant alteration (Table 1). Despite the upper teeth retraction suggests that occurs an increase of the nasolabial angle, this result was not observed.

Some authors assign this result to nasal growth, occurring a down inclination of the columella and the pronasal, reducing the nasolabial angle. Theses authors assert that the nasolabial angle is formed by soft tissue (pronasal) and cartilage (columella), which continues to grow forth as well as the soft tissue of the upper lip and observed that only a small statistically insignificant change occurred of nasal base retraction (subnasal), therefore, if the projection of the upper lip tends to reduce, while the base nasal projection remains the same, the nasolabial angle must become more obtuse.[1,7,30]

Kocadereli[16] and Uehara et al[28] observed mean values statistically equal of the nasolabial angle both for patients that did not experience dental extraction and those who were submitted to extractions of four premolars. Tadic and Woods[26] also did not find statistically significant alteration of the nasolabial angle in patients treated with extraction of upper first premolars.

However, Freitas et al[8] observed an increase of the nasolabial angle in cases treated with extraction of four premolars in a proportion of increase of nasolabial angle in 1,49° for each millimeter of retraction on upper teeth which also was confirmed by other authors.[27] Scott Conley and Jernigan[25] also found statistically significant alterations of the nasolabial angle which had an increase of 6.38°.

Erdinç et al[7] observed that the nasolabial angle reduced significantly in groups treated with extraction of four premolars and in groups without extractions these alterations were insignificant.

Despite the generalized idea that extractions cause an increase of the nasolabial angle, the results from this work are in agreement with latest conclusions of works mentioned above.

CLINICAL CONSIDERATIONS

The obtained results showed that profile alterations occur as effect of orthodontic treatment. However, each patient must be individually analyzed so the professional can plan the treatment and instruct the patient about these aspects. Concomitantly, it allows the clinician a greater predictability of possible alterations that the treatment will cause and thus increase the percentage of success in this type of treatment and the patient's satisfaction.

The lower lip retrusion is an essential data when planning the treatment and its positioning must be evaluated in the beginning of treatment and verified if it is affected by the positioning of upper incisors, for this will lead to lower lip retrusion and the patient must be aware. Generally this detail go unnoticed by the clinician, for he only reports the upper lip retrusion due the chosen treatment does not include extraction on the lower arch.

CONCLUSION

Based on the evaluated sample and the used methodology, the alterations caused by extraction of two premolars on Class II division 1 malocclusion were:

» Maxillary retrusion, improvement of the maxillomandibular relation, increase of the anteroinferior facial height, upper incisors retrusion, vestibularization, protrusion and extrusion of lower incisors, besides the reduction of overbite and overjet.

» The profile alterations were: Reduction of the facial convexity and upper lip retrusion.

REFERENCES

1. Basciftci FA, Uysal T, Buyukerkmen A, Demir A. The influence of extraction treatment on Holdaway soft-tissue measurements. Angle Orthod. 2004;74(2):167-73.
2. Bowbeer GR. The 6th key to facial beauty and TMJ health. Funct Orthod. 1987;4(4):10-11, 13-15.
3. Bowman SJ. More than lip service: facial esthetics in orthodontics. J Am Dent Assoc. 1999;130(8):1173-81.
4. Bravo LA, Canut JA, Pascual A, Bravo B. Comparison of the changes in facial profile after orthodontic treatment, with and without extractions. Br J Orthod. 1997;24(1):25-34.
5. Chua AL, Lim JY, Lubit EC. The effects of extraction versus nonextraction orthodontic treatment on the growth of the lower anterior face height. Am J Orthod Dentofacial Orthop. 1993;104(4):361-8.
6. Eirew HL. An orthodontic challenge. Int J Orthod. 1976;14(4):21-5.
7. Erdinc AE, Nanda RS, Dandajena TC. Profile changes of patients treated with and without premolar extractions. Am J Orthod Dentofacial Orthop. 2007;132(3):324-31.
8. Freitas MR, Henriques JFC, Pinzan A, Janson GRP, Siqueira VCV. Estudo longitudinal das alterações do ângulo naso-labial, em jovens com Classe II, 1ª divisão, que se submeteram ao tratamento ortodôntico corretivo. Ortodontia. 1999;32(1):8-16.
9. Gottlieb EL, Nelson AH, Vogels DS 3rd. 1990 JCO study of orthodontic diagnosis and treatment procedures. 1. Results and trends. J Clin Orthod. 1991;25(3):145-56.
10. Graber T, Vanarsdall R Jr. Ortodontia: princípios e técnicas atuais. 3a ed. Rio de Janeiro: Guanabara Koogan; 2000.
11. Janson G, Barros SE, de Freitas MR, Henriques JF, Pinzan A. Class II treatment efficiency in maxillary premolar extraction and nonextraction protocols. Am J Orthod Dentofacial Orthop. 2007;132(4):490-8.
12. Janson G, Brambilla Ada C, Henriques JF, de Freitas MR, Neves LS. Class II treatment success rate in 2- and 4-premolar extraction protocols. Am J Orthod Dentofacial Orthop. 2004;125(4):472-9.
13. Janson G, Camardella LT, Araki JD, de Freitas MR, Pinzan A. Treatment stability in patients with Class II malocclusion treated with 2 maxillary premolar extractions or without extractions. Am J Orthod Dentofacial Orthop. 2010;138(1):16-22.
14. Janson G, Leon-Salazar V, Leon-Salazar R, Janson M, de Freitas MR. Long-term stability of Class II malocclusion treated with 2- and 4-premolar extraction protocols. Am J Orthod Dentofacial Orthop. 2009;136(2):154.e1-10; discussion 154-5.
15. Janson G, Maria FR, Barros SE, Freitas MR, Henriques JF. Orthodontic treatment time in 2- and 4-premolar-extraction protocols. Am J Orthod Dentofacial Orthop. 2006;129(5):666-71.
16. Kocadereli I. Changes in soft tissue profile after orthodontic treatment with and without extractions. Am J Orthod Dentofacial Orthop. 2002;122(1):67-72.
17. Mailankody J. Enigma of Class II molar finishing. Am J Orthod Dentofacial Orthop. 2004;126(6):a15-16; author reply a16-17.

18. McNamara JA Jr. Components of class II malocclusion in children 8-10 years of age. Angle Orthod. 1981;51(3):177-202.

19. Merrifield LL, Cross JJ. Directional forces. Am J Orthod. 1970;57(5):435-64.

20. Oliveira GF, Almeida MR, Almeida RR, Ramos al Alterações dentoesqueléticas e do perfil facial em pacientes tratados ortodonticamente com extração de quatro primeiros pré-molares. Rev Dent Press Ortod Ortop Facial. 2008;13(2):105-14.

21. Paiva J, Rino Neto J, Batista K. Análise do lábio superior após o tratamento ortodôntico. Ortodontia. 2004;37(2):8-13.

22. Proffit WR. Forty-year review of extraction frequencies at a university orthodontic clinic. Angle Orthod. 1994;64(6):407-14.

23. Proffit WR, Phillips C, Tulloch JF, Medland PH. Surgical versus orthodontic correction of skeletal Class II malocclusion in adolescents: effects and indications. Int J Adult Orthodon Orthognath Surg. 1992;7(4):209-20.

24. Rains MD, Nanda R. Soft-tissue changes associated with maxillary incisor retraction. Am J Orthod. 1982;81(6):481-8.

25. Scott Conley R, Jernigan C. Soft tissue changes after upper premolar extraction in Class II camouflage therapy. Angle Orthod. 2006;76(1):59-65.

26. Tadic N, Woods MG. Incisal and soft tissue effects of maxillary premolar extraction in Class II treatment. Angle Orthod. 2007;77(5):808-16.

27. Talass MF, Talass L, Baker RC. Soft-tissue profile changes resulting from retraction of maxillary incisors. Am J Orthod Dentofacial Orthop. 1987;91(5):385-94.

28. Uehara SY, et al Perfil facial após tratamento de Classe II-1 com ou sem extrações. RGO: Rev Gaúch Odontol. 2007;55(1):61-8.

29. Waldman BH. Change in lip contour with maxillary incisor retraction. Angle Orthod. 1982;52(2):129-34.

30. Zierhut EC, Joondeph DR, Artun J, Little RM. Long-term profile changes associated with successfully treated extraction and nonextraction Class II division 1 malocclusions. Angle Orthod. 2000;70(3):208-19.

2

Stability of molar relationship after non-extraction Class II malocclusion treatment

Darwin Vaz de Lima[1], Karina Maria Salvatore de Freitas[2], Marcos Roberto de Freitas[3],
Guilherme Janson[3], José Fernando Castanha Henriques[3], Arnaldo Pinzan[4]

Objective: This study aimed to evaluate the stability of molar relationship after non-extraction treatment of Class II malocclusion. **Methods:** The sample comprised 39 subjects (16 females, 23 males) with initial Class II malocclusion treated with no extractions, using fixed appliances. Mean age at the beginning of treatment was 12.94 years, at the end of treatment was 15.14 years and at post-retention stage was 21.18 years. Mean treatment time was 2.19 years and mean time of post-treatment evaluation was 6.12 years. To verify the influence of the severity of initial Class II molar relationship in stability of molar relationship, the sample was divided into two groups, one presenting a ½-cusp or ¾-cusp Class II molar relationship, and the other with full-cusp Class II molar relationship. In dental casts from initial, final and post-retention stages, molar, first and second premolars and canine relationships were measured. Data obtained were analyzed by dependent ANOVA, Tukey and Pearson's correlation tests, as well as independent *t* test between the two groups divided by severity of initial molar relationship. **Results:** There was a non-statistically significant 0.12 mm relapse of molar relationship. The initial severity of Class II molar relationship was not correlated to relapse in the post-retention period. When compared, the two groups showed no difference in relapse of molar relationship. **Conclusion:** It was concluded that correction of Class II molar relationship is stable and initial severity does not influence relapse of molar relationship.

Keywords: Corrective orthodontics. Angle Class II malocclusion. Treatment outcomes.

[1] Professor, Specialization Course in Orthodontics, UNORP.
[2] Post-Doctor in Orthodontics, University of Toronto. Head Professor of the
Master Course in Orthodontics, UNINGÁ.
[3] Professor of Orthodontics, FOB-USP.
[4] Associate Professor of Orthodontics, FOB-USP.

» The author reports no commercial, proprietary or financial interest in the products
or companies described in this article.

Karina Maria Salvatore de Freitas
Rua Jamil Gebara, 1-25, apto. 111 - Bauru / SP, Brazil – CEP: 17.017-150
E-mail: kmsf@uol.com.br

INTRODUCTION

Class II malocclusion does not self-correct in growing patients.[8,17] The Class II skeletal pattern is established early and remains until puberty if no orthodontic intervention is performed.[8]

To this date, several authors have discussed the relationship of the initial malocclusion characteristics with the effectiveness of orthodontic treatment[22,31,40] and the stability of the corrections obtained.[7,33,43]

Normally, orthodontic treatment takes a long time and uses complex techniques, usually achieving good results; however, these results may be lost in varying degrees after the removal of appliances and retainers.[38] Orthodontic relapse includes crowding or spacing of teeth, and loss of overbite, overjet correction, and loss of Class II molar relationship correction.

Orthodontic changes of the position of the first permanent molars have a great tendency to relapse.[24] Some authors affirm that Class I molar relationship is more stable compared to others and, over time, the mandibular molar tends to distalize in patients with Class II malocclusion.[17] For Uhde, Sadowsky and Be-Gole,[39] changes that occur in molar relationship are always towards Class II relation. The changes are of small magnitude and independent of the type of initial malocclusion and the type of treatment. Other authors suggest that, in the long-term, there is minimal relapse in molar relationship and that changes in incisor position and intercuspation of the posterior teeth are statistically significant, although not considered clinically significant.[12,39]

The stability of Class II malocclusion has been widely studied, however, few studies that have actually evaluated relapse and stability of the correction of Class II molar relationship in models. The studies are mostly directed to a particular type of appliance or treatment protocol.

In this context, the objective of this study was to evaluate the stability of molar relationship in cases with initial Class II malocclusion, treated orthodontically without extractions, correlating with factors such as the severity of initial Class II molar relationship, treatment, retention and post-retention times. Moreover, the objective was to compare the post retention stability of molar relationship between two groups divided according to the severity of the initial Class II molar relationship.

MATERIAL AND METHODS

For the present retrospective study, the sample was obtained from the records of the Department of Orthodontics, Bauru Dental School, University of São Paulo.

The inclusion criteria comprised the following characteristics:
» Angle Class II malocclusion, treated without extractions.
» Presence of erupted permanent teeth up to first molars, at the beginning of orthodontic treatment.
» Absence of tooth agenesis and supernumerary teeth.
» No anomalies in size and / or shape of the teeth.
» Absence of rotations of the maxillary and mandibular molars in the initial models, which could influence variable measurement.
» Orthodontic treatment with fixed appliances, which may include the use of headgear and / or Class II intermaxillary elastics.
» Complete orthodontic records, including study models of pre and post treatment and post retention records.

All patients in the sample were Caucasian, of both genders. The study models of the pretreatment (T_1 - initial), posttreatment (T_2 – final) and post-retention phases (T_3 - post-retention at least 2 years after the end of treatment) were used.

The sample was composed of a total of 39 patients, 16 females and 23 males. The mean age at pretreatment was 12.94 ± 1.21 years, the mean age at the end of treatment was 15.14 ± 1.38 years, and the mean age at post-retention was 21.18 ± 2.65 years. The mean treatment time was 2.19 ± 0.83 years. The mean post-treatment time evaluation, (between the final and post-retention stages) was 6.30 ± 2.60 years. At the end of active orthodontic treatment all patients used a removable Hawley plate retainer in the maxillary arch and a bonded fixed retainer from canine to canine in the mandibular arch. The retainers were used, on average, 1.62 ± 0.49 years.

To evaluate the influence of the severity of the initial Class II molar relationship in the stability of molar relationship, the sample was divided into two groups: Group 1, 16 patients presenting half-cusp or ¾-cusp initial Class II molar relationship. The mean age at pretreatment was 13.27 ± 1.11 years, the mean age at the end of treatment was 15.10 ± 1.35 years and the mean age at post-retention was 20.18 ± 2.03 years. The mean treatment time was 1.83 ± 0.49 years, the mean retention time was 1.58 ± 0.55 years and the mean time between posttreatment and post-retention phases was 5.29 ± 1.57 years. Group 2 consisted of 23 patients with a complete initial Class II molar relationship. The mean age at pretreatment was 12.71 ± 1.25 years, the mean age at the end of treatment was 15.17 ± 1.42 years and the mean age at post-retention was 21.87 ± 2.84 years. The mean treatment time was 2.45 ± 0.94 years, the mean retention time was 1.69 ± 0.46 years and the mean time between posttreatment and post-retention phases was $6.70 \pm$ of 2.46 years.

The orthodontic records of the selected sample were used to obtain some relevant data for this work. Clinical records were examined for therapeutic procedures at pre and posttreatment, and the posttreatment follow-ups. The date of removal of retainers was also observed. These data, together with the patient's date of birth, allowed accurate determination of the total time of treatment, control, posttreatment, post-retention, retention time and age of the patients in the studied phases.

The study models concerning initial, final and post-retention stages of each patient were evaluated. Study models were photographed with a D-80 camera, with 105 mm close-up lens (AF-S VR Micro Nikkor 105 mm f/2.8G IF-ED, Nikon Corporation, Japan) and circular flash (Nikon Corporation, Japan) with 300 dpi (dots per inch). From each study model, two lateral photographs were obtained, one on the right side and one on the left, with the buccal surfaces of posterior teeth parallel to each other. All photographs were obtained with the same distance between the object and the lens (31.4 cm), to avoid magnification.

The digital images were inserted into a computer and analyzed with Dolphin Imaging software version 10 (Dolphin Imaging and Management Solutions, Chatsworth, CA, USA). This program magnifies each image by means of their size in dpi. For each variable, two points are marked and the distance between them was calculated by the software. The accuracy of measurements was 0.01 mm. For the statistical analysis, the mean right and left sides of each measurement was obtained. The calculated variables are presented in the following topics.

Molar relationship

The molar relationship was measured from the tip of the mesiobuccal cusp of the maxillary first molar to the mesiobuccal groove of the mandibular first molar (Fig 1). The average of right and left sides was used.

Second premolar relationship

The relationship of the second premolars was measured from the tip of the buccal cusp of the maxillary second premolar to the distal anatomical contact point between the mandibular second premolar and the mesial of the mandibular first molar (Fig 2). The average of right and left sides was used.

First premolar relationship

The relationship of first premolars was measured from the tip of the buccal cusp of the maxillary first premolar to the distal anatomical contact point of the mandibular first premolar and mesial of the mandibular second premolar (Fig 3). The average of right and left sides was used.

Canine relationship

The canine relationship was measured from the cusp tip of the maxillary canine to the anatomical contact point between the distal mandibular canine and the mesial of the mandibular first premolar (Fig 4). The average of right and left sides was used.

Statistical analysis
Method error

The intra-examiner error was evaluated by taking new measurements of the initial, final and post-retention study models of 15 patients randomly selected, performing a total of 45 pairs of models. The first and second measurements were performed with a time interval of one month. The formula proposed by Dahlberg[11] ($Se^2 = \Sigma\ d^2/2n$) was applied to estimate the magnitude of casual errors, while systematic errors were analyzed by applying the paired t test, according to Houston.[19]

Statistical treatment

Descriptive statistics were performed for the variables at the initial (T_1), final (T_2) and post-retention (T_3) phases, and for the differences between initial and final, (characterizing treatment correction), and

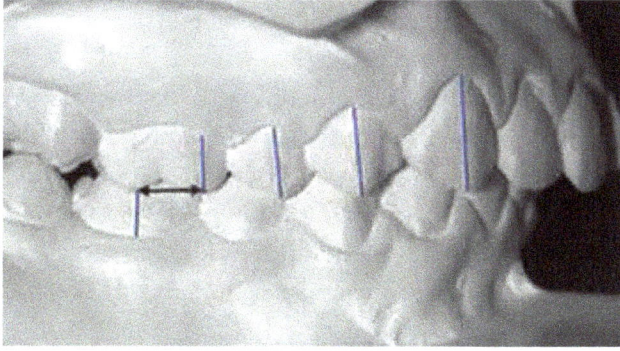

Figure 1 - Molar relationship measurement.

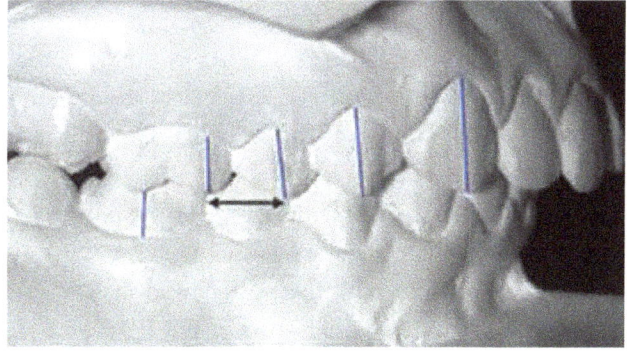

Figure 2 - Second pre-molars relationship measurement.

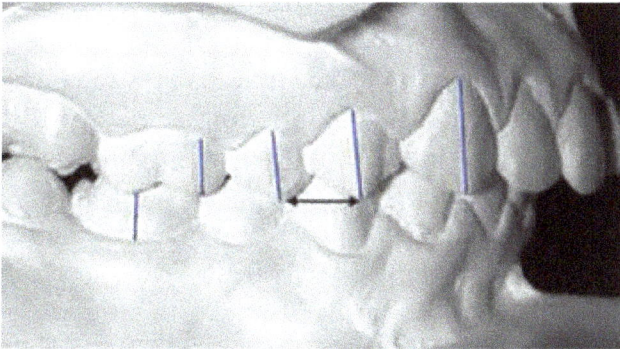

Figure 3 - First pre-molars relationship measurement.

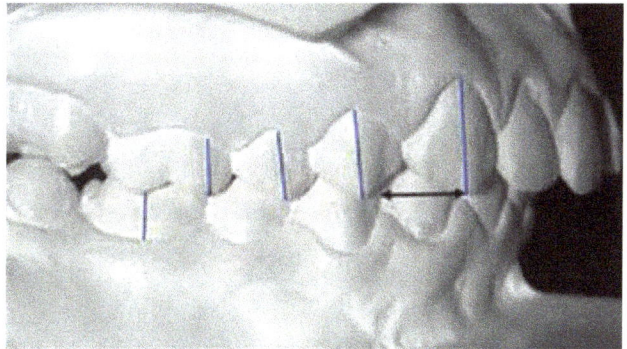

Figure 4 - Canines relationship measurement.

between the final and post-retention stages, (characterizing the change during post-retention). There was also descriptive statistics of the ages at initial, final and post-retention stages and the duration of treatment, retention and post-retention evaluation.

To evaluate variable changes between phases, the dependent ANOVA for repeated measures (repeated measures ANOVA) was used and in the presence of a significant result, Tukey's test was applied subsequently.

The Pearson correlation coefficient was calculated to verify the presence of correlation between molar relationship relapse with: severity of initial Class II relationship, treatment time, retention time and time of post-retention evaluation.

To better evaluate the influence of the initial Class II molar relationship severity on the stability of molar relationship, the sample was divided into two groups: Group 1 with ½-cusp or ¾-cusp initial molar Class II relationship, and Group 2, with initial complete Class II molar relationship. Therefore, the independent t test was applied for all variables between these two groups.

All tests were performed with the STATISTICA software (Statistica for Windows, Release 6.0, Copyright StatSoft, Inc. 2001), adopting a significance level of 5%.

RESULTS

Table 1 presents the results of the evaluation of systematic and casual errors, by evaluating the paired t test and Dahlberg' formula,[11] applied to all studied variables.

The descriptive statistics results (mean, standard deviation, minimum, maximum and number) of the variables molar relationship (MR), second premolars relationship (2PMR), first premolars relationship (1PMR) and canine relationship (CR) in every evaluated stage (T_1, T_2 and T_3) and periods (T_2-T_1 and T_3-T_2) are shown in Tables 2 to 5.

Table 6 shows the results of the analysis of variance (ANOVA) and Tukey's test for the variables molar relationship, relationship of first and second premolars and canines, at the initial, final and post-retention stages.

Table 7 presents the results of the Pearson correlation test to evaluate the correlation of the severity of Class II relationship with the post-retention relapse.

Table 8 shows the test results of the Pearson correlation test to determine the correlation of relapse and treatment time, retention time and time of post-retention evaluation.

Table 9 presents the results of the independent t test between groups 1 (½-cusp or ¾-cusp Class II) and 2 (complete Class II).

DISCUSSION
Methods

From the medical records of each patient general data such as date of birth, gender, type of appliance and mechanics used, date of beginning and end of treatment, duration of the use of the retainers, date of post-retention evaluation were collected. With these data, treatment, retention and posttreatment evalua-

tion times, age at the beginning and end of treatment, and at post-retention stage was assessed.

The choice of the methodology to be used should be based on the objective of the study. Since the purpose of this study was to evaluate the stability and relapse of molar relationship in the post-retention stage, the best method for evaluating molar relationship are study models. Although this method does not allow the clinical and radiographic analysis, the study models alone provide information related to diagnosis and orthodontic treatment.[6,15] Furthermore, it has been shown that there is a poor association among the occlusal characteristics and the morphology obtained in the lateral cephalograms and better prediction of orthodontic results can be obtained by occlusal indexes than by cephalometrics.[1] The fact that occlusal characteristics do not always reflect craniofacial morphology was evidenced by Pancherz, Zieber and Hoyer,[35] who observed similar cephalometric characteristics when comparing Class II, division 1 and 2, contradicting the widespread idea that the severe overbite of Class II division 2 malocclusion is related to a more horizontal skeletal pattern of this malocclusion.[21] Although this

Table 1 - Results of t test and Dahlberg formula, applied to the variables molar relationship, second premolar relationship, first premolar relationship and canine relationship, for estimation of systematic and casual errors, respectively (n=45).

Variables	1st. Measurement		2nd. Measurement		Dahlberg	p
	Mean	SD	Mean	SD		
MR	2.03	1.80	2.08	1.88	0.21	0.183
2PMR	3.47	2.05	3.54	2.05	0.26	0.056
1PMR	3.35	2.15	3.40	2.16	0.16	0.099
CR	4.40	2.29	4.43	2.21	0.27	0.530

Table 3 - Results of the descriptive statistical analysis for the variable second premolar relationship (2PMR), in all stages and periods evaluated.

Variables	Mean	SD	Minimum	Maximum	n
2PMR T_1	5.89	1.73	2.50	9.15	39
2PMR T_2	1.39	0.83	0.20	3.55	39
2PMR T_3	1.60	0.94	0.00	4.25	39
2PMR T_2-T_1	-4.50	1.65	-8.20	-0.95	39
2PMR T_3-T_2	0.21	0.90	-1.60	2.85	39

Table 2 - Results of the descriptive statistical analysis for the variable molar relationship (MR), in all stages and periods evaluated.

Variables	Mean	SD	Minimum	Maximum	n
MR T_1	4.65	1.52	1.85	8.40	39
MR T_2	0.50	0.70	0.00	3.05	39
MR T_3	0.62	0.74	0.00	2.80	39
MR T_2-T_1	-4.14	1.47	-7.15	-0.85	39
MR T_3-T_2	0.12	0.78	-2.10	2.50	39

Table 4 - Results of the descriptive statistical analysis for the variable first premolars relationship (1PMR), in all stages and periods evaluated.

Variables	Mean	SD	Minimum	Maximum	n
1PMR T_1	5.88	1.64	2.30	9.75	39
1PMR T_2	1.03	0.78	0.00	2.80	39
1PMR T_3	1.33	0.82	0.00	3.35	39
1PMR T_2-T_1	-4.85	1.71	-9.40	-0.30	39
1PMR T_3-T_2	0.30	0.73	-1.15	2.05	39

Table 5 - Results of the descriptive statistical analysis for the variable canine relationship (CR), in all stages and periods evaluated.

Variables	Mean	SD	Minimum	Maximum	n
CR T_1	7.22	1.64	2.75	10.45	39
CR T_2	2.32	0.94	0.55	4.70	39
CR T_3	2.28	1.04	0.20	5.55	39
CR T_2-T_1	-4.89	1.65	-8.85	0.60	39
CR T_3-T_2	-0.04	0.89	-1.80	2.50	39

Table 7 - Results of the Pearson's correlation test to verify the correlation of the severity of the Class II relationship with the post-retention relapse.

Correlations	r	p
MR T_1 x MR T_3	0.107	0.515
MR T_1 x MR T_3-T_2	-0.173	0.292
2PMR T_1 x 2PMR T_3	0.143	0.382
2PMR T_1 x 2PMR T_3-T_2	-0.159	0.331
1PMR T_1 x 1PMR T_3	-0.012	0.938
1PMR T_1 x 1PMR T_3-T_2	-0.172	0.293
CR T_1 x CR T_3	-0.049	0.763
CR T_1 x CR T_3-T_2	-0.354	0.026*

* Statistically significant difference for $p < 0.05$.

Table 6 - Results of the analysis of variance (ANOVA) and Tukey tests for the variables molar relationship, first and second premolars relationship and canine relationship (n=39), between the initial, final and post-retention stages (same letters mean no statistically significant difference).

Variables	Initial (T_1) Mean ± SD	Final (T_2) Mean ± SD	Post-retention (T_3) Mean ± SD	p
MR	4.65 ± 1.52 [a]	0.50 ± 0.70 [b]	0.62 ± 0.74 [b]	0.000*
2PMR	5.89 ± 1.73 [a]	1.39 ± 0.83 [b]	1.60 ± 0.94 [b]	0.000*
1PMR	5.88 ± 1.64 [a]	1.03 ± 0.78 [b]	1.33 ± 0.82 [b]	0.000*
CR	7.22 ± 1.64 [a]	2.32 ± 0.94 [b]	2.28 ± 1.04 [b]	0.000*

* Statistically significant difference for $p < 0.05$.

Table 8 - Results of the Pearson's correlation test to verify the correlation of the relapse with treatment time, retention time and time of post-retention evaluation.

Correlations	r	p
MR T_3-T_2 x TREATT	-0.205	0.210
MR T_3-T_2 x RETENT	-0.006	0.968
MR T_3-T_2 x POSTR	-0.373	0.019*

* Statistically significant difference for $p < 0.05$.

Table 9 - Results of independent t test, between the groups divided in ½-cusp or ¾-cusp Class II and complete Class II.

Variables	Group 1 – ½-cusp or ¾-cusp Class II (n=16) Mean	SD	Group 2 – Complete Class II (n=23) Mean	SD	p
ID T_1	13.27	1.11	12.71	1.25	0.164
ID T_2	15.10	1.35	15.17	1.42	0.895
ID T_3	20.18	2.03	21.87	2.84	0.048*
TREATT	1.83	0.49	2.45	0.94	0.021*
RETENT	1.58	0.55	1.65	0.46	0.685
POSTR	5.29	1.57	6.70	2.46	0.051
MR T_1	3.53	1.03	5.43	1.31	0.000*
MR T_2	0.25	0.39	0.67	0.82	0.064
MR T_3	0.48	0.78	0.72	0.71	0.339
MR T_2-T_1	-3.28	1.17	-4.75	1.36	0.001*
MR T_3-T_2	0.23	0.75	0.04	0.81	0.460
2PMR T_1	4.52	0.90	6.84	1.52	0.000*
2PMR T_2	0.91	0.62	1.72	0.81	0.001*
2PMR T_3	1.33	0.95	1.79	0.92	0.141
2PMR T_2-T_1	-3.61	1.17	-5.11	1.67	0.003*
2PMR T_3-T_2	0.42	0.76	0.06	0.98	0.230
1PMR T_1	4.50	1.08	6.85	1.23	0.000*
1PMR T_2	0.64	0.61	1.31	0.77	0.006*
1PMR T_3	1.17	0.79	1.45	0.83	0.303
1PMR T_2-T_1	-3.86	1.40	-5.53	1.59	0.001*
1PMR T_3-T_2	0.53	0.63	0.13	0.75	0.096
CR T_1	6.00	1.73	8.07	0.89	0.000*
CR T_2	1.96	0.83	2.58	0.95	0.043*
CR T_3	2.23	0.84	2.31	1.18	0.804
CR T_2-T_1	-4.04	1.77	-5.49	1.29	0.005*
CR T_3-T_2	0.26	0.88	-0.26	0.85	0.067

* Statistically significant difference for $p < 0.05$.

study did not use occlusal indexes, molar relationship measurement, a characteristic that can be well observed in study models, was used.[6,9]

Andrews[4] defined the six keys to normal occlusion based exclusively on the information contained in 120 study models, and these six keys are valuable parameters to obtain an ideal static occlusion. Similarly, the occlusal evaluation is an important research tool regarding the results of orthodontic treatments.[2,7,43] Therefore, this study performed the measurement of molar relationship on study models, a method that is simple and objective, and has previously been used in several studies.[10,12,23,39]

All measurements were made from photographs of the study models of the three phases for each patient. The study models were photographed with a D-80 camera, with a 105 mm close-up lens and circular flash (Nikon Corporation, Japan) with 300 dpi. The use of this lens prevents any distortion of the image. From each model, two lateral photographs were obtained, one of the right side and one of the left, with the buccal surfaces of the posterior teeth parallel to each other. The digital images were inserted into a computer and analyzed with Dolphin Imaging software version 10 (Dolphin Imaging and Management Solutions, Chatsworth, CA, USA). This program magnifies each image by means of the size in dpi, to be informed by the examiner. For each variable, two points are marked and the distance between them is thus calculated by the software. The accuracy of measurements was 0.01 mm. For the statistical analysis, the average of the right and left sides of each of the measures was obtained.

The main advantage of this measurement method is that the images, once inserted in the Dolphin software, can be magnified on the computer screen, or even displayed with a multimedia projector, and the points marked with the aid of a mouse connected to the computer. This possibility of image magnification greatly facilitates the visualization of the point to be marked, minimizing the possible methodological errors, as shown in Table 1.

According to Houston,[19] for an accurate analysis, the object of study should be reevaluated a minimum of 25 times. Thus, to evaluate the intra-examiner error, new measurements of the studied variables (molar relationship, relationship of second premolars, re-lationship of first premolars and canine relationship, Figures 1, 2, 3 and 4, respectively) were performed on study models of 15 patients randomly selected from the total sample, a total of 45 pairs of models, measured one month after the first measurement. The results of the two measurements were then subjected to the formula proposed by Dahlberg,[11] to obtain the casual errors. To obtain the systematic errors, the paired t test was applied.

The results demonstrated the absence of systematic errors. Casual errors were minimum and hence acceptable (Table 1). The greatest casual error occurred for the canine relationship (CR), with value of 0.27 mm. The absence of significant systematic errors and the minimum value of the casual errors observed in this study may result from both the standardization and accuracy of the measurements, and also by the simplicity and objectivity of the measurement used, making this method very reliable and reproducible.

Sample

Since the main objective of this study was to evaluate the stability of molar relationship in the long-term, the selection of the sample was performed aiming to eliminate the largest possible number of factors that could influence the results. Therefore, to evaluate the stability of molar relationship, and also the relationships of first and second premolars and canines, it was necessary to standardize the initial characteristics and the several factors related to the orthodontic treatment. Therefore, the initial malocclusion was calibrated, regarding the type and minimum severity, the treatment protocol used, and the type of appliance.

Therefore, the basic criteria for sample selection was initially Angle Class II malocclusion, with molar relationship of at least half-cusp Class II.[42] Cases could not present rotation of the maxillary and mandibular molars in the initial models, which could influence the measurement of the variables. In addition, all patients should have been treated with fixed orthodontic appliances[14,37] in both maxillary and mandibular arches, without extractions.[14,20,37] All patients used headgear in the maxillary arch and Class II elastics during orthodontic treatment.

Cases treated previously with functional, fixed and removable appliances, and with intraoral distalizers were excluded, which may influence the interpretation of the results of this study. It is known that the relapse of the skeletal changes of functional orthopedic appliances occurs after removal of the appliances, and this could influence the results.[32,34] In addition, distalizers also perform a quick distalization of the maxillary molars and generally cause a distal tipping of the crown of these teeth, relapse may be increased in these cases, due to these factors.[27,30]

The presence of permanent teeth erupted up to the first molars and the absence of supernumerary teeth and agenesis constituted criteria of sample selection, since the absence of permanent teeth, the presence of supernumerary and some anomalies related to the shape of the teeth can interfere with the normal development of the occlusion, producing malocclusions that require correction with a different orthodontic mechanics, increasing the complexity and difficulty of the orthodontic treatment, and stability.[6,25]

The sample consisted of a total of 41 patients, selected from the records of the Discipline of Orthodontics, treated by Graduate students (from the Department of Pediatric Dentistry, Orthodontics and Public Health, Bauru Dental School). Only those cases that had complete orthodontic records were selected, with all the forms properly completed, presenting the study models from initial, final and at least two years posttreatment stages.

The time of posttreatment evaluation, in the post-retention stage, is reasonable to observe the stability, one of the purposes of this study, because, according to Al Yami, Kuijpers-Jagtman and van't Hof,[3] about half of the total relapse occurs in the first two years after the end of treatment, with good stability for most of the characteristics in the period of more than five years posttreatment.

The sample selection did not involve the factor quality of finishing, which did not serve as a criterion for exclusion or inclusion. However, assessing the Class II cases treated without extractions in FOB-USP, Barros[6] found that even those cases where there is need for greater patient cooperation,[20,41] were finished, in general, in an acceptable manner. Furthermore, it has been previously demonstrated that the quality of finishing is not related to the long-term results of orthodontic treatments, and an excellent finishing does not guarantee stability.[13,29,33]

RESULTS
Molar relationship

The measurement of the initial Class II molar relationship showed a mean value of 4.65 mm, and was reduced to 0.50 mm after treatment. For the post-retention evaluation, in the long-term, 0.62 mm was found (Table 2). This demonstrates a correction with treatment of 4.14 mm and a minimum relapse of only 0.12 mm (Table 2). As shown in Table 6, after performing the ANOVA and Tukey tests, a statistically significant correction with treatment and stability in the post-retention period could be noted, since there was no statistically significant difference in the molar relationship between the final and post-retention stages. In other words, the molar relationship showed to be stable in the post-retention phase.

The results of this study are in agreement with previous findings in the literature.[10,12,23,39]

Canut and Arias,[10] evaluating Class II division 2 cases, found a mean of post-retention relapse of molar relationship of 0.6 mm, and all patients had a good molar occlusion in the post-retention phase. The authors considered the molar relationship stable at the end of the post-retention period.

Kim and Little[23] found even an improvement in molar relationship in the post-retention period evaluating Class II division 2 cases. At the end of treatment, the cases had a mean value of 1.3 mm for the molar relationship and, in post-retention stage, this value reduced to 1.2 mm, suggesting an improvement in the molar relationship of 0.1 mm.

Uhde, Sadowsky and BeGole,[39] evaluating Class I and Class II cases in the post-retention stage, reported that the mean change in molar relationship is always in relation to the Class II, however, these changes are not relevant, (about 0.50 mm). However, besides including Class I and Class II cases, which directly influences the results, the authors also included cases treated with and without extractions.

However, Fidler et al[12] found a significant relapse of molar relationship between the final and post-retention stages. However, although statistically significant, this relapse had low values of 0.34 mm for the molar relationship on the right side and 0.33 mm on the left side. Perhaps this difference with the present study was due to the fact that the authors selected cases with Class II malocclusion treated successfully at the end of treatment, and in the present study, the final treatment outcome of the Class II was not considered for the sample selection.

The literature shows stability of the molar relationship, especially in Class II, division 2 cases. Regarding the Class II division 1 malocclusion, this study showed slightly better results than those found in the literature.[12]

Second premolar relationship

The initial measurement of the second premolars relationship presented a mean value of 5.89 mm, being reduced to 1.39 mm after treatment. For the post-retention evaluation, in the long-term, 1.60 mm was found (Table 3). This demonstrates a correction of 4.50 mm, and a relapse of 0.21 mm (Table 3). As shown in Table 6, after performing the ANOVA and Tukey tests, a statistically significant correction with treatment and stability in the post-retention period could be noted, since there was no statistically significant difference of the second premolars relationship between the final and post-retention stages.

The study of Kim and Little[23] showed the same trend, however, in the final stage, the value of the premolars relationship was slightly higher than normal, and this value remained higher in the posttreatment stage. The initial value of the Class II premolars relationship was 4.6 mm, being corrected to 2.2 mm at the end of treatment and relapsed to 2.5 mm in the post-retention stage.

First premolar relationship

The initial measurement of the first premolars relationship presented a mean value of 5.88 mm, being reduced to 1.03 mm after treatment. For the post-retention evaluation, in the long-term, 1.33 mm was found (Table 4). This demonstrates a correction of 4.85 mm, and a relapse of 0.30 mm (Table 4). As shown in Table 6, after performing the ANOVA and Tukey tests, a statistically significant correction with treatment and stability in the post-retention period could be noted, since there was no statistically significant difference in the first premolars relationship between the final and post-retention stages.

Canine relationship

The initial measurement of the canine relationship presented a mean value of 7.22 mm, being re-

duced to 2.32 mm after treatment. For the post-retention evaluation, in the long-term, 2.28 mm was found (Table 5). This shows a correction of 4.89 mm, and an improvement in the post-retention period of 0.04 mm (Table 5). As shown in Table 6, after performing the ANOVA and Tukey tests, a statistically significant correction with treatment and a complete stability in the post-retention period could be noted, since there was no statistically significant difference of the canine relationship between the final and post-retention stages, and even a small improvement could be seen.

Kim and Little[23] found results similar to the present study. The initial Class II canine relationship had value of 5.3 mm, and at the end it was corrected to 1.6 mm and remained stable, showing the same value of 1.6 mm in the post-retention stage.

Correlations

To verify the correlation between the severity of the Class II relationship with the post-retention relapse, and the relapse of Class II molar relationship with treatment time, retention time and time of post-retention evaluation, the Pearson correlation test was used (Tables 7 and 8).

There was a correlation of the initial canine relationship with relapse (Table 7).

There was correlation of molar relationship relapse with the time of post-retention evaluation (Table 8). However, this correlation was negative, indicating that the longer the time of post-retention evaluation, the lower the relapse of molar relationship. This finding seems unreasonable; however, since patients were mostly young, at the end of orthodontic treatment, they still showed growth in the post-retention stage. As the growth tends to improve the relationship of skeletal bases,[18] it is natural that the if time has passed until the post-retention evaluation, the patient will have more growth, favoring the stability of the correction of the Class II molar relationship.

Intergroups comparison

To check the influence of the severity of the Class II molar relationship in the initial stability of the molar relationship, the sample was divided into two groups: Group 1 with initial half-cusp or ¾-cusp Class II molar relationship, and Group 2, with initial complete Class II molar relationship. Therefore the independent *t* test was applied for all variables between these two groups.

There was compatibility between the two groups for the initial and final ages, and only the post-retention age showed a statistically significant difference (Table 9). Subjects in Group 2 (complete Class II) had an older age in the post-retention stage than the subjects in Group 1. However, despite the complete Class II group had presented an older age in the post-retention stage, the time of post-retention evaluation of this group was not statistically significant higher than the group with ½-cusp and ¾-cusp Class II. The retention time was also compatible between the two groups studied (Table 9).

Regarding treatment time, the group with complete Class II showed longer treatment than the ½-cusp and ¾-cusp Class II group, and this difference was statistically significant (Table 9). This was expected since it is known that the severity of malocclusion, especially the severity of the Class II, when treated without extractions, can significantly increase treatment time.[6,20,40]

Regarding the initial molar relationship, as group selection was based on the severity of this relationship, a significant difference between the groups, was expected (Table 9). Obviously, the complete Class II group had a significantly higher value than the group with less severity. The molar relationship at the end of treatment and at the post-retention stage did not differ between the two groups (Table 9). There was also a difference in the amount of correction with treatment, which also was expected, because if the Class II molar relationship was more severe in Group 2, a greater correction of this relationship was really necessary in this group (Table 9). The molar relationship relapse between the two groups did not present a statistically significant difference, however, it was observed that the molar relationship presented a relapse of 0.23 mm in the group with less severity and only 0.04 mm in the group with greater severity. This evidence reinforces the findings of this study that there is no relationship of the initial Class II severity with molar relationship relapse.

The same pattern of results was observed for the first and second premolars and canine relationship. There were statistically significant differences be-

tween the two groups for these relationships in the initial (T_1) and final stage (T_2) and the change with treatment (T_2-T_1) (Table 9). For the relationships at the beginning of treatment, as explained above for the molar relationship, this result was expected due to the greater Class II severity in Group 2. Thus, it was also expected that the correction with treatment was greater, as confirmed by the results. However, there was also a significant result for these relationships at the end of treatment. Group 2, with complete Class II, presented a deficient finishing for the premolars and canine relationships.

A very important factor to be considered is the need for patient cooperation. The successful Class II malocclusion treatment without extractions is extremely connected to patient cooperation. It should be noted that a severe initial malocclusion, demands greater need for patient cooperation to achieve a satisfactory final result.[6,42] According to Barros,[6] the treatment of a complete Class II without extraction, in relation to two maxillary premolar extractions, requires approximately twice the degree of patient compliance.

Due to the fact that Group 2 includes only complete Class II malocclusion cases, it could be assumed that the greater severity of molar relationship at the beginning of treatment and hence the greatest amount of correction during treatment would influence the maintenance of long-term results.[28] However, this association was not confirmed by the present study, since both groups had a stability without statistically significant differences for the molar, premolar and canine relationships.

Araki[5] also found no major posttreatment changes in the group where the change of molar relationship was higher during treatment, and speculated that it probably occurred due to the proper retention of the dental relations obtained.

By studying the stability in the long-term posttreatment of Class II malocclusion by means of the Herbst appliance, Hansen, Pancherz and Hägg[16] observed that, when the maxilla and the mandible are well connected in a stable Class I relationship, the strength of the maxillary growth can be transmitted to the mandible and vice versa. For this reason, it is essential to finish treatment with the best possible intercuspation.

FINAL CONSIDERATIONS

It is considered that the stability of the correction of dental relationships, such as molar and canine relationships, are primary goals of a successful orthodontic treatment.

The stability of dental relationships is the most important aim to be achieved,[36] because relapse was clearly considered, in a clinical assessment of dentists and patients, as the cause of dissatisfaction in relation to orthodontic treatment. The posttreatment changes of the skeletal characteristics have secondary importance, since they are not visible in the clinical evaluation, but should also be aimed, because these changes may reflect changes in tooth position.[5]

The present study demonstrated a relative occlusal stability of the molar, second and first premolars and canine relationships, as the posttreatment changes were minimal. This is a very important data for planning and treating the cases, because, apart from the cephalometric data of the patients, it is known that at least the occlusal relationship, considered as the most important, is almost maintained in the long-term.

It is also important to highlight that there is a wide individual variability of stability and relapse, since it has a multifactorial cause, and there are several factors related to it, such as craniofacial growth, patient compliance with the use of retainers.[26]

CONCLUSIONS

According to the studied sample and to the methodology used, it can be concluded that:

» There was a non significant relapse of molar relationship, on average 0.12 mm. The relapses of premolars and canine relationships were also not significant.

» There was a significant correlation only between molar relationship relapse and time of post-retention evaluation.

» When the sample was divided into two groups, with half-cusp and ¾-cusp Class II and with complete Class II at the beginning of treatment, no difference in the relapses of molar, premolars and canine relationships could be found .

» The Class II molar relationship correction remained stable and the initial severity did not influence molar relationship relapse.

REFERENCES

1. Ackerman JL, Proffit WR. Soft tissue limitations in orthodontics: treatment planning guidelines. Angle Orthod. 1997;67(5):327-36.

2. Al Yami EA, Kuijpers-Jagtman AM, Vant Hof MA. Assessment of biological changes in a nonorthodontic sample using the PAR index. Am J Orthod Dentofacial Orthop. 1998;114(2):224-8.

3. Al Yami EA, Kuijpers-Jagtman AM, Vant Hof MA. Stability of orthodontic treatment outcome: follow-up until 10 years postretention. Am J Orthod Dentofacial Orthop. 1999;115(3):300-4.

4. Andrews LF. The six keys to normal occlusion. Am J Orthod. 1972;62(3):296-309.

5. Araki JDV. Comparação cefalométrica da estabilidade do tratamento da má oclusão de Classe II realizado sem e com a extração de dois pré-molares superiores [dissertação]. Bauru (SP): Universidade de São Paulo; 2007.

6. Barros SEC. Avaliação do grau de eficiência do tratamento da Classe II realizado sem extrações e com extrações de dois pré-molares superiores [dissertação] Bauru (SP): Universidade de São Paulo; 2004.

7. Birkeland K, Furevik J, Bøe OE, Wisth PJ. Evaluation of treatment and posttreatment changes by the PAR Index. Eur J Orthod. 1997;19(3):279-88.

8. Bishara SE, Hoppens BJ, Jakobsen JR, Kohout FJ. Changes in the molar relationship between the deciduous and permanent dentitions: a longitudinal study. Am J Orthod Dentofacial Orthop. 1988;93(1):19-28.

9. Brambilla AC. Comparação dos resultados oclusais do tratamento de Classe II realizado com extrações de dois pré-molares, com a terapêutica utilizando as extrações de quatro pré-molares [dissertação]. Bauru (SP): Universidade de São Paulo; 2002.

10. Canut JA, Arias S. A long-term evaluation of treated Class II division 2 malocclusions: a retrospective study model analysis. Eur J Orthod. 1999;21(4):377-86.

11. Dahlberg G. Statistical methods for medical and biological students. New York: Interscience; 1940.

12. Fidler BC, Artun J, Joondeph DR, Little RM. Long-term stability of Angle Class II, division 1 malocclusions with successful occlusal results at end of active treatment. Am J Orthod Dentofacial Orthop. 1995;107(3):276-85.

13. Freitas KM, Janson G, Freitas MR, Pinzan A, Henriques JF, Pinzan-Vercelino CR. Influence of the quality of the finished occlusion on postretention occlusal relapse. Am J Orthod Dentofacial Orthop. 2007;132(4):428.e9-14.

14. Graber TM, Vanarsdall RLJ. Orthodontics: current principles and techniques. St. Louis: Mosby; 1994.

15. Han UK, Vig KW, Weintraub JA, Vig PS, Kowalski CJ. Consistency of orthodontic treatment decisions relative to diagnostic records. Am J Orthod Dentofacial Orthop. 1991;100(3):212-9.

16. Hansen K, Pancherz H, Hagg U. Long-term effects of the Herbst appliance in relation to the treatment growth period: a cephalometric study. Eur J Orthod. 1991;13(6):471-81.

17. Harris EF, Behrents RG. The intrinsic stability of Class I molar relationship: a longitudinal study of untreated cases. Am J Orthod Dentofacial Orthop. 1988;94(1):63-7.

18. Harris EF, Vaden JL, Dunn KL, Behrents RG. Effects of patient age on postorthodontic stability in Class II, division 1 malocclusions. Am J Orthod Dentofacial Orthop. 1994;105(1):25-34.

19. Houston WJB. The analysis of errors in orthodontic measurements. Am J Orthod. 1983;83(5):382-90.

20. Janson G, Barros SE, Freitas MR, Henriques JF, Pinzan A. Class II treatment efficiency in maxillary premolar extraction and nonextraction protocols. Am J Orthod Dentofacial Orthop. 2007;132(4):490-8.

21. Karlsen AT. Craniofacial characteristics in children with Angle Class II div. 2 malocclusion combined with extreme deep bite. Angle Orthod. 1994;64(2):123-30.

22. Kim JC, Mascarenhas AK, Joo BH, Vig KW, Beck FM, Vig PS. Cephalometric variables as predictors of Class II treatment outcome. Am J Orthod Dentofacial Orthop. 2000;118(6):636-40.

23. Kim TW, Little RM. Postretention assessment of deep overbite correction in Class II Division 2 malocclusion. Angle Orthod. 1999;69(2):175-86.

24. Litowitz R. A study of the movements of certain teeth during and following orthodontic treatment. Angle Orthod. 1948;18(3):113-31.

25. Little RM. Stability and relapse of mandibular anterior alignment: University of Washington studies. Semin Orthod. 1999;5(3):191-204.

26. Little RM, Wallen TR, Riedel RA. Stability and relapse of mandibular anterior alignment — first premolar extraction cases treated by traditional edgewise orthodontics. Am J Orthod. 1981;80(4):349-65.

27. Mavropoulos A, Karamouzos A, Kiliaridis S, Papadopoulos MA. Efficiency of noncompliance simultaneous first and second upper molar distalization: a three-dimensional tooth movement analysis. Angle Orthod. 2005;75(4):532-9.

28. Nashed RR, Reynolds IR. A cephalometric investigation of overjet changes in fifty severe Class II division I malocclusions. Br J Orthod. 1989;16(1):31-7.

29. Nett BC, Huang GJ. Long-term posttreatment changes measured by the American Board of Orthodontics objective grading system. Am J Orthod Dentofacial Orthop. 2005;127(4):444-50.

30. Ngantung V, Nanda RS, Bowman SJ. Posttreatment evaluation of the distal jet appliance. Am J Orthod Dentofacial Orthop. 2001;120(2):178-85.

31. O'Brien KD, Robbins R, Vig KW, Vig PS, Shnorhokian H, Weyant R. The effectiveness of Class II, division 1 treatment. Am J Orthod Dentofacial Orthop. 1995;107(3):329-34.

32. Omblus J, Malmgren O, Pancherz H, Hägg U, Hansen K. Long-term effects of Class II correction in Herbst and Bass therapy. Eur J Orthod. 1997;19(2):185-93.

33. Ormiston JP, Huang GJ, Little RM, Decker JD, Seuk GD. Retrospective analysis of long-term stable and unstable orthodontic treatment outcomes. Am J Orthod Dentofacial Orthop. 2005;128(5):568-74.

34. Pancherz H, Ruf S, Kohlhas P. Effective condylar growth and chin position changes in Herbst treatment: a cephalometric roentgenographic long-term study. Am J Orthod Dentofacial Orthop. 1998;114(4):437-46.

35. Pancherz H, Zieber K, Hoyer B. Cephalometric characteristics of Class II division 1 and Class II division 2 malocclusions: a comparative study in children. Angle Orthod. 1997;67(2):111-20.

36. Sadowsky C, Sakols EI. Long-term assessment of orthodontic relapse. Am J Orthod. 1982;82(6):456-63.

37. Salzmann JA. Practice of Orthodontics. Philadelphia: J. B. Lippincott Company; 1966.

38. Thilander B. Orthodontic relapse versus natural development. Am J Orthod Dentofacial Orthop. 2000;117(5):562-3.

39. Uhde MD, Sadowsky C, Begole EA. Long-term stability of dental relationships after orthodontic treatment. Angle Orthod. 1983;53(3):240-52.

40. Valarelli FP. Relação entre o grau de severidade e o sucesso do tratamento sem extração da má oclusão de Classe II [tese]. Bauru (SP): Universidade de São Paulo; 2006.

41. Vig KW, Weyant R, Vayda D, O'Brien K, Bennett E. Orthodontic process and outcome: efficacy studies — strategies for developing process and outcome measures: a new era in orthodontics. Clin Orthod Res. 1998;1(2):147-55.

42. Wheeler TT, McGorray SP, Dolce C, Taylor MG, King GJ. Effectiveness of early treatment of Class II malocclusion. Am J Orthod Dentofacial Orthop. 2002;121(1):9-17.

43. Woods M, Lee D, Crawford E. Finishing occlusion, degree of stability and the PAR index. Aust Orthod J. 2000;16(1):9-15.

3

Comparative cephalometric study of Class II malocclusion treatment with Pendulum and Jones jig appliances followed by fixed corrective orthodontics

Mayara Paim Patel[1], José Fernando Castanha Henriques[2], Renato Rodrigues de Almeida[3], Arnaldo Pinzan[4], Guilherme Janson[2], Marcos Roberto de Freitas[2]

Objective: The purpose of this study was to cephalometrically compare the skeletal and dentoalveolar effects in the treatment of Class II malocclusion with Pendulum and Jones jig appliances, followed by fixed corrective orthodontics, and to compare such effects to a control group. **Methods:** The sample was divided into three groups. Group 1: 18 patients treated with Pendulum, Group 2: 25 patients treated with Jones jig, and Group 3: 19 young subjects with untreated Class II malocclusions and initial mean age of 12.88 years. The chi-square test was applied to assess severity and gender distribution. Groups 1 and 2 were compared to the control group by means of the one-way ANOVA and Tukey tests in order to differentiate treatment changes from those occurred by craniofacial growth. **Results:** There were no significant changes among the three groups with regard to the components of the maxilla and the mandible, maxillomandibular relationship, cephalometric and tegumental pattern. Buccal tipping of mandibular incisors was significantly greater in the experimental groups and increased mesial angulation of the maxillary second molars was found in the Jones jig group. In the experimental groups, dental relationship, overbite and overjet were corrected. **Conclusion:** It can be stated that the distalization achieved its purpose of correcting the Class II.

Keywords: Angle Class II malocclusion. Corrective orthodontics. Molar tooth.

[1] PhD in Orthodontics, College of Dentistry – Bauru/ University of São Paulo (USP).

[2] Full professor, Department of Pediatric Dentistry, Orthodontics and Collective Health, College of Dentistry – Bauru/ University of São Paulo (USP).

[3] Full professor, Department of Orthodontics, College of Dentistry – Bauru/ University of São Paulo (USP) and UNOPAR

[4] Full professor, Department of Pediatric Dentistry, Orthodontics and Collective Health, College of Dentistry – Bauru/ University of São Paulo (USP).

» The authors report no commercial, proprietary or financial interest in the products or companies described in this article.

Mayara Paim Patel
Rua Francisco Leitão, 115 – Bairro Pinheiros – São Paulo/SP — Brazil
CEP: 05414-025 – E-mail: mayarapaim@hotmail.com

INTRODUCTION

Intraoral distalizers differ in terms of insertion site,[4] mechanism of action and anchorage reinforcement.[15] The Jones jig appliance is inserted buccally and acts through a nickel titanium spring anchored in the second premolars.[14] The Pendulum appliance is palatally positioned, anchored in the first and second premolars and its force is dissipated through TMA springs.[12]

The intraoral distalization performed with fixed intraoral devices is only the first phase of a treatment that will be finalized with fixed corrective mechanics. There are few studies in the literature that scientifically assess the results of both phases of treatment;[3,6,7,20] most studies only assess the results of distalization.[9,10,12,15,16,17,21] Therefore, it is essential to perform a study assessing and comparing the results of corrective orthodontic treatment initiated by intraoral maxillary molar distalization with different intraoral distalization appliances.

MATERIAL AND METHODS

Initially, the research project was evaluated and approved by the College of Dentistry – Bauru/ University of São Paulo (USP) Institutional Review Board .

Three groups with Class II malocclusion were compared: Group 1: comprised 18 patients (initial mean age of 13.92 years), 6 males and 12 females. A normal molar relationship was obtained from maxillary molar distalization performed with the Pendulum appliance and maintained by the nightly use of cervical headgear (KHG) associated with corrective fixed appliances.

The mean treatment time was 4.55 years (Table 1). Group 2: comprised 25 patients (initial mean age of 12.09 years), 14 males and 11 females. Class II correction was achieved with the Jones jig appliance and maintained by the nightly use of medium-high headgear traction (helmet jeans), during corrective orthodontic treatment. The mean duration of orthodontic treatment was 4.09 years (Table 1).

Group 3: comprised 19 young subjects with untreated Class II malocclusion (control group), 10 males and 9 females (initial mean age of 12.88 years) and followed up for a mean period of 3.71 years (Table 1). This sample was selected from a group of young subjects that had been annually radiographed and accompanied by the Department of Orthodontics, School of Dentistry – Bauru/ University of São Paulo (USP). All patients had been referred for orthodontic treatment, however, some of them opted for late intervention and others had no interest in the treatment.

The cephalometric variables analyzed were based on the orthodontic literature[3,6,8,11,22] and aimed at promoting a comparative study, allowing discussion of the results obtained (Fig 1).

At first, chi-square tests were used to assess severity and gender distribution (Tables 2 and 3). The three groups were assessed and cephalometrically compared in order to observe the effects of orthodontic treatment and to differentiate them in terms of the changes promoted by craniofacial growth and development (Fig 1). Thus, one-way ANOVA and Tukey tests were used.

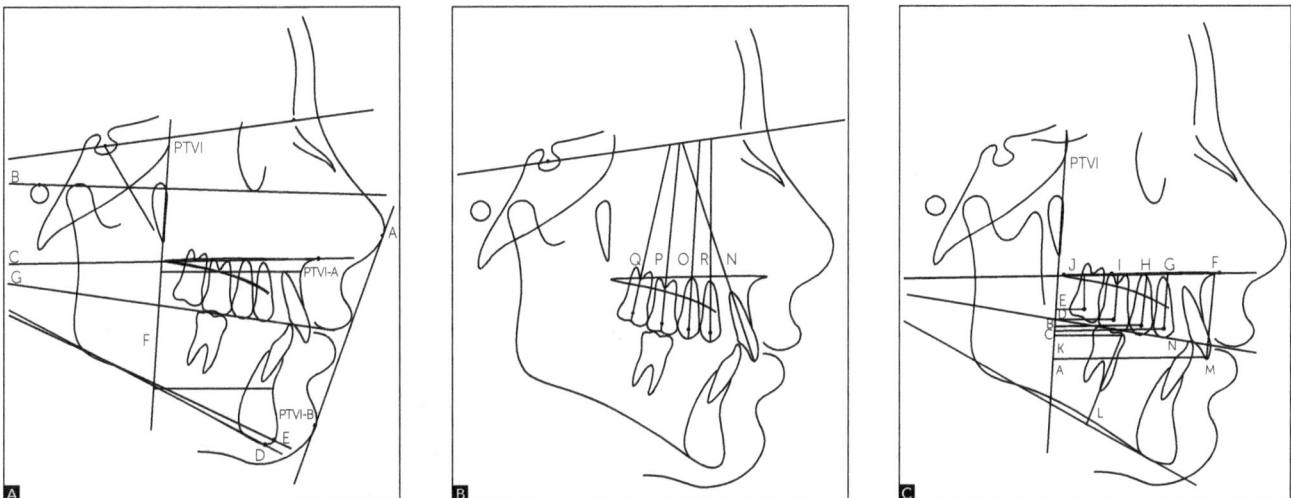

Figure 1 - A) Lines and Planes: A = Line E; B = Frankfort Plane; C = Palatal Plane; D = Mandibular Plane (Go-Me); E = Mandibular Plane (Go-Gn); F = Pterygoid vertical line (PTVI); G = Occlusal Plane; **B)** Dental angular measurements: N = SN.1; R = SN.4; O = SN.5; P = SN.6; Q = SN.7. **C)** Dental linear measurements: A = PTVI-1; B = PTVI-4; C = PTVI-5; D = PTVI-6; E = PTVI-7; F, = PP-1; G, = PP-4; H = PP-5; I = PP-6; J = PP-7; K = PTVI- ; L = GoMe - , M = Overjet; N = Overbite.

Table 1 - Compatibility of the mean initial and final ages as well as the observation mean time of the young patients in the three groups (ANOVA).

VARIABLE (Y)	Group 1 (Pendulum) N = 18		Group 2 (Jones jig) N = 25		Group 3 (Control) N = 19		P
	Mean ± SD		Mean ± SD		Mean ± SD		
Pretreatment age	13.92ᴬ	1.71	12.90ᴬ	1.43	12.88ᴬ	1.47	0.063
Posttreatment age	18.48ᴬ	1.33	16.99ᴮ	1.87	16.60ᴮ	2.31	0.008*
Observation time (T₃-T₁)	4.55ᴬ	0.79	4.09ᴬ	0.99	3.71ᴬ	1.63	0.110

* Statistically significant for P < 0.05
Different letters stand for statistically significant difference.

Table 2 - Number of female and male subjects for each group and result of the chi-square test.

Group	Sex		Total
	Male	Female	
1 – Pendulum	6 (33.3%)	12 (66.7%)	18
2 – Jones jig	14 (56%)	11 (44%)	25
3 – Control	10 (52.6%)	9 (47.4%)	19
Total	30	32	62
$\chi^2 = 2.35$; gl = 2; P = 0.3087			

* Statistically significant difference for P < 0.05
Different letters stand for statistically significant difference.

Table 3 - Comparison of Class II malocclusion severity among groups and chi-square test results.

Group	Molar relationship				Total
	¼ Class II	½ Class II	¾ Class II	Full-cusp Class II	
1 – Pendulum	1 (5.6%)	7 (38.8%)	5 (27.8%)	5 (27.8%)	18
2 – Jones jig	11 (44%)	7 (28%)	3 (12%)	4 (16%)	25
3 – Control	9 (47.4%)	5 (26.3%)	3 (15.8%)	2 (10.5%)	19
Total	21	19	11	11	62
$\chi^2 = 9.76$; gl=6; P = 0.1350					

* Statistically significant difference for P < 0.05
Different letters stand for statistically significant difference.

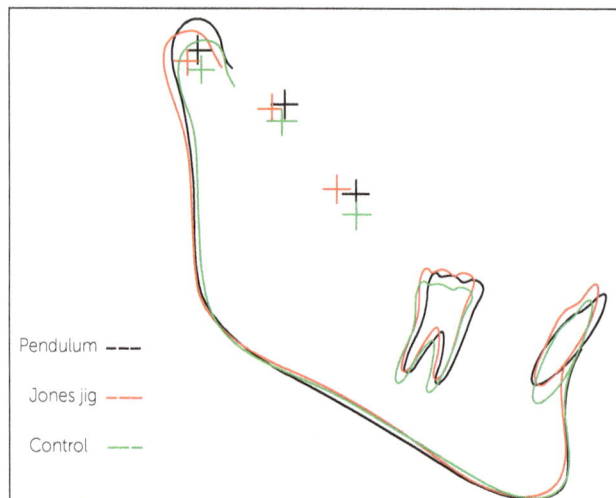

Pendulum ---

Jones jig ———

Control ———

Figure 2 - Comparison between Pendulum and Jones jig appliances and the control group.

RESULTS

Initially, the groups were compared in order to quantify any potential differences existing prior to orthodontic treatment. Out of the 43 variables analyzed, only 10 presented statistically significant differences, demonstrating that the sample had approximately 77% of initial cephalometric compatibility (Table 4).

Changes during treatment as well as changes occurring during the growth and development period were obtained by means of establishing the difference between treated patients' initial and final mean values. Table 4 shows the results of one-way ANOVA and Tukey tests performed among the initial cephalometric measurements mean values of the three groups.

The components related to the maxilla, mandible, maxillomandibular relationship, vertical pattern and soft tissue did not present statistically significant differences (Table 5).

Greater mesial movement of maxillary second molars was observed in the Jones jig group. Buccal tipping of mandibular incisors was greater in the Pendulum group than in the control group. Additionally, greater protrusion of these incisors was observed in the experimental groups (Fig 2). The mandibular first molars showed similar mesial movement for all the three groups; however, greater extrusion was observed in the Jones jig group when compared to the Pendulum and control groups (Table 5).

There was a significant difference in molar relationship, with a significant change for the experimental groups, which resulted in correction of the Class II. Conversely, the initial malocclusion remained in the control group (Table 5).

DISCUSSION

There are few comparatives studies assessing the first (maxillary molars distalization) and the second phase of treatment (corrective orthodontic treatment).[3,6,7,8] Thus, the aim of this study was to compare the changes at the end of the corrective orthodontic treatment, which was initialized by the distalization of the maxillary molars by two different intraoral distalization appliances. Additionally, it compared such changes to the control group.

Assessment of the characteristics related to the groups proved that there was compatibility in terms of initial age and treatment/observation times. On the other hand, the final age was statistically and

Table 4 - ANOVA and Tukey test results: means and standard deviation of initial cephalometric measurements mean values taken to assess compatibility among groups as well as values of the significance probability level (P) - (T$_1$).

Variable	Group 1 (Pendulum) n = 18	Group 2 (Jones Jig) n = 25	Group 3 (Control) n= 19	p
Maxillary Component (Mean ± SD)				
SNA (degrees)	83.13 ± 3.34^A	82.35 ± 4.13^A	81.14 ± 2.51^A	0.223
Co-A (mm)	86.66 ± 4.53^A	82.10 ± 4.86^B	81.68 ± 5.05^B	0.003*
PTVI-A (mm)	49.98 ± 2.34^A	47.82 ± 4.17^A	47.91 ± 3.03^A	0.090
Mandibular Component (Mean ± SD)				
SNB (degrees)	78.84 ± 2.77^A	78.82 ± 3.09^A	78.20 ± 2.01^A	0.702
Co-Gn (mm)	108.13 ± 4.50^A	104.86 ± 5.07^{AB}	102.72 ± 5.17^B	0.005*
P-NB (mm)	2.25 ± 1.76^A	1.56 ± 1.28^A	1.94 ± 1.21^A	0.283
PTVI-B (mm)	47.70 ± 3.04^A	46.87 ± 5.47^A	47.41 ± 4.55^A	0.833
Maxillomandibular Relationship (Mean ± SD)				
ANB (degrees)	4.28 ± 1.36^A	3.53 ± 3.08^A	2.94 ± 2.18^A	0.251
NAP (degrees)	6.29 ± 3.23^A	5.50 ± 7.12^A	4.06 ± 5.33^A	0.482
Vertical Component (Mean ± SD)				
FMA (degrees)	28.17 ± 5.14^A	29.87 ± 4.43^A	27.00 ± 3.20^A	0.096
SN.PP (degrees)	6.07 ± 3.54^A	6.22 ± 3.98^A	7.29 ± 3.15^A	0.522
SN.GoGn (degrees)	29.64 ± 5.17^A	31.54 ± 4.05^A	29.89 ± 3.34^A	0.273
SN.GoMe (degrees)	33.06 ± 5.28^A	34.64 ± 4.13^A	32.85 ± 3.12^A	0.309
NS.Gn (degrees)	65.30 ± 3.00^A	66.26 ± 3.61^A	65.40 ± 2.23^A	0.516
Occlusal plane (degrees)	8.51 ± 3.79^A	9.77 ± 4.13^A	9.54 ± 3.07^A	0.535
LAFH (mm)	62.31 ± 3.78^A	61.81 ± 5.19^A	58.37 ± 3.30^B	0.011*
Maxillary Dentoalveolar Component (Mean ± SD)				
SN.1 (degrees)	103.04 ± 6.60^A	107.84 ± 5.90^B	104.66 ± 4.96^{AB}	0.028*
PTVI-1 (mm)	55.96 ± 2.77^A	55.44 ± 4.95^A	54.71 ± 3.24^A	0.623
PP-1 (mm)	27.41 ± 2.29^A	26.87 ± 2.74^A	25.81 ± 2.01^A	0.127
1.NA (degrees)	19.89 ± 5.81^A	25.48 ± 6.09^B	23.72 ± 5.50^{AB}	0.011*
1-NA (mm)	3.29 ± 2.03^A	4.94 ± 2.86^A	4.50 ± 2.31^A	0.101
SN.4 (degrees)	81.29 ± 4.07^A	82.76 ± 4.99^A	80.06 ± 4.09^A	0.145
PTVI-4 (mm)	38.04 ± 2.28^A	36.20 ± 3.74^{AB}	35.16 ± 3.20^B	0.028*
PP-4 (mm)	19.28 ± 2.30^A	19.09 ± 2.42^A	18.31 ± 1.85^A	0.363
SN.5 (degrees)	79.33 ± 3.12^A	78.49 ± 5.46^A	77.99 ± 4.07^A	0.655
PTVI-5 (mm)	31.58 ± 2.42^A	29.80 ± 3.71^A	29.01 ± 3.32^A	0.056
PP-5 (mm)	18.81 ± 2.28^A	18.67 ± 2.42^A	17.60 ± 1.67^A	0.175
SN.6 (degrees)	66.70 ± 2.84^A	65.70 ± 4.65^A	66.98 ± 4.48^A	0.645
PTVI-6 (mm)	23.29 ± 2.37^A	21.68 ± 3.61^A	20.93 ± 3.59^A	0.092
PP-6 (mm)	17.10 ± 2.31^A	16.84 ± 2.27^A	15.72 ± 1.53^A	0.103
SN.7 (degrees)	52.96 ± 5.64^{AB}	50.92 ± 6.31^B	56.65 ± 5.02^A	0.007*
PTVI-7 (mm)	13.29 ± 2.36^A	11.98 ± 3.02^A	11.71 ± 3.05^A	0.201
PP-7 (mm)	13.57 ± 2.36^A	11.37 ± 3.76^{AB}	10.29 ± 3.01^B	0.009*
Mandibular Dentoalveolar Component (Mean ± SD)				
1.NB (degrees)	26.53 ± 4.64^A	25.64 ± 5.99^A	24.41 ± 4.50^A	0.463
1-NB (mm)	3.94 ± 2.07^A	4.45 ± 2.20^A	3.37 ± 1.39^A	0.198
PTVI- (mm)	22.22 ± 3.78^A	20.99 ± 4.27^A	21.28 ± 4.05^A	0.611
GoMe- (mm)	28.18 ± 2.01^A	27.69 ± 2.62^A	26.63 ± 2.10^A	0.117
Soft Tissue (Mean ± SD)				
NLA (degrees)	107.06 ± 11.07^{AB}	103.13 ± 10.35^A	114.09 ± 11.11^B	0.005*
E-Ls (mm)	2.38 ± 2.19^A	2.05 ± 2.71^A	2.68 ± 2.07^A	0.683
E-Li (mm)	1.46 ± 3.05^A	0.06 ± 2.38^A	1.14 ± 1.88^A	0.151
Dental Relationships (Mean ± SD)				
Molar Relationship (mm)	0.03 ± 1.17^A	-0.42 ± 1.02^{AB}	-0.93 ± 0.74^B	0.016*
Overjet (mm)	4.43 ± 1.15^A	4.67 ± 1.55^A	4.48 ± 1.95^A	0.867
Overbite (mm)	5.00 ± 1.70^A	3.92 ± 1.48^A	4.04 ± 1.53^A	0.069

* Statistically significant difference for P < 0.05.
Different letters stand for statistically significant difference.

Table 5 - ANOVA and Tukey test results: means and standard deviation of cephalometric measurements means.(ANOVA – T_3-T_1)

Variable	Group 1 (Pendulum) n = 18	Group 2 (Jones Jig) n = 25	Group 3 (Control) n = 19	P
Maxillary Component (Mean ± SD)				
SNA (degrees)	-1.07 ± 1.75[A]	0.02 ± 1.85[A]	-0.67 ± 3.43[A]	0.329
Co-A (mm)	1.22 ± 3.27[A]	1.41 ± 3.59[A]	3.20 ± 3.43[A]	0.151
PTVI-A (mm)	0.73 ± 2.40[A]	1.15 ± 2.29[A]	1.08 ± 3.62[A]	0.878
Mandibular Component (Mean ± SD)				
SNB (degrees)	-0.26 ± 1.73[A]	0.74 ± 2.28[A]	-0.35 ± 2.24[A]	0.169
Co-Gn (mm)	4.77 ± 5.82[A]	5.98 ± 4.21[A]	4.92 ± 3.31[A]	0.626
P-NB (mm)	0.61 ± 0.98[A]	0.46 ± 0.84[A]	0.25 ± 0.81[A]	0.473
PTVI-B (mm)	1.36 ± 3.62[A]	2.03 ± 2.70[A]	1.69 ± 5.09[A]	0.851
Maxillomandibular Relationship (Mean ± SD)				
ANB (degrees)	-0.81 ± 2.02[A]	-0.72 ± 2.19[A]	-0.11 ± 3.03[A]	0.796
NAP (degrees)	-2.30 ± 4.68[A]	-2.00 ± 4.79[A]	-1.07 ± 6.81[A]	0.771
Vertical Component (Mean ± SD)				
FMA (degrees)	0.46 ± 2.55[A]	1.72 ± 2.62[A]	0.31 ± 4.48[A]	0.298
SN.PP (degrees)	0.21 ± 1.83[A]	0.24 ± 3.11[A]	1.05 ± 3.22[A]	0.578
SN.GoGn (degrees)	0.46 ± 2.29[A]	0.23 ± 2.45[A]	1.16 ± 5.47[A]	0.689
SN.GoMe (degrees)	0.18 ± 2.14[A]	0.40 ± 2.20[A]	1.27 ± 4.89[A]	0.552
NS.Gn (degrees)	0.93 ± 1.51[A]	0.63 ± 2.14[A]	1.40 ± 2.93[A]	0.541
Occlusal plane (degrees)	-0.05 ± 2.80[A]	1.70 ± 3.32[A]	-1.22 ± 5.47[A]	0.057
LAFH (mm)	3.63 ± 3.01[A]	5.60 ± 2.82[A]	3.48 ± 5.38[A]	0.128
Maxillary Dentoalveolar Component (Mean ± SD)				
SN.1 (degrees)	1.68 ± 7.01[A]	-1.63 ± 6.65[A]	-1.87 ± 4.32[A]	0.147
PTVI-1 (mm)	1.40 ± 3.64[A]	1.26 ± 3.12[A]	1.63 ± 4.49[A]	0.947
PP-1 (mm)	0.58 ± 1.78[A]	1.68 ± 1.48[A]	1.07 ± 3.12[A]	0.273
1.NA (degrees)	2.79 ± 6.63[A]	-1.63 ± 6.77[A]	-1.43 ± 4.74[A]	0.051
1-NA (mm)	0.98 ± 2.40[A]	0.12 ± 2.55[A]	-0.18 ± 2.33[A]	0.322
SN.4 (degrees)	-0.29 ± 5.47[A]	-1.83 ± 4.69[A]	0.59 ± 3.23[A]	0.210
PTVI-4 (mm)	1.24 ± 2.87[AB]	2.20 ± 2.09[A]	2.10 ± 4.49[A]	0.587
PP-4 (mm)	1.80 ± 1.41[A]	2.13 ± 1.24[A]	1.63 ± 2.81[A]	0.673
SN.5 (degrees)	-1.43 ± 6.11[A]	1.76 ± 4.61[A]	0.06 ± 3.05[A]	0.095
PTVI-5 (mm)	1.20 ± 2.83[A]	2.22 ± 2.00[A]	1.81 ± 4.56[A]	0.587
PP-5 (mm)	1.86 ± 1.48[A]	2.10 ± 1.33[A]	1.95 ± 2.75[A]	0.915
SN.6 (degrees)	-0.77 ± 6.67[A]	1.55 ± 4.85[A]	0.20 ± 5.65[A]	0.409
PTVI-6 (mm)	0.61 ± 2.68[A]	1.82 ± 1.89[A]	1.98 ± 4.60[A]	0.356
PP-6 (mm)	2.10 ± 1.57[A]	2.39 ± 1.54[A]	2.36 ± 3.06[A]	0.896
SN.7 (degrees)	1.59 ± 6.53[AB]	5.44 ± 7.31[A]	-0.76 ± 5.81[B]	0.010*
PTVI-7 (mm)	0.75 ± 2.73[A]	1.42 ± 1.91[A]	1.47 ± 4.00[A]	0.695
PP-7 (mm)	2.37 ± 2.16[A]	4.40 ± 2.89[A]	4.32 ± 3.90[A]	0.074
Mandibular Dentoalveolar Component (Mean ± SD)				
1.NB (degrees)	6.18 ± 6.72[A]	2.52 ± 5.56[AB]	-0.73 ± 3.28[B]	0.001*
1-NB (mm)	1.70 ± 1.64[A]	1.41 ± 1.89[A]	0.06 ± 0.85[B]	0.004*
PTVI- (mm)	2.27 ± 2.68[A]	2.83 ± 2.23[A]	2.42 ± 3.14[A]	0.774
GoMe- (mm)	2.04 ± 1.60[A]	3.76 ± 2.37[B]	1.90 ± 1.85[A]	0.004*
Soft Tissue (Mean ± SD)				
NLA (degrees)	2.06 ± 9.01[A]	1.60 ± 7.54[A]	2.36 ± 8.51[A]	0.975
E-Ls (mm)	1.56 ± 1.01[A]	1.91 ± 1.53[A]	1.03 ± 2.03[A]	0.199
E-Li (mm)	0.28 ± 1.24[A]	0.74 ± 1.21[A]	1.40 ± 2.63[A]	0.165
Dental Relationships (Mean ± SD)				
Molar relationship (mm)	-2.62 ± 1.29[A]	-2.36 ± 1.36[A]	-0.22 ± 1.24[B]	0.000*
Overjet (mm)	-1.35 ± 1.37[AB]	-1.90 ± 1.69[A]	-0.14 ± 2.00[B]	0.005*
Overbite (mm)	-2.47 ± 1.68[A]	-1.56 ± 1.51[A]	-0.13 ± 1.94[B]	0.000*

* Statistically significant difference for P < 0.05
Different letters stand for statistically significant difference.

significantly different, representing a trend of an older age in group 1. However, most studies in the literature consider compatibility of initial age and treatment time,[2,5] only, which is considered as sufficient to characterize a reliable sample compatibility.[7]

Changes during treatment for the variables of both maxillary and mandibular components were similar among the three groups (Table 5), and improvements in the maxillomandibular relationship were observed. However, this change was more significant in the experimental groups and it is justified by the treatment performed. Conversely, although this improvement was less significant in the control group, it was due to craniofacial growth. The results prove that intraoral distalization appliances do not interfere in craniofacial growth and development.[6,19,21]

Assessment of the vertical skeletal variables in the initial stage, except for the lower anterior face height (LAFH), demonstrates that the measurements showed no statistically significant difference among groups. Changes happening as a result of treatment and growth were statistically similar for the three groups; however, they were numerically higher in the Jones jig group. The different changes for the Jones jig and control groups occurred due to the extrusion of first and second premolars during treatment, in other words, although not significant, extrusion of these teeth was slightly higher in the Jones jig group than in the control group (Table 5).

Results demonstrate that the three groups showed clockwise mandibular rotation, which confirms the downward displacement of the mandible, as observed during the post-distalization stage of several studies.[3,6,7,8,10,21] Assuming that this change occurred as a result of maxillary premolars and molars extrusion due to loss of anchorage and the distalization effect, it is thought that during corrective treatment, correction of extrusions will occur and the rotation will be reversed as a consequence. However, according to Taner-Sarisoy and Darendeliler,[23] most orthodontic mechanics, if not all, are extrusive and this extrusion increases the LAFH during treatment, keeping it increased during the retention period. Moreover, an increase in LAFH due to craniofacial growth and development is common.[18] Therefore, it can be stated that mandibular rotation is related to changes in the distalization phase,[3,8,21] the corrective orthodontic mechanics[23] and craniofacial growth and development.[18]

During the observation period, changes in the nasolabial angle were similar in the three groups. This finding demonstrates that the treatment protocol used does not interfere in the tegumental profile; therefore, the facial characteristics are maintained in the experimental groups.[8]

When assessing the maxillary dentoalveolar component, it was observed that only the maxillary second molars showed significant changes, i.e., at treatment onset, the Jones jig group presented the second molars more distally angulated than the control group, and during treatment, this group also showed a greater mesial angulation in relation to the control group. This initial position can be explained by the difference in the mean initial age that, although not significant, was lower in the Jones jig than in the control group (Table 1); hence, the second molars were more below the occlusal plane, showing a more distal position.

Regarding the positioning of the mandibular incisors, a minor change was observed in the control group, while the Pendulum and Jones jig groups presented greater buccal tipping and protrusion of the mandibular incisors, certainly related to the use of Class II rubber bands and overjet correction, which occurred as a consequence of the compensation of the mandibular teeth (Fig 2).

As for the vertical positioning of the mandibular molars, significant extrusion was greater in the Jones jig group than in the Pendulum and control groups. This change was related not only to the use of Class II rubber bands, but also to the end of eruption, since, at the beginning of treatment, the mandibular molars were more below the occlusal plan in comparison to the Pendulum group because patients were slightly younger and had greater potential for eruption.[13]

The molar relationship at treatment onset showed a statistically significant difference between the Pendulum and control groups, confirming the trend of greater severity of the Pendulum group. As expected, during observation of the change in molar relationship in the course of treatment, the experimental groups presented significative Class II correction when compared to the control group in which malocclusion remained. Therefore, it appears that the treatment successfully decreased anteroposterior interarch discrepancy, which reveals the contribution of this therapy in the correction of the Class II molar relationship and accentuated overjet.

The literature[3,7,8] proves that intraoral distalization appliances followed by fixed corrective orthodontics are effective in the correction of Class II and that there is stability of about 82% of the occlusal results achieved in the long-term.[1]

Overjet and overbite were similar in the three groups at treatment onset; however, there was a correction in the treated groups during treatment, which was not observed in the control group. This difference was expected since patients in the experimental groups were subjected to corrective treatment and individuals in the control group, in which malocclusion remained at the end of the observation period, the overjet and overbite also remained, i.e., the Class II malocclusion does not correct itself.

Despite the distinct insertion sites among the appliances assessed, i.e., palatal and buccal, no changes were related to this difference, since orthodontic treatment with fixed appliance acts with the purpose of neutralizing the specific effects of intraoral distalization and finalizing the corrective treatment.

CONCLUSIONS

Intraoral distalization appliances followed by fixed corrective orthodontics do not interfere in the cephalometric pattern and tegumental profile, as demonstrated by the results which are similar to the control group with regard to the components of both the maxilla and the mandible, maxillomandibular relationship, craniofacial and tegumental pattern. The mandibular incisors showed significant protrusion and buccal tipping in the experimental groups and the maxillary second molars showed more mesial angulation in the Jones jig group. Finally, correction of Class II malocclusion, overjet and overbite were observed in the Pendulum and Jones jig groups, and in the control group, the initial malocclusion remained at the end of the observation period.

REFERENCES

1. Alessio Jr L. Avaliação longitudinal da estabilidade do tratamento da má oclusão de Classe II com o aparelho Pendulum seguido pelo aparelho fixo [tese]. Bauru (SP): Universidade de São Paulo; 2009.

2. Angelieri F. Comparação dos efeitos cefalométricos promovidos pelos aparelhos extrabucal cervical e pendulum [tese]. Bauru (SP): Universidade de São Paulo; 2005.

3. Angelieri F, Almeida RR, Almeida MR, Fuziy A. Dentoalveolar and skeletal changes associated with the pendulum appliance followed by fixed orthodontic treatment. Am J Orthod Dentofacial Orthop. 2006;129(4):520-7.

4. Antonarakis GS, Kiliaridis S. Maxillary molar distalization with noncompliance intramaxillary appliances in Class II malocclusion. A systematic review. Angle Orthod. 2008;78(6):1133-40.

5. Brandão AG. Estudo cefalométrico comparativo das alterações promovidas pelos aparelhos de protração mandibular e Pendulum, associados ao aparelho fixo, no tratamento da má oclusão de Classe II, 1ª divisão [tese]. Bauru (SP): Universidade de São Paulo; 2006.

6. Brickman CD, Sinha PK, Nanda RS. Evaluation of the Jones jig appliance for distal molar movement. Am J Orthod Dentofacial Orthop. 2000;118(5):526-34.

7. Burkhardt DR, McNamara JA Jr, Baccetti T. Maxillary molar distalization or mandibular enhancement: a cephalometric comparison of comprehensive orthodontic treatment including the pendulum and the Herbst appliances. Am J Orthod Dentofacial Orthop. 2003;123(2):108-16.

8. Chiu PP, McNamara JA Jr, Franchi L. A comparison of two intraoral molar distalization appliances: Distal Jet versus pendulum. Am J Orthod Dentofacial Orthop. 2005;128(3):353-65.

9. Fuziy A, Rodrigues de Almeida R, Janson G, Angelieri F, Pinzan A. Sagittal, vertical, and transverse changes consequent to maxillary molar distalization with the pendulum appliance. Am J Orthod Dentofacial Orthop. 2006;130(4):502-10.

10. Ghosh J, Nanda RS. Evaluation of an intraoral maxillary molar distalization technique. Am J Orthod Dentofacial Orthop. 1996;110(6):639-46.

11. Haydar S, Uner O. Comparison of Jones jig molar distalization appliance with extraoral traction. Am J Orthod Dentofacial Orthop. 2000;117(1):49-53.

12. Hilgers JJ. The pendulum appliance for Class II non-compliance therapy. J Clin Orthod. 1992;26(11):706-14.

13. Iseri H, Solow B. Continued eruption of maxillary incisors and first molars in girls from 9 to 25 years, studied by the implant method. Eur J Orthod. 1996;18(3):245-56.

14. Jones RD, White JM. Rapid Class II molar correction with an open-coil jig. J Clin Orthod. 1992;26(10):661-4.

15. Kinzinger GS, Gross U, Fritz UB, Diedrich PR. Anchorage quality of deciduous molars versus premolars for molar distalization with a pendulum appliance. Am J Orthod Dentofacial Orthop. 2005;127(3):314-23.

16. Kinzinger G, Syrée C, Fritz U, Diedrich P. Molar distalization with different pendulum appliances: in vitro registration of orthodontic forces and moments in the initial phase. J Orofac Orthop. 2004;65(5):389-409.

17. Lopes RSR. Avaliação cefalométrica das alterações dentoesqueléticas e tegumentares em jovens com má oclusão de Classe II tratados com distalizadores Distal Jet [tese]. Bauru (SP): Universidade de São Paulo; 2007.

18. Martins DR, Janson G, Almeida RR, Pinzan A, Henriques JFC, Freitas MR. Atlas de crescimento craniofacial. São Paulo: Ed. Santos; 1998.

19. Papadopoulos MA, Mavropoulos A, Karamouzos A. Cephalometric changes following simultaneous first and second maxillary molar distalization using a non-compliance intraoral appliance. J Orofac Orthop. 2004;65(2):123-36.

20. Patel MP. Estudo cefalométrico comparativo do tratamento da má oclusão de Classe II com os distalizadores Pendulum e Jones jig seguidos do aparelho fixo corretivo [tese]. Bauru (SP): Universidade de São Paulo; 2010.

21. Patel MP, Janson G, Henriques JF, Almeida RR, Freitas MR, Pinzan A, et al. Comparative distalization effects of Jones jig and pendulum appliances. Am J Orthod Dentofacial Orthop. 2009;135(3):336-42.

22. Runge ME, Martin JT, Bukai F. Analysis of rapid maxillary molar distal movement without patient cooperation. Am J Orthod Dentofacial Orthop. 1999;115(2):153-7.

23. Taner-Sarisoy L, Darendeliler N. The influence of extraction orthodontic treatment on craniofacial structures: evaluation according to two different factors. Am J Orthod Dentofacial Orthop. 1999;115(5):508-14.

Class II malocclusion treatment using high-pull headgear with a splint

Helder B. Jacob[1], Peter H. Buschang[2], Ary dos Santos-Pinto[3]

Objective: To systematically review the scientific evidence pertaining to the effectiveness of high-pull headgear in growing Class II subjects. **Methods:** A literature survey was performed by electronic database search. The survey covered the period from January 1966 to December 2008 and used Medical Subject Headings (MeSH). Articles were initially selected based on their titles and abstracts; the full articles were then retrieved. The inclusion criteria included growing subjects between 8 to 15 years of age, Class II malocclusion treatment with high-pull headgear, and a control group with Class II malocclusion. References from selected articles were hand-searched for additional publications. Selected studies were evaluated methodologically. **Results:** Four articles were selected; none were randomized controlled trials. All of the articles clearly formulated their objectives and used appropriate measures. The studies showed that high-pull headgear treatment improves skeletal and dental relationship, distal displacement of the maxilla, vertical eruption control and upper molars distalization. One of the studies showed a slight clockwise rotation of the palatal plane; the others showed no significant treatment effect. The mandible was not affected by the treatment. **Conclusion:** While there is still a lack of strong evidence demonstrating the effects of high-pull headgear with a splint, other studies indicate that the AP relations improve due to distalization of the maxilla and upper molars, with little or no treatment effects in the mandible. Greater attention to the design should be given to improve the quality of such trials.

Keywords: Orthodontics. Angle Class II malocclusion. Treatment results.

[1] PhD in Orthodontics, Araraquara Dental School/São Paulo State University-UNESP, Araraquara, SP, Brazil. Post-doc in Orthodontics, Texas A&M Health Science Center.
[2] Professor, Baylor College of Dentistry, Texas A&M Health Science Center.
[3] Professor, Department of Orthodontics, Araraquara Dental School, São Paulo State University-UNESP, Araraquara, SP, Brazil

Helder Baldi Jacob
3302 Gaston Ave – Baylor College of Dentistry
Department of Orthodontics
75206 Dallas/TX – USA
E-mail: hjacob@bcd.tamhsc.edu

INTRODUCTION

Class II malocclusion can be dental and/or skeletal, involving mandibular deficiency, maxillary excess, or a combination of both.[1,2] Hyperdivergent patients with Class II malocclusion typically present with numerous three-dimensional skeletal and dental problems.[3] They exhibit retrognathic mandibles,[4] long anterior facial heights,[3] large mandibular plane angle,[4] large gonial angles,[3] and greater than average anterior facial height ratio.[5,6,7] Dentally, they often present with open bite[9] and overerupted incisors and molars in both arches.[3]

Orthodontists have attempted to address the vertical dimension of growing hyperdivergent patients in various ways (e.g. bite-blocks, extraction therapy, vertical-pull chin, etc.), with high-pull headgear being perhaps the most common approach. The use of extraoral high-pull forces to modify maxilla growth has a long history. The type of extraoral traction device, as well as the magnitude of force applied and the direction of pull, have been shown to be important considerations.[8,9] High-pull headgear has been shown to modify maxillary growth;[10] when attached to a splint directs maxillary growth towards a more posterosuperior direction.[11,12] To date, the treatment effects of high-pull headgear have not been systematically studied.

The purpose of this study was to systematically review clinical studies that have evaluated how high-pull headgear treatment with a splint affects growing Class II hyperdivergent patients. The review will foccused on:

» Changes in the amount and direction of skeletal growth.
» Control of maxillary and mandibular molar eruption.
» Improvements of the vertical and AP skeletal relationship.

MATERIAL AND METHODS

In order to identify all studies that examined treatment with high-pull headgear in patients with Class II malocclusion, a literature survey was performed using PubMed and Scopus databases. The survey covered the period from January 1966 to December 2008. Using the Medical Subject Heading (MeSH) term "orthodontics", crossed with the MeSH terms "malocclusion, Class II malocclusion" and "extraoral traction appliance", a total of 442 studies were identified. Only randomized controlled trials (RCTs) or non-randomized controlled trials (using untreated Class II hyperdivergent patients as controls) were included (Table 1). At the first view no distinction was made between high-pull headgear with a maxillary splint or banded molars. The reference list of each article was hand-searched for additional relevant publications that may have been missed in the database searches.

Following the recommendations by Petrén et al,[13] the articles were described based on the following: study design, sample size, male and female distribution, mean age of groups, type of orthodontic treatment, treatment duration, success, and authors' conclusion (Table 2).

To document the methodological soundness of each article, a modified version of the quality evaluation described by Antczak et al[14,15] was used (Table 3). The adequacy of sample was determined based on post-hoc power analyses of the primary variable used in each study to evaluate the AP treatment effects on the maxilla. The total quality score was based on assigning 1 point for each "Yes" in the Table, zero points for each "No", and 1 point for each controlled clinical trial (CCT). Prospective and retrospective studies were given one and zero points, respectively. The total number of points possible was 10.

Modified pitchfork diagrams were used to summarize the rotations, displacements and tooth movements associated with the high-pull headgear treatments. Rotations were based on the angular changes of the palatal and mandibular planes. The horizontal and vertical displacements of the maxilla and mandible were based on cranial base superimpositions. Tooth migration and eruption was based on maxillary and mandibular superimpositions. Estimates were based on averages of the four studies that provided tooth movements based on maxillary and mandibular superimpositions.

Table 1 - Inclusion and exclusion criteria used to select the articles.

Inclusion criteria	Exclusion criteria
• Meta-analyses, randomized clinical trials, prospective and retrospective studies	• Case reports, case series, descriptive studies, opinion articles or abstracts
• Articles published from January 1966 and December 2008	• Studies with casts
• Studies with Class II malocclusion	• Not human studies or laboratorial studies
• Studies with growing patients 8-15 years	• Adjunctive treatments
• Studies with extraoral high-pull headgear, using maxillary splints or banded molars	• Full or partially banded appliances
	• Subjects with TMJ diseases
• Cephalometric data provided	• No control group or control group with normal malocclusion

Table 2 - Summarized data of the studies included in the review.

Authors and year	Study design	Sample size	Male (%)	Age	Orthodontic treatment	Treatment duration	Success	Authors' conclusion
Caldwell et al[12] (1984)	CCT	47 HG 52 CG	HG: 45% CG: 52%	HG: M=10.23(y) F=10.19(y) CG: M=10.36(y) F=10.21(y)	Maxillary splint appliance	Between 4 and 20(m)	Not declared (100% - implicit)	The maxillary dentition was both tipped and displaced distally, and downward development was inhibited or even slightly reversed
Martins et al[18] (2008)	CCT	17 HG 17 CG	HG: 24% CG: 47%	HG: 8.61(y) CG: 8.9(y)	Maxillary splint appliance	HG: 1.70(y) CG: 1.40(y)	Not declared (100% - implicit)	The HG corrected the Class II primarily by dentoalveolar changes
Orton et al[19] (1992)	CCT	26 HG 26 CG	HG: 42% CG: 42%	HG: 11.4(y) CG: 11(y)	Maxillary splint appliance	HG: 1.1(y) CG: 1.7(y)	Not declared (100% - implicit)	Slight maxillary restraint in both sagittal and vertical planes was obtained showing that principal effect was in the maxillary teeth
Üner, Yücel-Eroğlu[20] (1996)	CCT	13 HG 13 CG	HG: 46% CG: 46%	HG: 10.76y CG: 10.39(y)	Maxillary splint appliance	HG: 11.00(m) GC: 11.31(m)	84%	The HG revealed that the splint had both orthopedic and orthodontic effects on the growth pattern of the dentoskeletal structures

Table 3 - Quality evaluation of the 6 selected studies (CCT: control clinical trial).

Authors and year	Objective clearly formulated	Study design	Adequacy of selection description	Adequate sample size	Appropriate measurement method	Retrospective / prospective study	Appropriate statistical analysis	Description of method error analysis	Blind measurement	Quality score / total
Caldwell et al[12] (1984)	Yes	CCT	No	Yes	Yes	Retrospective	No	No	No	4
Martins et al[18] (2008)	Yes	CCT	Yes	Yes	Yes	Prospective	Yes	Yes	No	7
Orton et al[19] (1992)	Yes	CCT	Yes	Yes	Yes	Retrospective	Yes	No	No	6
Üner, Yücel-Eroğlu[20] (1996)	Yes	CCT	Yes	Yes	Yes	Retrospective	Yes	Yes	No	7

RESULTS

Based on the information provided in the titles and abstracts of the 442 articles identified, 17 of the studies were pre-selected (Fig 1). The main reasons for exclusion were: Different types of appliances used (e.g. high-pull headgear associated with functional appliance or bonded brackets), the direction of force application (cervical or combination traction), no cephalometric data provided, and case reports. Of the 17 studies identified, only 4 used untreated Class II control.[12,18-20]

Sample sizes of the treatment groups ranged from 13 to 47, with comparable numbers of controls (Table 2). While the sex ratio ranged from 24 to 46% of males, none of the studies analyzed sex differences. Pretreatment ages and treatment durations ranged from 8.6 to 11.4 years and 4 to 20 months, respectively. All four selected studies compared maxillary orthopedic splint versus no treatment.

Three of the studies implied a 100% success Class II correction; the Üner and Yücel-Eroğlu[20] study reported an 84% success rate.

The quality evaluation scores of the four studies ranged from 4 to 7 (Table 2). None of the articles were RCT; all studies were controlled clinical trials. None of the articles blinded the measurement process. Only one of the studies was prospective and only two described the methods used for the error analysis. Three of the studies adequately described the selection of their subjects and three used appropriate statistical techniques. All of the articles clearly formulated their objectives and all used appropriate measures.

Treatment effects produced by high-pull headgear

Treatments consistently improved the AP skeletal relationships (with the ANB angle decreasing from 0.9 to 1.5 degrees and the Wits decreasing from 0.6 to 1.5 mm), decreased overjet (2.6 to 6.5 mm), and corrected the Class II malocclusions (Table 4).

Maxillary treatment effects

Although the studies used different criteria to measure the anteroposterior displacement, they all reported statistically significant posterior displacement of the maxilla (ranging from 0.1 to 0.5 mm) for the treated group, versus anterior displacement for the untreated controls (Fig 2). Of the three studies that evaluated the palatal plane angle, just one study showed statistically significant clockwise rotation between the treated and control groups (Fig 3).

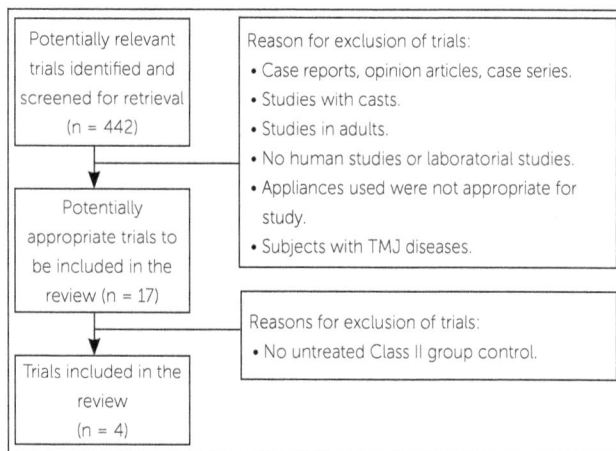

Figure 1 - Flow diagram summarizing literature search.

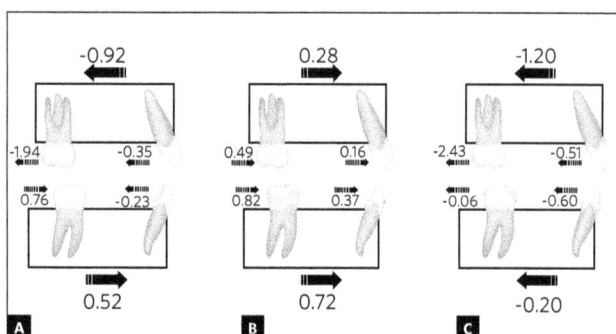

Figure 2 - Modified pitchforks of average horizontal (mm) changes reported for (A) patient treated with headgear and (B) matched untreated controls, along with (C) differences between high-pull headgear and controls.

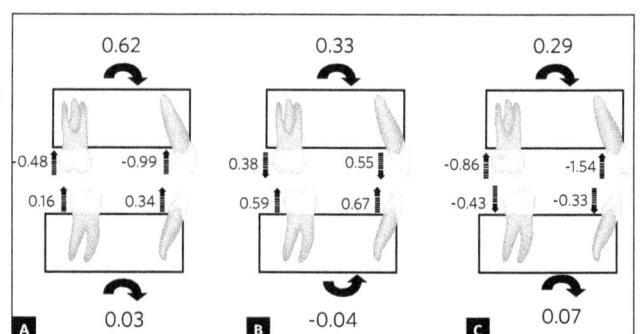

Figure 3 - Modified pitchforks of average vertical (mm) and angular (degrees) changes reported for (A) patient treated with headgear and (B) matched untreated controls, along with (C) differences between high-pull headgear and controls.

Table 4 - Treatment effects based on significant differences between patients and untreated controls.

Authors and year	Antero-posterior relationships	Skeletal-maxillary changes	Dental-maxillary changes	Skeletal-mandibular changes	Dental-mandibular changes
Caldwell et al[12] (1984)	Decreased ANB; decreased overjet	Posterior displacement; backward rotation of palatal plane	Distalized molars; intruded molars; retroclined incisor; intruded incisors	Anterior displacement NS; backward mandibular rotation	Mesialized molar NS; extruded molar NS; incisor retroclined
Martins et al[18] (2008)	Greater decreased ANB and Wits than expected	Posterior displacement; palatal plane angle NE	Distalized molars; intrusion NE; retroclined incisors	Anterior displacement NS; mandibular rotation NS	Mesialized molar NS; incisor proclined NS; vertical NE
Orton et al[19] (1992)	Reduction of ANB; decreased overjet	Posterior displacement; backward rotation of the palatal plane	Distalized molars; intruded molars; retroclined incisors; intruded incisors	Anterior displacement NS; mandibular rotation NS	Mesialized molar NS; extruded molars; incisor retroclined NS
Üner and Yücel-Eroğlu[20] (1996)	Correction of Class II molar relations; decreased overjet	Posterior displacement; NS in palatal plane rotation	Distalized molars; molar intrusion NS; proclined incisors; intruded incisors	Anterior displacement NS; mandibular rotation NS	Molar movements NS; incisors retroclined

(NS=no significant group differences; NE=not evaluated).

All of the studies reported significant distalization of the maxillary molar (ranging between 0.5 and 3.3 mm) and two showed maxillary molar intrusion (between 0.4 and 0.7 mm). The control groups typically showed mesial drift and eruption of the maxillary molars (Figs 2 and 3). Three studies reported statistically significant retroclination (between 4.4 and 11.0 degrees) and intrusion of the maxillary incisors (between 0.2 and 2.1 mm).

Treatment effects on the mandible

All four articles showed no treatment effect on the AP position of the mandible (Fig 2). All studies evaluated the mandibular plane rotation and reported no significant differences between the treated and control groups (Figs 2 and 3).

All studies reported similar amounts of mesial movement of the mandibular molars (ranging between 0.8 mm and 1.2 mm) for the treated and control groups (Fig 2). Of the three studies that evaluated the vertical movements of the molars, all showed no treatment effects, but just one showed relative molar extrusion (Fig 3). Of the four articles that evaluated the incisors, three showed incisor retroclination (ranging from 0.2 to 1.9 degrees), and one showed incisor proclination (1.0 degree) with no significant difference between both groups.

DISCUSSION

The goal of orthopedic headgear treatment is to correct the dental malocclusion, normalize AP skeletal relationships, and improve, or prevent worsening of the vertical skeletal relationships. The results clearly showed improvement of the dental and AP skeletal relationships. The ANB and Wits appraisal decreased in the treated group; Class II correction was successful in 3 of the studies. Based on the mandibular plane angle, the vertical skeletal relations were generally maintained.

High-pull headgear treatment restricted the forward growth of the maxilla. Based on SNA changes, there was, on average, approximately 1.1 degree posterior repositioning of the maxilla in the treated subjects, compared to slight anterior repositioning for the untreated controls. Studies consistently report that headgears used to correct Class II malocclusions are generally effective in redirecting the maxillary growth posteriorly[10,21,22] or in limiting the forward growth of the maxilla.[23]

High-pull headgear appears to produce a slight clockwise rotation of the palatal plane. However, this effect was small (less than 0.8 degrees on average) and inconsistent across studies of high-pull headgear. Other studies evaluating the effects of combined, cervical or high-pull headgear have also reported a lack of consistent results.[10,23] Clockwise rotation of the palatal plane might be expected considering that the headgear forces are directly through the posterior maxilla, resulting in relatively greater inferior displacement of the anterior maxilla. If the force is applied in the canine area, high-pull headgear has been shown to decrease the palatal plane angle.[24]

Bowden[8,9] previously emphasized how important the point of force application was for understanding changes of the palatal plane angle. If the force vector passes through the center of resistance of the maxilla, which is approximately located at the superior and posterior part of the zygomato-maxillary suture,[25,26] no moment will be created and no rotation should be expected. If however, the force vector pass posterior to the center of resistance, clockwise rotation of the maxilla might be expected. The direction and moment created will depend upon the shortest perpendicular distance from the force vector to the center of resistance.

Dentoalveolar changes were largely responsible for the correction of the Class II malocclusions. The maxillary molars were moved and tipped distally. Based on the averages derived from the studies, distal molar movement accounted for approximately 2.1 mm (between 84% and 100%) of the correction. Headgears generally maintain or move the maxillary first molars distally.[23,28] Vertically, high-pull headgear is used to control the vertical movements of the maxillary molars, and may even intrude them slightly, whereas cervical headgear has little or no effects on vertical molar changes.[10,22-25]

Although, on average, the maxillary incisors were retroclined and intruded, there was great variability (from -1.7 to -4.5 mm in horizontal direction and from -2.1 to 0.2 mm in vertical direction) in the changes reported in the six studies evaluated. The literature is also inconsistent in terms of incisor changes for headgear studies in general.[27] The variability could be attributed to differences in the force directions and study appliances used.

There were only very limited effects of the appliance on the mandible. Mandibular sagittal changes were effectively similar in the treated and untreated groups. Of the studies that evaluated the AP position of the mandible, all four reported no treatment effect.

As such, headgear improves the sagittal intermaxillary relationship almost exclusively by holding the maxilla. This effect on sagittal intermaxillary relationship is in contrast to functional appliances, which have shown improve sagittal intermaxillary relationship with treatment effects on the mandible.[27,28] Slight clockwise rotation of the mandible occurred in only one study, indicating adequate vertical control. Compared with cervical headgear, the high-pull headgear therapy appears to provide better vertical control.[29]

With respect to mandibular tooth movements, the studies showed retroclination of the incisors. This can be explained by anterior contact of these teeth with the acrylic splint that covers the maxillary incisors, exerting a distal force on the incisors. When upper molars are intruded with the high-pull headgear, the lower molar extruded might be expected in order to maintain occlusal contact.[10,22] The lack of significant extrusion in the lower molars in the studies reviewed is associated with the maxillary splints that were used, acting like a bite block to maintain the position of the lower molars. Treatment had no effect on the mesial movements of the mandible molars.

CONCLUSION

While there is a lack of strong evidence demonstrating the effects of high-pull headgear with a splint, based on the information provided in this systematic review of four clinically controlled trials evaluating the effects of high-pull headgear on subjects with Class II malocclusions, the following conclusions could be drawn:

1. High-pull headgear displaced the maxilla posteriorly and slightly rotated the palatal plane clockwise.
2. The upper molars were distalized and the vertical position was maintained by high-pull headgear. Treatment effects on the lower incisors were inconsistent.
3. High-pull headgear treatment consistently improved the AP skeletal relationships, but not the vertical skeletal relationships.
4. Greater attention to the design and report of studies should be given to improve the quality of such trials.

REFERENCES

1. McNamara JA. Components of Class II malocclusion in children 8-10 years of age. Angle Orthod. 1981;51(3):177-202.
2. Proffit WR, Fields HW, Ackerman JL, Sinclair PM, Thomas PM, Tulloch JFC. Contemporary orthodontics. St. Louis: Mosby-Year Book; 1993.
3. Buschang PH, Sankey W, English JD. Early treatment of hyperdivergent open-bite malocclusions. Semin Orthod. 2002;8:130-40.
4. Isaacson JR, Isaacson RJ, Speidel TM, Worms FW. Extreme variation in vertical facial growth and associated variation in skeletal and dental relations. Angle Orthod. 1971;41(1):219-29.
5. Cangialosi T. Skeletal morphologic features of anterior open-bite. Am J Orthod. 1984;85(1):28-36.
6. Fields H, Proffit W, Nixon W, Phillips C, Stanek E. Facial pattern differences in long-faced children and adults. Am J Orthod. 1984;85(3):217-23.
7. Nanda S. Patterns of vertical growth in the face. Am J Orthod Dentofacial Orthop. 1988;93(2):103-16.
8. Bowden DE. Theoretical considerations of headgear therapy: a literature review. Br J Orthod. 1978;5:145-52.
9. Bowden DE. Theoretical considerations of headgear therapy: a literature review 2. Br J Orthod. 1978;5(4):173-81.
10. Brown P. A cephalometric evaluation of high-pull molar headgear and face-bow neck strap therapy. Am J Orthod. 1978;74(6):621-32.
11. Boecler PR, Riolo ML, Keeling SD, Tenhave TR. Skeletal changes associated with extraoral appliance therapy: an evaluation of 200 consecutively treated cases. Angle Orthod. 1989;59(4):263-70.
12. Caldwell SF, Hymas TA, Timm TA. Maxillary traction splint: a cephalometric evaluation. Am J Orthod. 1984;85(5):376-84.
13. Petrén S, Bondemark L, Soderfeld B. A systematic review concerning early orthodontic treatment of unilateral posterior crossbite. Angle Orthod. 2003;73(5):588-96.
14. Antczak AA, Tang J, Chalmers TC. Quality assessment of randomized control trials in dental research. I. Methods. J Periodontal Res. 1986;21:305-14.
15. Antczak AA, Tang J, Chalmers TC. Quality assessment of randomized control trials in dental research. II. Results: periodontal research. J Periodontal Res. 1986;21:315-21
16. Baumrind S, Korn EL, Isaacson RJ, West EE, Molthen R. Quantitative analysis of the orthodontic and orthopedic effects of maxillary traction. Am J Orthod. 1983;84(5):384-98.
17. Firouz M, Zernik J, Nanda R. Dental and orthopedic effects of high-pull headgear in treatment of Class II, division 1 malocclusion. Am J Orthod Dentofacial Orthop. 1992;102(3):197-205.
18. Martins RP, Martins JCR, Martins LP, Buschang PH. Skeletal and dental components of Class II correction with the bionator and removable headgear splint appliances. Am J Orthod Dentofacial Orthop. 2008;134(6):732-41.
19. Orton HS, Slattery DA, Orton S. The treatment of severe "gummy" Class II division 1 malocclusion using the maxillary intrusion splint. Eur J Orthod. 1992;14(3):216-23.
20. Üner O, Yucel-Eroğlu E. Effects of a modified maxillary orthopaedic splint: a cephalometric evaluation. Eur J Orthod. 1996;18(3):269-86.
21. Melsen B. Effects of cervical anchorage during and after treatment: an implant study. Am J Orthod. 1978;73(5):526-40.
22. Üçem TT, Yüksel S. Effects of different vectors of forces applied by combined headgear. Am J Orthod Dentofacial Orthop. 1998;113(3):316-23.
23. O'Reilly MT, Nanda SK, Close J. Cervical and oblique headgear: A comparison of treatment effects. Am J Orthod Dentofacial Orthop. 1993;103(6):504-9.
24. Barton JJ. High-pull headgear versus cervical traction: a cephalometric comparison. Am J Orthod. 1972;62(5):517-29.
25. Teuscher UM. A growth related concept for skeletal Class II treatment. Am J Orthod. 1978;74(3):258-75.
26. Teuscher UM. Appraisal of growth and reaction to extraoral anchorage. Am J Orthod. 1986;89(2):113-21.
27. Keeling SD, Wheeler TT, King GJ, Garvan CW, Cohen DA, Cabassa S, et al. Anteroposterior skeletal and dental changes after early Class II treatment with bionators and headgear. Am J Orthod Dentofacial Orthop. 1998;113(1):40-50.
28. Türkkahraman H, Sayin MÖ. Effects of activator and activator headgear treatment: comparison with untreated Class II subjects. Eur J Orthod. 2006;28(1):27-34.
29. Burke M, Jacobson A. Vertical change in high angle Class II, division 1 patients treated with cervical or occipital headgear. Am J Orthod Dentofacial Orthop. 1992;102(6):501-8.

5

Impact of malocclusion on the quality of life of children aged 8 to 10 years

Sônia Rodrigues Dutra[1], Henrique Pretti[2], Milene Torres Martins[3], Cristiane Baccin Bendo[2], Miriam Pimenta Vale[2]

Objective: The aim of the present cross-sectional study was to assess the impact of malocclusion on the quality of life of children aged 8 to 10 years attending public elementary schools in Belo Horizonte, State of Minas Gerais, Brazil. **Methods:** The Brazilian version of the Child Perceptions Questionnaire 8-10 (CPQ8-10) was used to evaluate oral health-related quality of life. The children were examined for the diagnosis of malocclusion using the Dental Aesthetic Index (DAI). The data were analyzed by bivariate and multivariate descriptive statistics using Poisson regression at a 5% significance level. A total of 270 children participated in the study. **Results:** Children with normal occlusion or mild malocclusion (DAI ≤25) were 56% less likely (95%CI: 0.258-0.758; $p=0.003$) to have their quality of life affected compared with children diagnosed with extremely severe malocclusion (DAI≥36). Children with a maxillary anterior overjet ≥ 3mm had higher CPQ_{8-10} mean scores (19.4; SD = 17.1) than those with an overjet < 3mm (13.6; SD = 11.7; $p=0.038$). **Conclusions:** Extremely severe malocclusion and pronounced maxillary anterior overjet were associated with a negative impact on quality of life.

Keywords: Mixed dentition. Malocclusion. Quality of life.

[1] Private practice (Belo Horizonte/MG, Brazil).

[2] Universidade Federal de Minas Gerais, Faculdade de Odontologia, Departamento de Odontopediatria e Ortodontia (Belo Horizonte/MG, Brazil).

[3] Universidade Estadual de Montes Claros, Curso de Odontologia (Montes Claros/MG, Brazil).

» The authors report no commercial, proprietary or financial interest in the products or companies described in this article.

Sônia Rodrigues Dutra
Av. Antônio Carlos, 6627 – Belo Horizonte/MG – CEP: 31.270-901, Brasil
E-mail: soniardutra@yahoo.com.br

INTRODUCTION

Quality of life is a concept that includes several domains, such as the subjective perception of physical, psychological, and social functions, in addition to a subjective sense of well-being.[1,2] Oral health is crucial for good quality of life[3] as it may have an impact on children's feeding, smiling, speaking, and socializing. Facial appearance influences self-esteem and emotional well-being, playing an important role in social interaction. Changes in these functions will consequently affect children's quality of life.[4]

Several authors have investigated the benefits of using more subjective criteria, such as an individual's perception of his/her health status and the impact of his/her disease on his/her quality of life, in the clinical assessments made by healthcare professionals. Clinical measures are important to determine a patient's normative need for treatment and associating them with information on the impact of oral changes in people's daily lives turns out to be useful.[2,5-8]

Normative indices —which are quite useful for the planning of public health services in orthodontics— have been used for assessing the severity of malocclusion. These indices allow determining the priority of care among extremely severe cases by the Brazilian Unified Health System, known as SUS.[9]

Malocclusion is a health problem that has received rapt attention, being the third most prevalent oral disease, outranked only by dental caries and periodontal disease.[9] Because of its high prevalence, malocclusion is regarded as a public health problem that may negatively interfere in patients' quality of life, hinder their social interaction, and affect their psychological well-being.[8] The same type of malocclusion has different psychosocial impacts.[10,11]

Numerous studies have assessed the impact of malocclusion on quality of life.[12-17] However, there is a paucity of studies on the impact of malocclusion on mixed dentition, especially studies that address the psychosocial factors that lead people to seek orthodontic treatment.[12] Most studies on the impact of malocclusion on quality of life have assessed adolescents and young adults.[14-17]

Previous studies involving children aged 8 to 10 years revealed that those children with malocclusion were more prone to have a negative impact on their quality of life than malocclusion-free individuals.[12,13] Some types of malocclusion also had a higher impact on quality of life.[12,13]

Accordingly, the aim of this study was to contribute to the formulation of public health policies in orthodontics. To achieve such goal, the study assessed the impact of malocclusion on the quality of life of children aged 8 to 10 years enrolled in public schools of Belo Horizonte, State of Minas Gerais, Brazil

MATERIAL AND METHODS

This cross-sectional study was conducted in Belo Horizonte, State of Minas Gerais, Brazil. A total of 270 children aged 8 to 10 years, of both sexes, were included in the study. Children with special needs or cognitive impairments reported by parents and teachers were excluded for the sample. Children with traumatic dental injuries or enamel development defects in permanent teeth were also excluded, as well as those who were wearing orthodontic appliances or with history of previous orthodontic treatment.

All of the participants were regularly enrolled in the city's public elementary schools, each of which belonged to one of the nine regional administrative units. Schools were selected from the list of all elementary schools in Belo Horizonte, provided by the State of Minas Gerais Department of Education. First, one public elementary school was randomly selected in each administrative district in Belo Horizonte. After that, the classes within the schools were selected. All 8-to-10-year-old students attending the selected classes were asked to participate. The sample was completed when the target number was reached.

The power of the sample was calculated based on the impact of malocclusion on quality of life, using EpiInfo software. The following parameters were used: 95% confidence interval; children with normal occlusion or mild malocclusion, n=157 (CPQ_{8-10} mean=13.5; SD=11.7); children with definite, severe and extremely severe malocclusion, n=113 (CPQ_{8-10} mean=20.4; SD=16.4). Using theses parameters, the power of the study was 96.9%.

The Brazilian version of the Child Perceptions Questionnaire 8-10 (CPQ_{8-10}) was applied to assess oral health-related quality of life. The responses to the questionnaire follow the 5-point Likert scale, with scores 0 to 4 for each item. The sum of scores can vary from 0 to 100. Score zero (0) indicates no impact of children's oral health on their quality of life, while Score 100 indicates the opposite, i.e., maximum impact of oral health on children's quality of life.[18]

The clinical examination was performed with wooden spatulas, and CPI (Community Periodontal Index) periodontal probes. The CPI periodontal probes were used to measure occlusal characteristics in millimeters. The children were evaluated by one calibrated dentist, who used the Dental Aesthetic Index (DAI) for malocclusion and the DMFT/deft (decayed, missing and filled teeth/decayed, indicated for extraction, and filled teeth) for dental caries, both recommended by the World Health Organization (WHO).[19] Oral examinations were performed in the classroom with the child sat on a chair near the window.

Calibration for DAI (malocclusion) and DMFT/deft (dental caries) included theoretical and clinical stages. The theoretical stage consisted of discussions about the diagnostic criteria for malocclusion and dental caries by means of photographs and plaster models. The calibration process was coordinated by experts in pediatric dentistry and orthodontics as golden standard.

The clinical stage was conducted with 20 children. Children were evaluated by the golden standard and the examiner. These children were not included in the total study sample. The same children were reexamined one month afterwards. The Cohen's kappa coefficient for interrater reliability was 0.81 for dental caries and 0.90 for malocclusion, whereas for intrarater reliability, it was 0.87 for dental caries and 0.91 for malocclusion (agreement between the examiner and the gold standard). The coefficients showed good and excellent agreement.

DAI scores less than or equal to 25 indicate normal occlusion or mild malocclusion with little or no orthodontic treatment need. Scores between 26 and 30 indicate definite malocclusion requiring elective treatment. Scores between 31 and 35 indicate severe malocclusion with highly desirable treatment. Scores equal to or greater than 36 indicate extremely severe or handicapping malocclusion with mandatory treatment.

Dental caries was included in the clinical examination and treated as confounding variable; its assessment was based on the DMFT/deft indices. DMFT/deft was used as a quantitative variable. And for an additional statistical analysis, this variable was dichotomized according to the presence or absence of cavitation caused by dental caries.

The pilot study was undertaken in a school that did not participate in the main study so as to test the methods and understand the tools used for data collection.

The Social Vulnerability Index (SVI) was used for the socioeconomic classification. The SVI is an area-based measure drafted for the city of Belo Horizonte and determines to what extent the population of each region of the city is vulnerable to social exclusion. The index is made up of five dimensions: environmental, cultural, economic, legal and security/survival. There are five different classes: Class I comprises the most socially vulnerable families and Class V comprises the least socially vulnerable families. In this study, the SVI was grouped into two categories for statistical purposes: Classes I and II were grouped in the category 'high social vulnerability', and Classes III to V were grouped in the category 'low social vulnerability'. As children usually live near their schools and study in a social environment similar to that of their homes, school districts were used for this classification.[12,20]

The statistical analyses were made by Statistical Package for the Social Sciences (SPSS for Windows, version 22.0, SPSS Inc., Chicago, IL, USA). The Kolmogorov-Smirnov test demonstrated that CPQ_{8-10} scores were not normally distributed. The data were analyzed by descriptive analysis using absolute and relative frequencies, means, and standard deviation. Mann-Whitney and Kruskal-Wallis tests were used for comparison of CPQ_{8-10} means with the independent variables. Bivariate Poisson regression was used to compare the CPQ_{8-10} means between the DAI categories (DAI≤ 25; DAI = 26 to 30; DAI = 31 to 35; DAI ≥ 36). Poisson regression with robust error variance was used for the multivariate analysis. The variables were inserted into the regression model according to their statistical significance ($p < 0.20$). The significance level was set at 5%.

This study was approved by the Research Ethics Committee of *Universidade Federal de Minas Gerais* (protocol #40521114.9.0000.5149). Only those children who granted authorization and obtained it from their parents/legal guardians participated in the study. Parents/ guardians and children read and signed an informed consent form prior to their participation in the study.

RESULTS

A total of 270 children aged 8 to 10 years attending public schools in Belo Horizonte were included in the study. Fifty percent of the children ($n = 135$) were male and 67.8% had non-cavitated caries lesions. From these, 175 (58.1%) children had normal occlusion or mild malocclusion; 75 (27.8%) children presented with definite malocclusion (DAI = 26 to 30); 31 (11.5%) children were diagnosed with severe malocclusion (DAI = 31 to 35), and seven (2.6%) children had extremely severe malocclusion (DAI ≥ 36) (Table 1).

Table 2 shows the frequency of each type of malocclusion. The most frequent types of malocclusion were anterior crowding in one segment (39.6%), anterior diastema in one segment (44.1%), maxillary anterior overjet ≥ 3 mm (24.0%), and one-half cusp molar relationship (24.1%).

Table 3 displays the results for the bivariate analysis between the DAI categories and dental caries on the CPQ_{8-10} scores. Children without malocclusion or with mild malocclusion (DAI ≤ 25) were 56% less likely (95%CI: 0.258-0.758; $p = 0.003$) to have a negative impact on their quality of life, compared with those children diagnosed with extremely severe malocclusion (DAI ≥ 36). Presence of untreated dental caries was associated with negative impact on quality of life ($p = 0.010$). Higher DMFT index was associated with higher CPQ_{8-10} scores ($p < 0.001$). Social vulnerability was not associated with quality of life ($p = 0.327$).

Table 1 - Sample frequency (n = 270) according to the variables; Belo Horizonte, Brazil, 2015.

Variables	Frequency n (%)
Sex	
Male	135 (50%)
Female	135 (50%)
Age (years)	
8	114 (42.2%)
9	109 (40.4%)
10	47 (17.4%)
Social vulnerability	
Low vulnerability	188 (69.6%)
High vulnerability	82 (30.4%)
Presence of untreated decayed teeth	
No	183 (67.8%)
Yes	87 (32.2%)
DMFT (mean and SD)	0.91 (1.49)
DAI	
≤ 25	157 (58.1%)
26-30	75 (27.8%)
31- 35	31 (11.5%)
≥ 36	07 (2.6%)

Note: SD = standard deviation; DMFT was used as a quantitative variable.

Table 2 - Frequency of the types of malocclusion; Belo Horizonte; Brazil, 2015.

Malocclusion	Frequency n (%)
Anterior crowding	
No crowding	96 (35.6%)
One crowded segment	107 (39.6%)
Two crowded segments	67 (24.8%)
Anterior spacing	
No spacing	51 (18.9%)
One segment with spacing	119 (44.1%)
Two segments with spacing	100 (37.0%)
Incisal diastema (mm)	
<2	227 (84.1%)
≥2	43 (15.9%)
Larger anterosuperior irregularity (mm)	
<2	212 (78.5%)
≥2	58 (21.5%)
Larger anteroinferior irregularity (mm)	
<2	213 (78.9%)
≥2	57 (21.1%)
Maxillary anterior overjet (mm)[1]	
<3	198 (73.3%)
≥3	65 (24.0%)
Mandibular anterior overjet (mm)	
Absent	247 (91.5%)
Present	23 (8.5%)
Anterior open bite (mm)	
Absent	250 (92.5%)
Present	20 (7.5%)
Anteroposterior molar relationship	
Normal	205 (75.9%)
One-half cusp	65 (24.1%)

Note: [1] Maxillary anterior overjet does not amount to 100% due to seven cases of anterior crossbite.

Table 4 shows the CPQ_{8-10} mean values according to the independent variables. Children with maxillary anterior overjet ≥ 3 mm had higher CPQ_{8-10} means (19.4; SD = 17.1) than those with an overjet <3 mm (13.6; SD = 11.7; $p = 0.038$). The other independent variables were not significantly associated with CPQ_{8-10} ($p > 0.05$).

Table 5 shows the results for the multivariate Poisson regression with robust error variance. The final model adjusted by incisal diastema, larger anteroinferior irregularity, social vulnerability and DMFT demonstrated that children with a maxillary anterior overjet ≥ 3 mm were 32% more likely (95% CI: 1.03-1.70; $p = 0.028$) to have a negative impact on their quality of life than those with a maxillary anterior overjet <3 mm.

Table 3 - Bivariate Poisson regression showing the influence of DAI categories, dental caries and social vulnerability on quality of life; Belo Horizonte; Brazil, 2015.

	CPQ_{8-10}		
	Mean (SD)	PR (95%CI)	p value
DAI (Malocclusion)			
DAI≤ 25 (Normal occlusion or mild malocclusion)	13.5 (11.7)	0.442 (0.258-0.758)	0.003
DAI= 26-30 (Definite malocclusion)	18.1 (15.6)	0.591 (0.339-1.031)	0.064
DAI= 31 - 35 (Severe malocclusion)	12.5 (10.5)	0.407 (0.224-0.740)	0.003
DAI≥36 (Extremely severe malocclusion)	30.6 (23.2)	1	
Presence of untreated decayed teeth			
No	13.7 (12.9)	0.758 (0.613-0.937)	0.01
Yes	18.1 (14.1)	1	
DMFT	-------	1.11 (1.06-1.63)	<0.001
Social vulnerability			
Low vulnerability	14.6 (13.0)	0.892 (0.710-1.121)	0.327
High vulnerability	16.3 (14.4)	1	

Note: CI = confidence interval; DAI = Dental Aesthetic Index; PR = prevalence ratio; SD = standard deviation; DMFT was used as a quantitative variable.

Table 4 - Mean and standard deviation of CPQ_{8-10} according to independent variables; Belo Horizonte; Brazil, 2015.

Variables	CPQ_{8-10} Mean (SD)	p value
Anterior crowding[2]		
No crowding	14.2 (12.6)	
One crowded segment	15.0 (12.6)	0.813
Two crowded segments	16.5 (15.8)	
Anterior spacing[2]		
No spacing	16.6 (15.8)	
One segment with spacing	14.5 (13.2)	0.627
Two segments with spacing	15.0 (12.5)	
Incisal diastema[1]		
<2	14.6 (13.5)	0.056
≥2	17.9 (13.1)	
Anterosuperior irregularity[1]		
<2	15.2 (13.8)	0.82
≥2	14.9 (12.2)	
Anteroinferior irregularity[1]		
<2	14.5 (13.4)	0.084
≥2	17.3 (13.5)	
Maxillary anterior overjet[1]		
<3mm	13.6 (11.7)	0.038
≥3mm	19.4 (17.1)	
Mandibular anterior overjet[1]		
Absent	15.2 (13.7)	0.866
Present	14.3 (10.6)	
Anterior open bite[1]		
Absent	14.7 (13.0)	0.27
Present	19.5 (18.3)	
Anteroposterior molar relationship[1]		
Normal	14.2 (12.4)	0.229
One-half cusp	18.0 (16.0)	

Note: [1] Mann-Whitney test; [2] Kruskal-Wallis test; SD = standard deviation.

Table 5 - Multivariate Poisson regression showing the influence of types of malocclusion and dental caries on quality of life; Belo Horizonte; Brazil, 2015.

Malocclusion	PR	95% CI	p value
Incisal diastema (in mm)			
<2	1	0.88-1.48	0.313
≥2	1.14		
Larger anteroinferior irregularity (in mm)			
<2	1	0.93-1.49	0.176
≥2	1.18		
Maxillary anterior overjet (in mm)			
<3mm	1	1.03-1.70	0.028
≥3mm	1.32		
Social vulnerability			
Low vulnerability	1	0.90-1.42	0.296
High vulnerability	1.13		
DMFT	1.09	1.05-1.15	<0.001

Note: PR = prevalence ratio; CI = confidence interval; DMFT was used as a quantitative variable.
Presence of untreated decayed teeth variable was not inserted in the multivariate model due to its high correlation with DMFT.

DISCUSSION

There is a growing interest among researchers in the influence of facial esthetics on the quality of life of children and adolescents. This study found that children with extremely severe malocclusion were more likely to have a negative impact on quality of life, corroborating the findings of other studies on the effect of malocclusion on quality of life conducted with children in the same age group (8 to 10 years).[12,13]

The bivariate analysis demonstrated that most types of malocclusion were not statistically associated with oral health-related quality of life. Studies report that tooth decay is associated with an impact on the quality of life,[3,12] by this reason dental caries was included in the clinical examination and treated as confounding variable. However, dental caries did not interfere in the results of malocclusion. Of the ten occlusal characteristics assessed by DAI, the present study demonstrated that only accentuated maxillary anterior overjet was associated with a negative impact on quality of life. Other studies carried out with children aged 8 to 10 years detected more occlusal characteristics statistically associated with an impact on quality of life.[12,13] One of this studies demonstrated that anterior segment spacing and anterior

mandibular overjet were associated with worse quality of life.[12] The other study found such association with upper anterior irregularity, anterior open bite and diastema.[13] These differences may be due to sample size and studied population. The present study was conducted with 270 children only from public schools, and one of these previous studies was carried out with a larger sample size (n=1,204) from public and private schools.[12] The other previous study was conducted with a smaller sample (n=102) only from public schools.[13]

The analysis of the results revealed that malocclusion (DAI >25) affected 41,9% of the children examined, while previous studies carried out with children of the same age group found that malocclusions affected 32,2%[12] and 61%[13] of the children examined. We should emphasize the difference in the sample size of the studies: 1,204 chidren,[12] 102 children[13] and 270 children in the present study.

It was not possible to compare the present results with many others carried out with children of the same age group since there is a paucity of studies on the impact of malocclusion on the mixed dentition,[12] specially studies that address the psychosocial factors that lead people to seek for orthodontic treatment.

Previous studies described the presence of several occlusal characteristics associated with a negative impact on quality of life,[14-17] including the presence of larger maxillary anterior overjet.[15,16,17] However, these results must be viewed with caution as the age range of participants was different from the one used in the present study. These studies were conducted with adolescents and young adults. Adolescents[13] tend to be more concerned with body image and it is important the approval from others of the same age group. Children[13] aged eight to ten years old are more concerned with the approval of adults. It is important to highlight that most studies on the impact of malocclusion on oral health-related quality of life have been conducted with adolescents and young adults.

The presence of malocclusion, mainly in the anterior region, may interfere with children's and adolescents' psychosocial well-being. DAI was the criterion for the diagnosis of malocclusion in this study as it uses a single score, being practical for epidemiologists,[21,22] and assesses occlusal characteristics that could potentially cause psychosocial impairment.[22]

DAI was designed for permanent dentition. There is no orthodontic index that is specific to mixed dentition. DAI could thus overestimate the need for orthodontic treatment, and this tends to occur more often with mixed dentition because of transient occlusal changes such as midline diastema, spacing between incisors, edge-to-edge molar relationship, among others.[23] Another transient change observed in mixed dentition is temporary primary crowding, which has spontaneous correction.[24] Consequently, these transient changes in mixed dentition may get the DAI score up, classifying malocclusion into a severity level that is not necessarily present. This is one of the limitations of the present study. Moreover, cross-sectional studies have limitations inherent to the design.

A previous study asserts that malocclusion does not self-correct from deciduous to mixed dentition, nor from mixed to permanent dentition,[24] thereby underscoring the importance of orthodontic assessment and diagnosis of children with mixed dentition. Therefore, it is paramount to make a distinction between transient changes and malocclusion at that stage. Early diagnosis aids with interceptive orthodontics and may prevent psychosocial distress in children with malocclusion.

An earlier study emphasized the importance of classifying malocclusion into severity levels in order to prioritize the treatment of more severe cases at healthcare units affiliated with SUS.[9] It is also essential that the assessment of oral health-related quality of life be included among normative criteria.[17] In the present study, the normative criterion for the diagnosis of malocclusion was combined with the children's self-perception of subjective need, yielding important results that may contribute to the referral of patients with malocclusion for treatment at public orthodontic health units since it was observed that Orthodontics Protocol used by SUS in Belo Horizonte city does not make it clear which children diagnosed with malocclusion should be referred to the orthodontic specialty. General clinical dentists can interpret the protocol in different ways so that children will not have the same opportunities to be referred to orthodontic treatment. To change the current reality, a standardization of the protocol must take place and this can be done by examining the children for the diagnosis of malocclusion using an orthodontic index combined with the children's self-perception of subjective need.

One of the advantages of combining children's self-perception with the clinical assessment made by the health professional lies with the definition of cases that are more likely to have a negative impact on quality of life, given that, according to some studies,[10,11] there are different psychosocial implications for a single type of malocclusion.

CONCLUSIONS

» Children diagnosed with extremely severe malocclusion and those with a pronounced maxillary anterior overjet experienced a larger impact on their quality of life.

» Malocclusion, especially in the anterior teeth, can compromise a child's psychosocial well-being.

» Further studies are needed with children addressing the impact of malocclusion in the mixed dentition.

Authors contribution

Conception or design of the study: SRD, HP, MTM, MPV. Data acquisition, analysis or interpretation: SRD, MTM, CBB. Writing the article: SRD, CBB. Critical revision of the article: SRD, MTM, CBB, MPV. Final approval of the article: SRD, MTM, CBB, MPV.

REFERENCES

1. Corless IB, Nicholas PK, Nokes KM. Issues in cross-cultural quality-of-life research. J Nurs Scholarsh. 2001;33(1):15-20.

2. Oliveira CM, Sheiham A. Orthodontic treatment and its impact on oral health-related quality of life in Brazilian adolescents. J Orthod. 2004 Mar;31(1):20-7; discussion 15.

3. Tesch FC, Oliveira BH, Leão A. Mensuração do impacto dos problemas bucais sobre a qualidade de vida de crianças: aspectos conceituais e metodológicos. Cad Saúde Pública. 2007;23(11):2555-64.

4. Yusuf H, Gherunpong S, Sheiham A. Validation of an English version of the Child-OIDP index, oral health-related quality of life measure for children. Health Qual Life Outcomes. 2006;4:38.

5. Broder HL, McGrath C, Cisneros GJ. Questionnaire development: face validity and item impact testing of child oral health impact profile. Community Dent Oral Epidemiol. 2007;35(1):8-19.

6. Feitosa S, Colares V, Pinkham J. The psychosocial effects of severe caries in 4-year-old children in Recife, Pernambuco, Brazil. Cad Saúde Pública. 2005;21(5):1550-6.

7. Locker D, Jokovic A, Stephens M, Kenny D, Tompson B, Guyatt G. Family impact of child oral and oro-facial conditions. Community Dent Oral Epidemiol 2002;30(6):438-48.

8. Marques LS, Ramos-Jorge ML, Paiva SM, Pordeus IA. Malocclusion: esthetic impact and quality of life among Brazilian schoolchildren. Am J Orthod Dentofacial Orthop. 2006 Mar;129(3):424-7.

9. Suliano AA, Rodrigues MJ, Junior AFC, Fonte PP, Porto-Carreiro CF. Prevalência de maloclusão e sua associação com alterações funcionais do sistema estomatognático entre escolares. Cad Saúde Pública. 2007;23(8):1913-23.

10. Feu D, Oliveira BH, Sales HX, Miguel JA. M. Más-oclusões e seu impacto na qualidade de vida de adolescentes que buscam tratamento ortodôntico. Ortodontia SPO. 2008;41(4):355-65.

11. Kiyak HA. Cultural and psychologic influences on treatment demand. Semin Orthod. 2000 Dec;6(4):242-8.

12. Sardenberg F, Martins MT, Bendo CB, Pordeus IA, Paiva SM, Auad SM, et al. Malocclusion and oral health-related quality of life in Brazilian school children A population-based study. Angle Orthod. 2013 Jan;83(1):83-9.

13. Martins-Júnior PA, Marques LS, Ramos-Jorge ML. Malocclusion: social, functional and emotional influence on children. J Clin Pediatr Dent. 2012 Fall;37(1):103-8.

14. Bernabé E, Flores-Mir C. Influence of anterior occlusal characteristics on self-perceived dental appearance in young adults. Angle Orthod. 2007 Sept;77(5):831-6.

15. Bernabe E, Oliveira CM, Sheiham A. Condition-specific sociodental impacts attributed to different anterior occlusal traits in Brazilian adolescents. Eur J Oral Sci. 2007 Dec;115(6):473-8.

16. Seehra J, Fleming PS, Newton T, DiBiase AT. Bullying in orthodontic patients and its relationship to malocclusion, self-esteem and oral health-related quality of life. J Orthod. 2011 Dec;38(4):247-56; quiz 294.

17. Johal A, Cheung MYH, Marcenes W. The impact of two different malocclusion traits on quality of life. Br Dent J. 2007;202(2):1-4.

18. Martins MT, Ferreira FM, Oliveira AC, Paiva SM, Vale MP, Allison PJ. Preliminary validation of the Brazilian version of the Child Perceptions Questionnaire 8-10. Eur J Paediatr Dent. 2009 Sept;10(3):135-40.

19. Cons NC, Jenny J, Kohout FJ, Freer TJ, Eismann D. Perceptions of occlusal conditions in Australia, the German Democratic Republic and the United States of America. Int Dent J. 1983 June;33(2):200-6.

20. Nahas MI, Ribeiro C, Esteves O, Moscovitch S, Martins VL. The map of social exclusion in Belo Horizonte: Methodology of building an urban management tool. Cad Cienc Soc. 2000;7:75-88.

21. Jenny J, Cons NC. Establishing malocclusion severity levels on the Dental Aesthetic Index (DAI) scale. Aust Dent J. 1996 Feb;41(1):43-6.

22. Jenny J, Cons NC. Comparing and contrasting two orthodontic indices, the Index of Orthodontic Treatment Need and the Dental Aesthetic Index. Am J Orthod Dentofacial Orthop. 1996 Oct;110(4):410-6.

23. Johnson M, Harkness M, Crowther P, Herbison P. A comparison of two methods of assessing orthodontic treatment need in the mixed dentition: DAI and IOTN. Aust Orthod J. 2000 July;16(2):82-7.

24. Almeida MR, Pereira ALP, Almeida RR, Almeida-Pedrin RR, Silva Filho OG. Prevalence of malocclusion in children aged 7 to 12 years. Dental Press J Orthod. 2011 July-Aug;16(4):123-31.

6

Global distribution of malocclusion traits

Maged Sultan Alhammadi[1,2], Esam Halboub[3], Mona Salah Fayed[4,5], Amr Labib[4], Chrestina El-Saaidi[6]

Objective: Considering that the available studies on prevalence of malocclusions are local or national-based, this study aimed to pool data to determine the distribution of malocclusion traits worldwide in mixed and permanent dentitions. **Methods:** An electronic search was conducted using PubMed, Embase and Google Scholar search engines, to retrieve data on malocclusion prevalence for both mixed and permanent dentitions, up to December 2016. **Results:** Out of 2,977 retrieved studies, 53 were included. In permanent dentition, the global distributions of Class I, Class II, and Class III malocclusion were 74.7% [31−97%], 19.56% [2−63%] and 5.93% [1−20%], respectively. In mixed dentition, the distributions of these malocclusions were 73% [40−96%], 23% [2−58%] and 4% [0.7−13%]. Regarding vertical malocclusions, the observed deep overbite and open bite were 21.98% and 4.93%, respectively. Posterior crossbite affected 9.39% of the sample. Africans showed the highest prevalence of Class I and open bite in permanent dentition (89% and 8%, respectively), and in mixed dentition (93% and 10%, respectively), while Caucasians showed the highest prevalence of Class II in permanent dentition (23%) and mixed dentition (26%). Class III malocclusion in mixed dentition was highly prevalent among Mongoloids. **Conclusion:** Worldwide, in mixed and permanent dentitions, Angle Class I malocclusion is more prevalent than Class II, specifically among Africans; the least prevalent was Class III, although higher among Mongoloids in mixed dentition. In vertical dimension, open bite was highest among Mongoloids in mixed dentition. Posterior crossbite was more prevalent in permanent dentition in Europe.

Keywords: Prevalence. Malocclusion. Global health. Population. Permanent dentition. Mixed dentition.

[1] Jazan University, College of Dentistry, Department of Preventive Sciences, Division of Orthodontics and Dentofacial Orthopedics (Jazan, Saudi Arabia).

[2] Ibb University, Faculty of Oral and Dental Medicine, Department of Orthodontics and Dentofacial Orthopedics (Ibb, Republic of Yemen).

[3] Jazan University, College of Dentistry, Department of Maxillofacial Surgery and Diagnostic Sciences (Jazan, Saudi Arabia).

[4] Cairo University, Faculty of Oral and Dental Medicine, Department of Orthodontics and Dentofacial Orthopedics (Cairo, Egypt).

[5] University of Malaya, Faculty of Dentistry, Department of Pediatric Dentistry and Orthodontics (Kuala Lumpur, Malaysia).

[6] Kyoto University, Graduate School of Medicine, Department of Global Health and Socio-epidemiology (Kyoto, Japan).

» The authors report no commercial, proprietary or financial interest in the products or companies described in this article.

Esam Halboub
Department of Maxillofacial Surgery and Diagnostic Sciences
College of Dentistry, Jazan University, Jazan, Saudi Arabia
E-mail: mhelboub@gmail.com

INTRODUCTION

Angle introduced his famous classification of malocclusion in 1899.[1] Now the World Health Organization estimates malocclusions as the third most prevalent oral health problem, following dental caries and periodontal diseases.[2]

Many etiological factors for malocclusion have been proposed. Genetic, environmental, and ethnic factors are the major contributors in this context. Certain types of malocclusion, such as Class III relationship, run in families, which gives a strong relation between genetics and malocclusion. Likewise is the ethnic factor, where the bimaxillary protrusion, for example, affects the African origin more frequently than other ethnicities. On the other hand, functional adaptation to environmental factors affects the surrounding structures including dentitions, bone, and soft tissue, and ultimately resulting in different malocclusion problems. Thus, malocclusion could be considered as a multifactorial problem with no specific cause so far.[3]

A search in the literature for studies on prevalence of malocclusion and related factors revealed that most of these epidemiological investigations were published between the 1940s and the 1990s. Thereafter, publications have been turned into focusing more on determination of treatment needs, treatment techniques and mechanisms, and treatment outcomes.[4]

Epidemiological studies play a pivotal role in terms of determining the size of the health problems, providing the necessary data and generating and analyzing hypotheses of associations, if any. Through these valuable information, the priorities are set and the health policies are developed.[5] Hence, the quality of these epidemiological studies must be evaluated crucially and it will be valuable to pool their results, whenever possible.

In this regard, there has been a continuous increase in conducting critical analyses for the published epidemiological health studies. The aim behind this is to generate a more precise and trusted evidence on the health problem under investigation using strict criteria for quality analysis. However, few have been conducted in orthodontics. The objective of the current study, therefore, was to present a comprehensive estimation on the prevalence of malocclusion in different populations and continents.

MATERIALS AND METHODS
Search method

A literature search in PubMed, Embase, and Google Scholar search engines was conducted up to December 2016. The following search terms were used: 'Prevalence', 'Malocclusion', 'Mixed dentition', and 'Permanent dentition'. In addition, an electronic search in websites of the following journals was conducted: Angle Orthodontist, American Journal of Orthodontics and Dentofacial Orthopedics, Journal of Orthodontics, and European Journal of Orthodontics.

Studies that fulfilled the following criteria were included:

1) Population-based studies.

2) Sample size greater than 200 subjects.

3) Studies that evaluated malocclusion during mixed and/ or permanent dentitions.

4) Studies that used Angle's classification of malocclusion.

5) Studies that considered the following definitions of the specified malocclusion characteristics: "abnormal overjet" if more than 3mm; "reverse overjet" when all four maxillary incisors were in a crossbite; "abnormal overbite" if more than 2.5 mm (for deep bite) and if less than 0 mm (for open bite); and "posterior crossbite" when affecting more than two teeth. The malocclusion traits included were: Angle Classification (Class I / II / III), overjet (increased / reversed), overbite (deep bite / open bite), posterior crossbite, based on the above mentioned definitions for these traits.

A study was excluded if it was conducted in a clinical/hospital-based setting and/or targeted malocclusion prevalence in primary dentition or in a population with specific medical problem.

Characteristics of all studies[6-58] analyzed were formulated similar to that used in analysis of epidemiological studies[59,60] (Table 1).

Critical appraisal of the included studies was done based on a modified version of STROBE checklist[61,62] comprising seven items related to: study design, study settings, participants criteria, sample size, variable description, and outcome measurements. The quality of the studies was categorized into weak (≤ 3), moderate (4 or 5) and high quality (≥ 6), as described in Table 2.

Table 1 - Characteristics of the included studies.

No	Author	Year	Sample	Age	Gender	Country	Region	Race	Population
1	Massler and Frankel[6]	1951	2758	14-18	M=1238, F=1520	America	America	Caucasian	Schoolchildren
2	Goose et al.[7]	1957	2956	7-15	Not mentioned	Britain	Europe	Caucasian	Schoolchildren
3	Mills[8]	1966	1455	8-17	M=719, F=736	America	America	Caucasian	Schoolchildren
4	Grewe et al.[9]	1968	651	9-14	M=322, F=329	America	America	Caucasian	Community
5	Helm[10]	1968	1700	6-18	M=742, F=958	Denmark	Europe	Caucasian	Schoolchildren
6	Thilander and Myrberg[11]	1973	6398	7-13	M=3093, F=3305	Sweden	Europe	Caucasian	Schoolchildren
7	Foster and Day[12]	1974	1000	12	Not mentioned	Britain	Europe	Caucasian	Schoolchildren
8	Ingervall et al.[13]	1978	389	21-54	M=389, F=0	Sweden	Europe	Caucasian	Military service
9	Helm and Prydso[14]	1979	1536	14-18	Not mentioned	Denmark	Europe	Caucasian	Schoolchildren
10	Lee et al.[15]	1980	2092	17-21	M=1281, F=811	Korea	Asia	Mongoloids	Community
11	Gardiner[16]	1982	479	10-12	Not mentioned	Libya	Africa	Caucasian	Community
12	De Muñiz[17]	1986	1554	12-13	M=655, F=899	Argentine	America	Caucasian	Schoolchildren
13	Kerosuo et al.[18]	1988	642	11-18	M=340, F=302	Tanzania	Africa	Africans	Schoolchildren
14	Woon et al.[19]	1989	347	15-19	Not mentioned	China	Asia	Mongoloids	Community
15	Al-Emran et al.[20]	1990	500	14	M=500, F=0	Saudia	Asia	Caucasian	Schoolchildren
16	El-Mangoury and Mostafa[21]	1990	501	18-24	M=231, F=270	Egypt	Africa	Caucasian	Community
17	Lew et al.[22]	1993	1050	12-14	Not mentioned	China	Asia	Mongoloids	Schoolchildren
18	Tang[23]	1994	201	20	Not mentioned	China	Asia	Mongoloids	Community
19	Harrison and Davis[24]	1996	1438	7-15	Not mentioned	Canada	America	Caucasian	Community
20	Ng'ang'a et al.[25]	1996	919	7-15	M=468, F=451	Kenya	Africa	Africans	Community
21	Ben-Bassat et al.[26]	1997	939	6-13	M=442, F=497	Israel	Asia	Caucasian	Schoolchildren
22	Proffit et al.[27]	1998	14000	8-50	Not mentioned	America	America	Caucasian	Community
23	Dacosta[28]	1999	1028	11-18	M=484, F=544	Nigeria	Africa	Africans	Community
24	Saleh[29]	1999	851	9-15	M=446, F=405	Lebanon	Asia	Caucasian	Schoolchildren
25	Esa et al.[30]	2001	1519	12-13	M=772, F=747	Malaysia	Asia	Mongoloids	Schoolchildren
26	Thilander et al.[31]	2001	4724	5-17	M=2371, F=2353	Colombia	America	Caucasian	Heath center
27	Freitas et al.[32]	2002	520	11-15	M=250, F=270	Brazil	America	Caucasian	Schoolchildren
28	Bataringaya[33]	2004	402	14	M=141, F=261	Uganda	Africa	Africans	Schoolchildren
29	Onyeaso[34]	2004	636	12-17	M=334, F=302	Nigeria	Africa	Africans	Schoolchildren
30	Tausche et al.[35]	2004	197	6-8	M=970, F=1005	Germany	Europe	Caucasian	Schoolchildren
31	Abu Alhaija et al.[36]	2005	1003	13-15	M=619, F=384	Jordan	Asia	Caucasian	Schoolchildren
32	Ali and Abdo[37]	2005	1000	7-12	M=501, F=499	Yemen	Asia	Caucasian	Schoolchildren
33	Behbehani et al.[38]	2005	1299	13-14	M=674, F=625	Kuwait	Asia	Caucasian	Schoolchildren
34	Ciuffolo et al.[39]	2005	810	11-14	M=434, F=376	Italy	Europe	Caucasian	Schoolchildren
35	Karaiskos[40]	2005	395	9	Not mentioned	Canada	America	Caucasian	Schoolchildren
36	Ahangar Atashi[41]	2007	398	13-15	Not mentioned	Iran	Asia	Caucasian	Community
37	Gelgör et al.[42]	2007	810	11-14	M=1125, F=1204	Turkey	Europe	Caucasian	Health center
38	Jonsson et al.[43]	2007	829	31-44	M=342, F=487	Iceland	Europe	Caucasian	Schoolchildren
39	Josefsson et al.[44]	2007	493	12-13	Not mentioned	Sweden	Europe	Caucasian	Schoolchildren
40	Ajayi[45]	2008	441	11-18	M=229, F=212	Nigeria	Africa	Africans	Schoolchildren
41	Mtaya[46]	2008	1601	12-14	M=632, F=969	Tanzania	Africa	Africans	Schoolchildren
42	Borzabadi-Farahani et al.[47]	2009	502	11-14	M=249, F=253	Iran	Asia	Caucasian	Schoolchildren
43	Daniel et al.[48]	2009	407	9-12	M=191, F=216	Brazil	America	Caucasian	Schoolchildren
44	Šidlauskas and Lopatiené[49]	2009	1681	7-15	M=672, F=1009	Lithuania	Europe	Caucasian	Schoolchildren
45	Alhammadi[50]	2010	1000	18-25	M=500, F=1000	Yemen	Asia	Caucasian	Schoolchildren
46	Bhardwaj et al.[51]	2011	622	16-17	M=365, F=257	India	Asia	Caucasian	Schoolchildren
47	Nainani and Relan[52]	2011	436	12-15	M=224, F=212	India	Asia	Caucasian	Schoolchildren
48	Bugaighis et al.[53]	2013	343	12-17	M=169, F=174	Libya	Africa	Caucasian	Schoolchildren
49	Kaur et al.[54]	2013	2400	13-17	M=1192, F=1208	India	Asia	Caucasian	Schoolchildren
50	Reddy et al.[55]	2013	2135	6-10	M=1009, F=1126	India	Asia	Caucasian	Schoolchildren
51	Bilgic F et al.[56]	2015	2329	12.5-16.2	M=1125, F=1204	Turkey	Europe	Caucasian	Schoolchildren
52	Gupta et al.[57]	2016	500	12-17	M=1125, F=1204	India	Asia	Caucasian	Schoolchildren
53	Narayanan et al.[58]	2016	2366	10-12	M=1281, F=1085	India	Asia	Caucasian	Schoolchildren

M = male; F = female.

Table 2 - STROBE -based quality analysis of the included studies.

No	Author	Study design	Setting	Participants	Sample size	Variables description	Outcome measurement	Statistical analysis	Total score
1	Massler and Frankel[6]	✓	✓	✓	X	✓	✓	✓	5
2	Goose et al.[7]	X	✓	✓	X	X	✓	✓	4
3	Mills[8]	X	✓	✓	X	✓	✓	✓	5
4	Grewe et al.[9]	X	✓	✓	X	✓	✓	✓	5
5	Helm[10]	✓	✓	✓	X	✓	✓	✓	6
6	Thilander and Myrberg[11]	✓	✓	✓	X	✓	✓	✓	6
7	Foster and Day[12]	X	X	✓	X	✓	✓	✓	4
8	Ingervall et al.[13]	X	X	✓	X	✓	✓	✓	4
9	Helm and Prydso[14]	X	✓	✓	✓	✓	✓	✓	6
10	Lee et al.[15]	X	✓	✓	X	✓	✓	✓	5
11	Gardiner[16]	X	✓	✓	X	✓	✓	✓	5
12	De Muñiz[17]	X	✓	✓	X	X	✓	✓	4
13	Kerosuo et al.[18]	X	✓	✓	X	✓	✓	✓	5
14	Woon et al.[19]	X	✓	✓	X	✓	✓	✓	5
15	Al-Emran et al.[20]	X	✓	✓	X	X	✓	✓	4
16	El-Mangoury and Mostafa[21]	X	✓	✓	X	X	✓	✓	4
17	Lew et al.[22]	X	✓	✓	X	✓	✓	✓	5
18	Tang[23]	X	✓	✓	X	✓	✓	✓	5
19	Harrison and Davis[24]	X	✓	✓	X	✓	✓	✓	5
20	Ng'ang'a et al.[25]	X	✓	✓	✓	X	✓	✓	6
21	Ben-Bassat et al.[26]	X	✓	✓	X	✓	✓	✓	5
22	Proffit et al.[27]	✓	✓	✓	X	✓	✓	✓	6
23	Dacosta[28]	X	✓	✓	X	✓	✓	✓	5
24	Saleh[29]	✓	✓	✓	X	X	✓	✓	5
25	Esa et al.[30]	X	✓	✓	✓	✓	✓	✓	6
26	Thilander et al.[31]	X	✓	✓	X	✓	✓	✓	5
27	Freitas et al.[32]	X	✓	✓	X	✓	✓	✓	5
28	Dataringaya[33]	✓	✓	✓	✓	✓	✓	✓	7
29	Onyeaso[34]	X	✓	✓	X	✓	✓	✓	5
30	Tausche et al.[35]	✓	✓	✓	X	✓	✓	✓	6
31	Alhaija et al.[36]	X	✓	✓	X	✓	✓	✓	5
32	Ali and Abdo[37]	X	✓	✓	X	✓	✓	✓	5
33	Behbehani et al.[38]	X	✓	✓	✓	✓	✓	✓	6
34	Ciuffolo et al.[39]	✓	X	✓	X	✓	✓	✓	5
35	Karaiskos[40]	X	✓	✓	X	✓	✓	✓	5
36	Ahangar Atashi[41]	X	✓	✓	X	✓	✓	✓	5
37	Gelgör et al.[42]	X	✓	✓	X	✓	✓	✓	5
38	Jonsson et al.[43]	✓	✓	✓	✓	✓	✓	✓	7
39	Josefsson et al.[44]	X	✓	✓	X	✓	✓	✓	5
40	Ajayi[45]	X	✓	✓	X	✓	✓	✓	5
41	Mtaya[46]	✓	✓	✓	✓	✓	✓	✓	7
42	Borzabadi-Farahani et al.[47]	✓	✓	✓	X	✓	✓	✓	6
43	Daniel et al.[48]	X	✓	✓	✓	✓	✓	✓	6
44	Šidlauskas and Lopatienė[49]	X	X	✓	X	✓	✓	✓	4
45	Alhammadi[50]	✓	✓	✓	X	✓	✓	✓	6
46	Bhardwaj et al.[51]	✓	✓	✓	X	X	✓	✓	5
47	Nainani and Relan[52]	✓	✓	✓	X	X	✓	✓	5
48	Bugaighis et al.[53]	X	✓	✓	X	✓	✓	✓	5
49	Kaur et al.[54]	X	✓	✓	X	✓	✓	✓	5
50	Reddy et al.[55]	✓	✓	✓	X	X	✓	✓	5
51	Bilgic F et al.[56]	✓	✓	✓	X	✓	✓	✓	6
52	Gupta et al.[57]	X	✓	✓	X	X	✓	✓	4
53	Narayanan et al.[58]	✓	✓	✓	X	X	✓	✓	5

Statistical analysis

Prevalence rates, by different variables, were presented as means and standard deviations (SD), with the minimum and maximum values. The data were checked for normal distribution using Kolmogorov-Smirnov test. As the distribution was not normal, analyses were conducted using non-parametric tests. Kruskal-Wallis test was used for comparisons between more than two groups. Mann-Whitney U test was used for pair-wise comparisons between groups whenever Kruskal-Wallis test was significant. Spearman's coefficient was calculated to determine the correlations, if any, between different variables. All tests were supposed to be two-tailed, and the power and the significance values were set at 0.8 and 0.05, respectively. Statistical analysis was performed with IBM® SPSS® Statistics for Windows software, version 21 (Armonk, NY: IBM Corp.)

RESULTS

Two thousands nine hundreds and seventy seven studies were found to be potentially relevant to the study. The flow diagram (Fig 1) describes the process of articles retrieval; 255 articles were excluded due to duplication. The main cause of dropping of the retrieved articles was removal of irrelevant titles (2,348). The final closely related were 374 articles published between years 1951 and 2016. After reading their abstracts, only 53 articles (Table 1) fulfilled the inclusion criteria and were included in the subsequent analyses.

The results of the critical appraisal of the included studies are presented in Table 2. The total quality score ranged from 4 to 7. Thirty eight studies (72%) were considered of moderate quality and fifteen (28%), of high quality. The most common drawbacks among all studies were failure to declare the study design (whether it is of cross-sectional, follow-up, etc.) and lack of sample size calculation.

In permanent dentition (Table 3), the global distributions of Class I, Class II, and Class III were 74.7%, 19.56% and 5.93%, respectively. Increased and reverse overjet was recorded in 20.14% and 4.56%, respectively. Regarding vertical malocclusions, the observed deep overbite and open bite were 21.98% and 4.93%, respectively. Considering the transverse occlusal discrepancies, the posterior crossbite affected 9.39% of the total examined sample.

Regarding the distribution of malocclusion in adults according to geographical location (Table 4), four continents classification system was considered, in which Americas are considered as one continent. In permanent dentition, Europe showed the highest prevalence of Class II and posterior crossbite (33.51% and 13.8%, respectively), and the lowest prevalence of Class I (60.38%). This was applied to mixed dentition regarding Class I and Class II. No statistically significant differences in prevalence of Class III, increased overjet, reversed overjet, deep bite and open bite between the four geographic areas were reported.

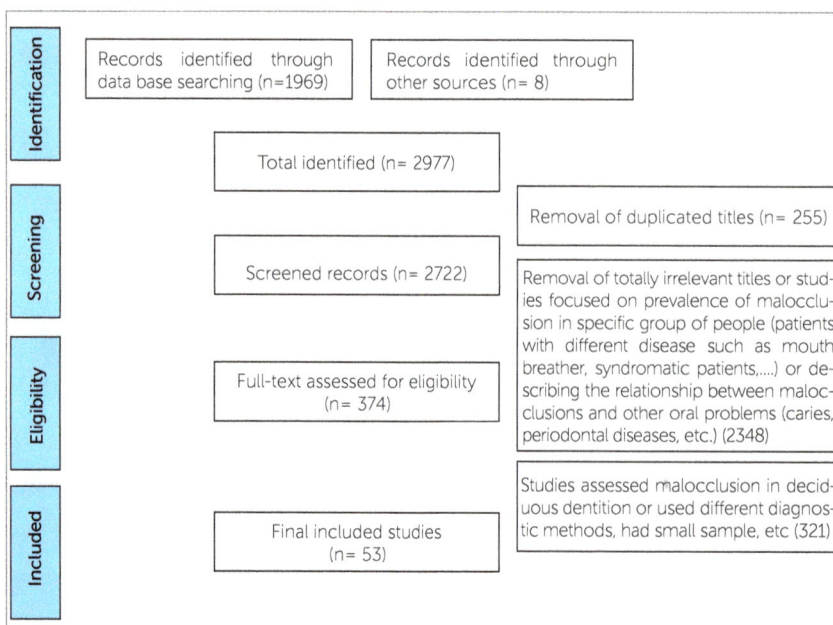

Figure 1 - Flowchart of the literature selection process.

Table 3 - Global prevalence of malocclusion in permanent and mixed dentitions

Dimension	Malocclusion form	Permanent dentition				Mixed dentition			
		Min	Max	Mean	SD	Min	Max	Mean	SD
Antero-posterior	Class I	31	96.6	74.7	15.17	40	96.2	72.74	16
	Class II	1.6	63	19.56	13.76	1.7	58	23.11	14.94
	Class III	1	19.9	5.93	4.69	0.7	12.6	3.98	2.75
	Increased overjet	1.6	48.4	20.14	11.13	9.4	35.7	23.01	7.56
	Reversed overjet	0	20.1	4.56	5.26	0.4	11.9	3.65	3.67
Vertical	Deep bite	2.2	56	21.98	14.13	3.5	57.1	24.34	14.54
	Open bite	0.1	15	4.93	3.97	0.29	25.1	5.29	5.9
Transverse	Posterior crossbite	4	32.2	9.39	5.04	3.72	29.1	11.72	7.22

Table 4 - Prevalence of malocclusion in different geographic locations.

Variable		Permanent dentition								P-value
		America		Africa		Asia		Europe		
		Mean	SD	Mean	SD	Mean	SD	Mean	SD	
Antero-posterior	Class I	78.53	8.56	83.68	12.48	78.93	9.77	60.39	16.76	0.019*
	Class II	15.25	7.06	11.45	9.08	12.26	4.28	33.51	17.73	0.016*
	Class III	6.23	2.68	4.75	4.6	6.32	6.46	6.2	2.75	0.5
	Increased overjet	16.67	5.61	21.4	13.91	19.79	10.5	20.79	12.38	0.9
	Reversed overjet	2.26	2.17	3.47	2.89	6.09	7	4.37	1.96	0.829
Vertical	Deep bite	11.13	6.41	25.83	18.96	23.83	12.95	21.56	13.33	0.227
	Open bite	5.03	4.32	6.34	3.12	4.01	3.86	4.92	4.82	0.378
Transverse	Posterior crossbite	7.08	2.24	7.9	1.78	8.27	2.65	13.08	7.93	0.029*
		Mixed dentition								
Antero-posterior	Class I	69.98	19.67	90	6.11	72.78	10.29	63.95	13.77	0.035*
	Class II	27.22	20.22	7.5	5.71	21.42	10.4	31.95	12.47	0.024*
	Class III	2.78	0.84	2.48	0.59	5.76	3.91	3.53	1.21	0.226
	Increased overjet	21.12	8.23	21.23	11.3	25.09	7.62	23.02	5.12	0.841
	Reversed overjet	3.9	5.01	5.25	4.22	4.35	3.63	1.33	0.9	0.348
Vertical	Deep bite	14.98	7.73	23.3	15.5	22.09	9.97	37.4	17.62	0.122
	Open bite	5.57	3.09	8.3	5.31	4.5	7.79	4.18	5.79	0.077
Transverse	Posterior crossbite	10.67	8.26	12.13	6.62	17.77	8.47	12.45	6.54	0.832

*: Significant at P ≤ 0.05.

In permanent stage of dentition by ethnic groups, the highest prevalences of Class I malocclusion and open bite (89.44% and 7.82%, respectively) were reported among African population, although the difference of the latter was not statistically significant. However, the highest prevalence of Class II (22.9%) was reported among Caucasians. Otherwise, no statistically significant differences were found in prevalence of Class III, increased overjet, reversed overjet, deep bite and posterior crossbite between the three main populations (Table 5).

The global distributions of Class I, Class II, and Class III in mixed dentition stage were 72.74%, 23.11% and 3.98%, respectively. The prevalence figures of increased and reverse overjet were 23.01% and 3.65%, respectively. Deep overbite and open bite cases were reported in 24.34% and 5.29%, respectively. Posterior crossbite represented 11.72% of the total pooled studies (Table 3).

Regarding prevalence of malocclusion in mixed dentition according to geographical location (Table 4), Africa showed the highest prevalence of Class I (90%)

but the lowest prevalence of Class II malocclusions (7.5%). The highest prevalence figures of Class II, Class III, and open bite malocclusions were reported in Europe (31.95%), Asia (5.76%), and Africa (8.3%), respectively. Deep bite was significantly higher in Europe (37.4%) compared to other geographical areas.

In mixed dentition, African population showed the highest prevalence of Class I (92.47%), but the lowest prevalence of Class II malocclusions (5.1%), while Caucasians showed the lowest prevalence of open bite (3.7%). Mongoloid showed significantly higher prevalence of Class III (10.95%). No significant differences in the prevalence of other malocclusions were found between different ethnicities (Table 5).

The prevalence of Class II was observed less frequently in permanent than in mixed dentition (19.56 ± 13.76 and 23.11 ± 14.94%, respectively), while the prevalence of Class III was observed more frequently in permanent than in mixed dentition (5.93 ± 4.96 and 3.98 ± 2.75, respectively).

Table 5 - Prevalence of malocclusion in different races

Variable		Permanent dentition						
		Africans		Caucasians		Mongoloids		P-value
		Mean	SD	Mean	SD	Mean	SD	
Antero-posterior	Class I	89.44	9.34	71.61	15.15	74.87	9.68	0.027*
	Class II	6.76	4.99	22.9	14.07	14.14	4.43	0.006*
	Class III	3.8	4.67	5.92	4	9.63	9.02	0.228
	Increased overjet	14.62	6.22	22.29	11.77	12.87	6.78	0.132
	Reversed overjet	3.5	2.93	3.99	5.11	10.87	6.68	0.122
Vertical	Deep bite	19.02	15.81	22.95	14.07	19.5	16.6	0.587
	Open bite	7.82	2.24	4.52	4.17	3.27	2.89	0.074
Transverse	Posterior crossbite	7.2	1.61	10.08	5.64	7.53	0.31	0.149
		Mixed dentition						
Antero-posterior	Class I	92.47	4.41	70.39	14.78	66.75	1.77	0.02*
	Class II	5.1	3.8	25.91	14.86	22.1	0.85	0.028*
	Class III	2.4	0.69	3.53	1.86	10.95	2.33	0.045*
	Increased overjet	16.4	7.21	23.62	7.3	27.45	11.67	0.305
	Reversed overjet	3.9	3.97	3.15	3.59	8.5	1.77	0.217
Vertical	Deep bite	26.37	17.43	24.35	15.13	21.25	10.11	1
	Open bite	10	5	3.7	3.77	14.15	15.49	0.035*
Transverse	Posterior crossbite	10.77	7.39	11.64	7.49	16.2 (one case)		0.689

*: Significant at P ≤ 0.05.

DISCUSSION

Global, regional and racial epidemiological assessment of malocclusions is of paramount importance, since it provides important data to assess the type and distribution of occlusal characteristics. Such data will aid in determining and directing the priorities in regards to malocclusion treatment need, and the resources required to offer treatment — in terms of work capacity, skills, agility and materials to be employed. In addition, assessment of malocclusion prevalence by different populations and locations may reflect existence of determining genetic and environmental factors. In line with that, the hypothesized tendency of changing prevalence of a specific type of malocclusion, such as Class II, from mixed to permanent dentition stage may give an indication about the effect of adolescent growth in correction of this problem. Finally, the availability of such global data will be important for educational purposes. Regional and/or racial-specific malocclusion may change the health policy toward developing the specialists' skills and offering the resources required for that malocclusion. It must be emphasized that the current study summarizes the global distribution of malocclusion in mixed and permanent dentitions based on data extracted from studies of moderate (72% of the included studies) to high (28%) quality. None of the included studies was of low quality.

The pooled global prevalence of Class I was the highest (74.7±15.17%), ranging from 31% (Belgium) to 96.6% (Nigeria). It was higher among Africans (89.44%), but equivalent among Caucasians and Mongoloids (71.61% and 74.87%, respectively). This pattern of distribution was reported for both dentitions with slight differences. Noteworthy, the prevalence of Class I in permanent dentition of Mongoloids tends to increase with pubertal growth, mostly due to the associated tendency for Class II correction in this race specifically.

The overall global prevalence of Class II was 19.56%. However, it was interesting to see a wide range from 1.6% (Nigeria) to 63% (Belgium). The lowest prevalence was reported for Africans 6.76% and the highest was reported for Caucasian (22.9%); the reported prevalence for Mongoloids was in-between (14.14%). The pattern of global distribution of Class II malocclusion by race was somewhat similar in mixed and permanent dentitions. With exception of African people (Africa), there is a tendency for correction of Class II with pubertal growth upon transition from mixed to permanent dentition.

Both, prevalence and growth correction of Class II, can be attributed to the genetic influence. Recent research emphasizes the pivotal role of genetic control over condylar cartilage and condylar growth.[63,64]

The global prevalence of Class III was the lowest among all Angle's classes of malocclusion (5.93±4.69%). The range was interestingly wide: 0.7% (Israel) to 19.9% (China). The corresponding figures for Caucasians, Africans and Mongoloids were 5.92, 3.8% and 9.63%, respectively. This pattern of global distribution of Class III applies to mixed and permanent dentitions. A tendency to develop this type of malocclusion appears to increase upon transition from mixed to permanent dentition among Africans and Caucasians, rather than among Mongoloids. The role of genetics must be emphasized. In fact, Class III malocclusion in Asians is mainly due to the mid-face deficiency, rather than mandibular prognathism.[65]

The positive correlation found between Class II and increased overjet is logical. Simply, this is due to the fact that the most prevalent Class II malocclusion globally is Class II division 1.[66] Similarly, the positive correlation of Class III malocclusion with reversed overjet is related to skeletal base discrepancy with minimal dentoalveolar compensation.[67]

The lowest prevalent malocclusion traits globally were reversed overjet and open bite (4.56 and 4.93, respectively). There is a high variation in prevalence of both traits as reported in the literature. Most of the studies reported that open bite trait is highly prevalent in African populations and low in Caucasian populations,[17,18,20,25] in contrast to the reversed overjet, which reported to be prevalent in Mongoloids. In general, both traits are genetically determined.[63,64]

An interesting finding was the higher prevalence of Class II malocclusion in the mixed dentition than in the permanent dentition. This could be explained by the fact that self-correction of a skeletal Class II problem might occur in the late mixed and early permanent dentition stage as a result of a potential mandibular growth spurt. However, a sound conclusion can't be drawn, as the present study was not prospective. In addition, the difference in leeway space between maxillary and mandibular arches, and residual growth in the permanent dentition stage could explain the higher prevalence of Class III malocclusion in the permanent dentition than in the mixed dentition, and the fact that the mandible might continue to grow till the mid-twenties.

The present pooled data showed a decrease in the prevalence of deep bite upon transition from mixed to permanent dentition. Thilander et al,[31] likewise, showed that increased overbite was more prevalent in the mixed dentition. Such an overbite reduction from the mixed to the permanent dentition is due to both occlusal stabilization involving full eruption of premolars and second molars, and the more pronounced mandibular growth.[35] This also explains the reduction in Class II cases as well as the increase in Class III cases (reverse overjet as well) during the period of changing dentition.

In addition to the importance of reporting global malocclusion, it is of an equal importance to report the worldwide orthodontic treatment needs. We planned to do so if the included studies had covered both issues. This was not the case, however, and hence we recommend addressing this latter issue with a similar systematic review.

CONCLUSIONS

1) Consistent with most of the included individual studies, Class I and II malocclusions were the most prevalent, while Class III and open bite were the least prevalent malocclusions.

2) African populations showed the highest prevalence of Class I and open bite malocclusions, while Caucasian populations showed the highest prevalence of Class II malocclusion.

3) Europe continent showed the highest prevalence of Class II among all continents.

4) Class III malocclusion was more prevalent in permanent dentition than mixed dentition, conversely finding for Class II, while all other malocclusions variables showed no difference between the two stages.

Author's Contribution (ORCID ⓘ)

Maged S. Alhammadi (MSA): 0000-0002-1402-0470 ⓘ
Esam Halboub (EH): 0000-0002-1894-470X ⓘ
Mona Saleh Fayed (MSF): 0000-0001-8124-6587 ⓘ
Amr Labib (AL): 0000-0003-1387-9571 ⓘ
Chrestina El-Saaidi (CES) 0000-0002-3993-9029 ⓘ

Conception or design of the study: MSA, AL. Data acquisition, analysis or interpretation: MSA, EH, MSF, AL, CES. Writing the article: MSA, EH, MSF. Critical revision of the article: MSA, EH, MSF, AL, CES. Final approval of the article: MSA, EH, MSF, AL, CES. Overall responsibility: MSA, EH.

REFERENCES

1. Angle EH. Classification of malocclusion. Dent Cosmos. 1899;41:248-64.
2. Guo L, Feng Y, Guo HG, Liu BW, Zhang Y. Consequences of orthodontic treatment in malocclusion patients: clinical and microbial effects in adults and children. BMC Oral Health. 2016 Oct 28;16(1):112.
3. Heimer MV, Tornisiello Katz CR, Rosenblatt A. Non-nutritive sucking habits, dental malocclusions, and facial morphology in Brazilian children: a longitudinal study. Eur J Orthod. 2008 Dec;30(6):580-5.
4. Brook PH, Shaw WC. The development of an index of orthodontic treatment priority. Eur J Orthod. 1989 Aug;11(3):309-20.
5. Foster TD, Menezes DM. The assessment of occlusal features for public health planning purposes. Am J Orthod. 1976 Jan;69(1):83-90.
6. Massler M, Frankel JM. Prevalence of malocclusion in children aged 14 to 18 years. Am J Orthod 1951;37(10):751-68.
7. Goose DH, Thompson, D.G., and Winter, F.C. Malocclusion in School Children of the West Midlands. Brit Dent J. 1957;102:174-8.
8. Mills LF. Epidemiologic studies of occlusion. IV. The prevalence of malocclusion in a population of 1,455 school children. J Dent Res. 1966;45:332-6.
9. Grewe JM, Cervenka J, Shapiro BL, Witkop CJ Jr. Prevalence of malocclusion in Chippewa Indian children. J Dent Res. 1968 Mar-Apr;47(2):302-5.
10. Helm S. Malocclusion in Danish children with adolescent dentition: an epidemiologic study. Am J Orthod. 1968 May;54(5):352-66.
11. Thilander B, Myrberg N. The prevalence of malocclusion in Swedish schoolchildren. Scand J Dent Res. 1973;81(1):12-21.

12. Foster TD, Day AJ. A survey of malocclusion and the need for orthodontic treatment in a Shropshire school population. Br J Orthod. 1974 Apr;1(3):73-8.
13. Ingervall B, Mohlin B, Thilander B. Prevalence and awareness of malocclusion in Swedish men. Community Dent Oral Epidemiol. 1978 Nov;6(6):308-14.
14. Helm S, Prydso U. Prevalence of malocclusion in medieval and modern Danes contrasted. Scand J Dent Res. 1979 Apr;87(2):91-7.
15. Lee KS CK, Ko JH, Koo CH. Occlusal variations in the posterior and anterior segments of the teeth. Korean J Orthod. 1980;10:70-9.
16. Gardiner JH. An orthodontic survey of Libyan schoolchildren. Br J Orthod. 1982 Jan;9(1):59-61.
17. Muniz BR. Epidemiology of malocclusion in Argentine children. Community Dent Oral Epidemiol. 1986 Aug;14(4):221-4.
18. Kerosuo H, Laine T, Kerosuo E, Ngassapa D, Honkala E. Occlusion among a group of Tanzanian urban schoolchildren. Community Dent Oral Epidemiol. 1988 Oct;16(5):306-9.
19. Woon KC, Thong YL, Abdul Kadir R. Permanent dentition occlusion in Chinese, Indian and Malay groups in Malaysia. Aust Orthod J. 1989 Mar;11(1):45-8.
20. al-Emran S, Wisth PJ, Boe OE. Prevalence of malocclusion and need for orthodontic treatment in Saudi Arabia. Community Dent Oral Epidemiol. 1990 Oct;18(5):253-5.
21. El-Mangoury NH, Mostafa YA. Epidemiologic panorama of dental occlusion. Angle Orthod. 1990 Fall;60(3):207-14.

22. Lew KK, Foong WC, Loh E. Malocclusion prevalence in an ethnic Chinese population. Aust Dent J. 1993 Dec;38(6):442-9.

23. Tang EL. The prevalence of malocclusion amongst Hong Kong male dental students. Br J Orthod. 1994 Feb;21(1):57-63.

24. Harrison RL, Davis DW. Dental malocclusion in native children of British Columbia, Canada. Community Dent Oral Epidemiol. 1996 June;24(3):217-21.

25. Ng'ang'a PM, Ohito F, Ogaard B, Valderhaug J. The prevalence of malocclusion in 13- to 15-year-old children in Nairobi, Kenya. Acta Odontol Scand. 1996 Apr;54(2):126-30.

26. Ben-Bassat Y, Harari D, Brin I. Occlusal traits in a group of school children in an isolated society in Jerusalem. Br J Orthod. 1997 Aug;24(3):229-35.

27. Proffit WR, Fields HW Jr, Moray LJ. Prevalence of malocclusion and orthodontic treatment need in the United States: estimates from the NHANES III survey. Int J Adult Orthodon Orthognath Surg. 1998;13(2):97-106.

28. Dacosta OO. The prevalence of malocclusion among a population of northern Nigeria school children. West Afr J Med. 1999 Apr-June;18(2):91-6.

29. Saleh FK. Prevalence of malocclusion in a sample of Lebanese schoolchildren: an epidemiological study. East Mediterr Health J. 1999 Mar;5(2):337-43.

30. Esa R, Razak IA, Allister JH. Epidemiology of malocclusion and orthodontic treatment need of 12-13-year-old Malaysian schoolchildren. Community Dent Health. 2001 Mar;18(1):31-6.

31. Thilander B, Pena L, Infante C, Parada SS, de Mayorga C. Prevalence of malocclusion and orthodontic treatment need in children and adolescents in Bogota, Colombia. An epidemiological study related to different stages of dental development. Eur J Orthod. 2001 Apr;23(2):153-67.

32. Freitas MR, Freitas DS, Pinherio FH, Freitas KMS. Prevalência das más oclusões em pacientes inscritos para tratamento ortodôntico na Faculdade de Odontologia de Bauru-USP. Rev Fac Odontol. 2002;10(3):164-9.

33. Bataringaya A. Survey of occlusal trait in an adolescent population in Uganda. Cabo: University of the Western Cape; 2004.

34. Onyeaso CO. Prevalence of malocclusion among adolescents in Ibadan, Nigeria. Am J Orthod Dentofacial Orthop. 2004 Nov;126(5):604-7.

35. Tausche E, Luck O, Harzer W. Prevalence of malocclusions in the early mixed dentition and orthodontic treatment need. Eur J Orthod. 2004 June;26(3):237-44.

36. Abu Alhaija ES, Al-Khateeb SN, Al-Nimri KS. Prevalence of malocclusion in 13-15 year-old North Jordanian school children. Community Dent Health. 2005 Dec;22(4):266-71.

37. Ali AH AM. Prevalence of Malocclusion in a Sample of Yemeni Schoolchildren: an epidemiological study. Abstracts Yemeni Health Med Res. 2005;44:44.

38. Behbehani F, Artun J, Al-Jame B, Kerosuo H. Prevalence and severity of malocclusion in adolescent Kuwaitis. Med Princ Pract. 2005 Nov-Dec;14(6):390-5.

39. Ciuffolo F, Manzoli L, D'Attilio M, Tecco S, Muratore F, Festa F, et al. Prevalence and distribution by gender of occlusal characteristics in a sample of Italian secondary school students: a cross-sectional study. Eur J Orthod. 2005 Dec;27(6):601-6.

40. Karaiskos N, Wiltshire WA, Odlum O, Brothwell D, Hassard TH. Preventive and interceptive orthodontic treatment needs of an inner-city group of 6- and 9-year-old Canadian children. J Can Dent Assoc. 2005 Oct;71(9):649.

41. Ahangar Atashi MH. Prevalence of Malocclusion in 13-15 Year-old Adolescents in Tabriz. J Dent Res Dent Clin Dent Prospects. 2007 Spring;1(1):13-8.

42. Gelgor IE, Karaman AI, Ercan E. Prevalence of malocclusion among adolescents in central anatolia. Eur J Dent. 2007 July;1(3):125-31.

43. Jonsson T, Arnlaugsson S, Karlsson KO, Ragnarsson B, Arnarson EO, Magnusson TE. Orthodontic treatment experience and prevalence of malocclusion traits in an Icelandic adult population. Am J Orthod Dentofacial Orthop. 2007 Jan;131(1):8.e11-8.

44. Josefsson E, Bjerklin K, Lindsten R. Malocclusion frequency in Swedish and immigrant adolescents--influence of origin on orthodontic treatment need. Eur J Orthod. 2007 Feb;29(1):79-87.

45. Ajayi EO. Prevalence of Malocclusion among School children in Benin City, Nigeria. J Biomed Res. 2008;7(1-2):58-65.

46. Mtaya M, Astrom AN, Brudvik P. Malocclusion, psycho-social impacts and treatment need: a cross-sectional study of Tanzanian primary school-children. BMC Oral Health. 2008 May 6;8:14.

47. Borzabadi-Farahani A, Borzabadi-Farahani A, Eslamipour F. Malocclusion and occlusal traits in an urban Iranian population. An epidemiological study of 11- to 14-year-old children. Eur J Orthod. 2009 Oct;31(5):477-84.

48. Daniel IB PF, Rogerio G. Prevalência de más oclusões em crianças de 9 a 12 anos de idade da cidade de Nova Friburgo (Rio de Janeiro). Rev Dental Press Ortod Ortop Facial. 2009;14(6):118-24.

49. Sidlauskas A, Lopatiene K. The prevalence of malocclusion among 7-15-year-old Lithuanian schoolchildren. Medicina (Kaunas). 2009;45(2):147-52.

50. Alhammadi M. The prevalence of malocclusion in a group of Yemeni adult population: an epidemiologic study [thesis]. Cairo: Cairo University; 2010.

51. Bhardwaj VK, Veeresha KL, Sharma KR. Prevalence of malocclusion and orthodontic treatment needs among 16 and 17 year-old school-going children in Shimla city, Himachal Pradesh. Indian J Dent Res. 2011 July-Aug;22(4):556-60.

52. Nainani JT, Relan S. Prevalence of Malocclusion in School Children of Nagpur Rural Region - An Epidemiological Study. J Dental Assoc. 2011;5:865-7.

53. Bugaighis I. Prevalence of malocclusion in urban libyan preschool children. J Orthod Sci. 2013 Apr;2(2):50-4.

54. Kaur H, Pavithra US, Abraham R. Prevalence of malocclusion among adolescents in South Indian population. J Int Soc Prev Community Dent. 2013 July;3(2):97-102.

55. Reddy ER, Manjula M, Sreelakshmi N, Rani ST, Aduri R, Patil BD. Prevalence of Malocclusion among 6 to 10 Year old Nalgonda School Children. J Int Oral Health. 2013 Dec;5(6):49–54.

56. Bilgic F, Gelgor IE, Celebi AA. Malocclusion prevalence and orthodontic treatment need in central Anatolian adolescents compared to European and other nations' adolescents. Dental Press J Orthod. 2015 Nov-Dec;20(6):75-81.

57. Gupta DK, Singh SP, Utreja A, Verma S. Prevalence of malocclusion and assessment of treatment needs in beta-thalassemia major children. Prog Orthod. 2016;17:7.

58. Narayanan RK, Jeseem MT, Kumar IA. Prevalence of Malocclusion among 10-12-year-old Schoolchildren in Kozhikode District, Kerala: An Epidemiological Study. Int J Clin Pediatr Dent. 2016 Jan-Mar;9(1):50-5.

59. Mattheeuws N, Dermaut L, Martens G. Has hypodontia increased in Caucasians during the 20th century? A meta-analysis. Eur J Orthod. 2004 Feb;26(1):99-103.

60. Polder BJ, Van't Hof MA, Van der Linden FP, Kuijpers-Jagtman AM. A meta-analysis of the prevalence of dental agenesis of permanent teeth. Community Dent Oral Epidemiol. 2004 June;32(3):217-26.

61. Vandenbroucke JP, von Elm E, Altman DG, Gotzsche PC, Mulrow CD, Pocock SJ et al. Strengthening the Reporting of Observational Studies in Epidemiology (STROBE): explanation and elaboration. Int J Surg. 2014;12:1500-24.

62. Kalakonda B, Al-Maweri SA, Al-Shamiri HM, Ijaz A, Gamal S, Dhaifullah E. Is Khat (Catha edulis) chewing a risk factor for periodontal diseases? A systematic review. J Clin Exp Dent. 2017;9:e1264-70.

63. Shibata S, Suda N, Suzuki S, Fukuoka H, Yamashita Y. An in situ hybridization study of Runx2, Osterix, and Sox9 at the onset of condylar cartilage formation in fetal mouse mandible. J Anat. 2006 Feb;208(2):169-77.

64. Hinton RJ. Genes that regulate morphogenesis and growth of the temporomandibular joint: a review. Dev Dyn. 2014 July;243(7):864-74.

65. Newman GV. Prevalence of malocclusion in children six to fourteen years of age and treatment in preventable cases. J Am Dent Assoc. 1956 May;52(5):566-75.

66. Silva Filho OG, Ferrari Junior FM, Okada Ozawa T. Dental arch dimensions in Class II division 1 malocclusions with mandibular deficiency. Angle Orthod. 2008 May;78(3):466-74.

67. Kim SJ, Kim KH, Yu HS, Baik HS. Dentoalveolar compensation according to skeletal discrepancy and overjet in skeletal Class III patients. Am J Orthod Dentofacial Orthop. 2014 Mar;145(3):317-24.

7

Malocclusion prevalence and orthodontic treatment need in central Anatolian adolescents compared to European and other nations' adolescents

Fundagul Bilgic[1], Ibrahim Erhan Gelgor[2], Ahmet Arif Celebi[3]

Objective: To determine the prevalence of malocclusion and orthodontic treatment need in a large sample of Central Anatolian adolescents and compare them with European-other nations' adolescents. **Methods:** The sample included 1125 boys and 1204 girls aged between 12 and 16 years with no previous orthodontic treatment history. Occlusal variables examined were molar relationship, overjet, overbite, crowding, midline diastema, posterior crossbite, and scissors bite. The dental health (DHC) and aesthetic components (AC) of the Index of Orthodontic Treatment Need (IOTN) were used as an assessment measure of the need for orthodontic treatment for the total sample. **Results:** The results indicated a high prevalence of Class I (34.9%) and Class II, Division 1 malocclusions (40.0%). Moreover, increased (18%) and reduced bites (14.%), and increased (25.1%) and reversed overjet (10.%) were present in the sample. **Conclusion:** Using the DHC of the IOTN, the proportion of subjects estimated to have great and very great treatment need (grades 4 and 5) was 28.%. However, only 16.7% of individuals were in need (grades 8-10) of orthodontic treatment according to the AC.

Keywords: Malocclusion. Orthodontic treatment need. IOTN.

[1] Assistant Professor, Mustafa Kemal University, Faculty of Dentistry, Department of Orthodontics, Hatay, Turkey.

[2] Professor, Kirikkale University, Faculty of Dentistry, Department of Orthodontics, Kirikkale, Turkey.

[3] Lecturer, Ishik University, Faculty of Dentistry, Department of Orthodontics, Erbil, Iraq.

» The authors report no commercial, proprietary or financial interest in the products or companies described in this article.

Fundagul Bilgic
Email: fundagulbilgic@hotmail.com

INTRODUCTION

On an increased basis, malocclusion is considered an expression of normal biologic variation, and treatment need is often based as much on psychosocial concerns as on proven oral health risks attributable to malocclusion.[1] The criteria for determining who is most likely to benefit from orthodontic treatment are controversial. These factors make it particularly difficult for the general dentist to determine for whom orthodontic treatment is clearly indicated, since the traditional pathway to orthodontic care starts at the general dentist's office.

Different populations have been investigated to provide epidemiological data of the prevalence of malocclusion.[2-7] As a common trend, quantitative variables along with Angle's classification were used in these reports. Additionally, treatment-need indexes were also used to determine orthodontic need based on esthetic impairment, potential for adverse effect on dental health, and deviation from normal occlusion.[8] The Index of Orthodontic Treatment Need (IOTN), involving the Dental Health Component (DHC) and the Aesthetic Component (AC), is the tool most frequently used for measuring treatment need.[9,10] Perhaps, being objective and synthetic, and allowing for comparisons between different population groups, are the most important aspects of this index.[7,11,12]

Certain European populations, such as the Swedish,[13] British,[14] German,[5,15] French[16] and Italian[6,7,17] have been examined extensively in regards to IOTN. However, there is little research and/or published data that evaluated together the prevalence of malocclusion[8,18] and orthodontic treatment need[19,20] in adolescents. Therefore, the aim of the present survey was to document the prevalence of individual traits of malocclusion, and to assess the need for orthodontic treatment in relation to sex by using the IOTN in a group of adolescent schoolchildren. It also aimed to compare the data provided with the findings of chiefly European patients as well as other surveys.

MATERIAL AND METHODS

Data were collected during an epidemiological survey, in the period of May, 2008 to December, 2012, from 2329 adolescents (1125 males and 1204 females) aged 12.5–16.2 years, randomly selected using a one-stage cluster sampling procedure in 13 state-funded secondary schools in Kirikale city which is located in the south area of the capital of Turkey. The schools were randomly selected from an initial pool of 27 schools that had been previously identified by the school district to avoid possible biases ensuing from social heterogeneity. Written parent informed consent forms were obtained for dental examinations. Family origin and registration information were examined in order to determine that the sample was a good representative of ancestry from the central part of the country. All male and female patients who met the following criteria were included in the sample: (1) age from 12 to 16 years; (2) secondary dentition present with no remaining deciduous teeth; (3) no multiple missing teeth; (4) presence of first permanent canines and molars; and (5) no previous history of orthodontic treatment. Each examination took place while the subject was seated in a standard, quiet classroom in the designated chairs. Clinical examination was carried out by one examiner who was previously calibrated. The examination lasted 20 minutes per child, following World Health Organization guidelines.[21]

Orthodontic variables

Patients with an occlusal pattern that deviated from the ideal Class I relationship, which is based on the buccal groove of the mandibular first molar settled on the mesiobuccal cusp of the maxillary first molar as described by Angle, (including crowding, spacing, rotations), were categorized as Class I malocclusion. Thus, the Class I normal category was limited to patients with occlusions that were ideal or near ideal. Patients with a different Angle classification of occlusion on each side were categorized into a single Class based on the predominant pattern of occlusion and/or canine relationship.[4,22]

For overbite and overjet, values between 0 and 4 mm were considered normal.[7] Posterior crossbite and scissors bite were registered as bilateral, right and left.[4,5] Crowding was recorded for the incisor and also posterior segments of each jaw (1-3 mm = mild; 4-6 mm = moderate; > 6 mm = severe).[4] Anterior diastema was diagnosed when there was a space of at least 1 mm between central incisors in either arch.[4]

Patients with a normal occlusion pattern had normal molar and canine relationships, no crowding or crossbites, normal overjet and overbite, well-balanced faces, and no history of previous orthodontic treatment.

Orthodontic treatment need

The findings served to determine orthodontic treatment need with reference to the IOTN[9,10] which consists of the DHC and the AC. Considerations as to no treatment need, borderline need, or great need were based on five grades in the DHC and 10 grades in the AC.

Statistical analysis

To test examiner reproducibility, 25 children were reexamined by Kappa's method four weeks after initial examination.[23] The ratio of the sample, as a maximum estimate of the proportion of individual traits of malocclusion in the whole population, was calculated for the total sample and for girls and boys separately. The number of subjects with diagnosed anomaly (n) and its prevalence (n/N x 100, in which N is the number of subjects examined) was determined. The differences between sex groups were assessed by means of chi-square test. Data were analyzed by SPSS software package (version 21.0, SPSS Inc., Chicago, Ill., USA). for IOTN DHC and AC grades. Level of significance was established at $p < 0.05$.

RESULTS

Kappa test indicated high reliability and reproducibility (0.73 - 0.80) for the parameters tested. Table 1 presents the prevalence of each occlusal trait in the total sample. Class I malocclusion was found in 812 subjects, which represented 34.9% of the 2329 individuals examined. Class II malocclusion was diagnosed in 1041

individuals, 40.0% of all patients were Division 1 and 4.7% of all patients were Division 2. Class III malocclusion was found in 240 subjects, 10.3% of the sample. Normal overbite was the most common (73.5%), mostly observed in girls ($p < 0.001$). Increased overbite was recorded in 18.3% of the sample, mostly observed in boys ($p < 0.05$). The prevalence of reduced bite value was found as 8.2%. Normal overjet was present in 1371 individuals (64.5%). Prevalence of increased overjet (25.1%) was found to be higher than negative overjet (10.4%). While crossbite was found more frequently, as much as of 4.0 % of the sample, scissors bite was rarely diagnosed in only 0.3% of the subjects.

Anterior crowding was present in 1638 individuals (66.2%) (Table 2); 17.9, 9.1 and 38.1% of those had crowding in the upper arch, lower arch and both arches, respectively. Moderate crowding was more common in both arches. Midline and spread diastemas were found in 14.8 and 12.9% of the sample, respectively. Diastemas were observed mostly in the upper arch (Table 2).

In the study group, the IOTN revealed no treatment need in 45.6% of the sample, when the DHC was used (mostly in boys ($p < 0.05$) and 43.1% when the AC was used. (Figs 1 and 2, and Tables 3 and 4). When borderline cases were taken into consideration, treatment need was diagnosed in 25.7% of the sample when the DHC was used and in 40.2% when the AC was used. The number of subjects with the need for orthodontic treatment was 648 (28.7%) when the DHC was used, and 376 (16.7%) when the AC was used.

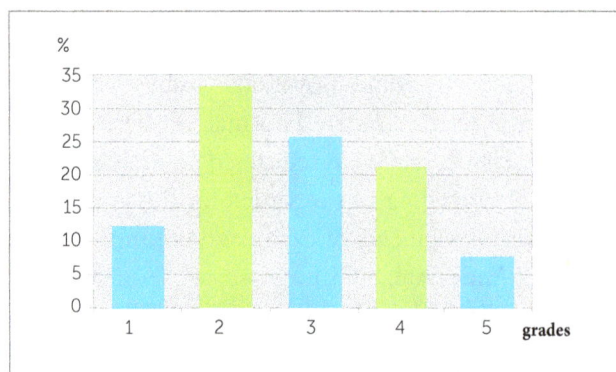

Figure 1 - Dental Health Component (DHC) grades of the Index of Orthodontic Treatment Need (IOTN) in Anatolian adolescents (Grades 1 and 2, no need; Grade 3, borderline need; Grades 4 and 5, definite need).

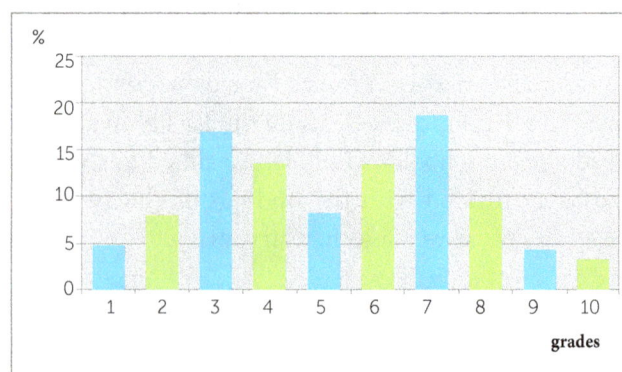

Figure 2 - Aesthetic component (AC) grades of the Index of Orthodontic Treatment Need (IOTN) in Anatolian adolescents (Grades 1-4, no need; Grade 5-7, borderline need; Grades 8-10, definite need).

Table 1 - Occlusal classifications.

			Boys		Girls		Total		p-value	
			n	%	n	%	n	%		
Occlusal anteroposterior relationships										
Normal occlusion			110	9.8	126	10.5	236	10.1	NS	0.63
Class I			404	35.9	408	33.9	812	34.9	NS	0.317
Class II, Division 1			448	39.8	483	40.1	931	40.0	NS	0.899
Class II, Division 2			56	5.0	54	4.5	110	4.7	NS	0.625
Class III			107	9.5	133	11.0	240	10.3	NS	0.246
Distribution of overbite										
Normal (0-4 mm)			802	71.2	913	75.8	1715	73.5	***	0.0001
Increased (> 4 mm)			227	20.2	197	16.4	424	18.3	*	0.018
Reduced (< 0 mm)			96	8.5	94	7.8	190	8.2	NS	0.098
Distribution of overjet										
Normal			731	65	770	64	1501	64.5	NS	0.866
Increased			281	25	304	25.2	585	25.1	NS	0.886
Negative			113	10	130	10.8	243	10.4	NS	0.588
Distribution of posterior crossbite and scissors bite										
	No finding		1021	90.8	1082	89.9	2103	90.3	NS	0.677
	Bilateral		41	3.6	52	4.3	93	4.0	NS	0.544
Crossbite	Unilateral	right	35	3.1	41	3.4	76	3.3	NS	0.890
		left	24	2.1	27	2.2	51	2.2	NS	0.970
	Bilateral		1	0.1	1	0.1	2	0.1	NS	0.957
Scissors bite	Unilateral	right	2	0.2	0	0.0	2	0.1	NS	0.949
		left	1	0.1	1	0.1	2	0.1	NS	0.889

NS: Not significant. *p < 0.05; ***p < 0.001.

Table 2 - Distribution of crowding and diastema.

		Boys		Girls		Total		p	
		n	%	n	%	n	%		
Crowding									
No crowding		383	34.0	428	35.5	811	34.8	NS	0.460
Upper arch, only	mild	140	12.4	120	10.0	260	11.2	NS	0.214
	moderate	55	4.9	60	5.0	115	4.9	NS	0.732
	severe	18	1.6	24	2.0	42	1.8	NS	0.810
Lower arch, only	mild	67	6.0	70	5.8	137	5.9	NS	0.845
	moderate	28	2.5	31	2.6	59	2.5	NS	0.760
	severe	8	0.7	9	0.7	17	0.7	NS	0.77
Both arches	mild	280	24.9	303	25.2	583	25.0	NS	0.981
	moderate	127	11.3	137	11.4	264	11.3	NS	0.831
	severe	19	1.7	22	1.8	41	1.8	NS	0.985
Diastema									
No finding		808	71.8	852	70.8	1660	71.3	NS	0.328
Upper arch	midline	140	12.4	156	13	296	12.7	NS	0.214
	spread	99	8.8	95	7.9	194	8.4	NS	0.632
Lower arch	midline	20	1.8	30	2.4	50	2.1	NS	0.870
	spread	58	5.2	71	5.9	129	5.5	NS	0.670

NS: Not significant.

Table 3 - DHC of IOTN statistics of boys and girls.

Occlusal anteroposterior relations-hips	Boys		Girls		Total			p-value
	n	%	n	%	n	%		
No need	531	48.3	492	42.8	1023	45.6	*	0.01
Borderline need	263	23.9	316	27.5	579	25.7	NS	0.054
Need	306	27.8	342	29.7	648	28.7	NS	0.328
Total	1100	100	1150	100	2250	100		

*,p < 0.05; NS: Not significant.

Table 4 - AC of IOTN statistics of boys and girls.

Occlusal anteroposterior relationships	Boys		Girls		Total			p-value
	n	%	n	%	n	%		
No need	492	44.6	478	41.6	970	43.1	NS	0.136
Borderline need	437	39.6	467	40.7	904	40.2	NS	0.699
Need	171	15.4	205	17.9	376	16.7	NS	0.142
Total	1100	100	1150	100	2250	100		

NS: Not significant.

DISCUSSION

Although many studies were published to describe the prevalence and types of malocclusion, when examining a certain population it is difficult to compare and contrast these findings, partly because of the varying methods and indexes used to assess and record occlusal relationships, age differences of the study populations, examiner subjectivity, specific objectives, and differing sample sizes.[22] Methodology used in this study was mostly collected from European studies,[4,6,7,22] and our results were discussed with the findings from different European geological regions due to close proximity and since there was limited information of individuals in the literature. The general consensus about treatment timing for malocclusions is that it should start around permanent dentition. At this stage, maxillary and mandibular development is almost completed and the malocclusion takes its final pattern. Given the characteristics of the sample, this paper demonstrated the occlusal traits of an untreated adolescent population at those ages.

With respect to the occlusal findings, Class I malocclusion was found in 34.9% of the sample. This Class I occlusion figure included individuals with incisor crowding and dental malalignment and thus did not imply ideal normal occlusion. The prevalence of Class II, Division 1 (40.0%), in the present study, was greater than the rates reported for English school children (12.5%),[24] Shropshire school population (27.2%),[25] adolescents in Bogotá (14.9%),[4] and Italian school adolescents (36.3%.[7] However, Lauc[26] on Hvar Island, and Josefsson et al[13] for a Swedish population, found that Class II malocclusion was more common in their population (greater than 45%), and explained this figure by a genetic influence on the incidence of Class II malocclusions. Early treatment in the primary or early mixed dentition has been recommended for Class III malocclusions.[4,27] The prevalence of Class III malocclusion determined in this study is 10.3%. However, Goose et al[28] (2.91%), Haynes[24] (2.5%), Foster and Day[25] (3.5%), Proffit et al[29] (5.7%), Thilander et al[4] (5.8%), Lauc[26] (4.8%), and Perillo et al[7] (4.3%) reported lower rates. The present study confirmed that the predominant anteroposterior relationship of the arches in adolescents was Class II, Division 1. Of the vertical anomalies, increased overbite was more than twice as frequent as anterior open bite. Our results were similar to the rates reported by Thilander et al[4] and Lauc[26] who also claimed that deep bite was often associated with a Class II malocclusion and more common in boys. However, higher ratios were found in Italian samples.[6,7] Increased overjet proved to be as high as increased overbite in this study; this is a reflection of the higher prevalence of Class II malocclusion among adolescents. Our findings agree with those of Thilander et al,[4] in Bogotanian adolescents, and Ciuffolo et al,[6] in Italian adolescents, in which high rates of increased overjet in the permanent dentition were reported. In a French sample, increased overjet was present in fewer subjects (6%).[3]

In this study, uni/bilateral posterior crossbite was more frequent than scissors bite and was observed in 9.5% of the sample. This rate was similar to the findings of Ciuffolo et al[6] and higher than Thilander et al.[4] Perillo et al[7] showed a higher percentage for crossbite and scissors bite (14.2 and 3.5%, respectively).

Crowding, in one or both arches, was the most frequent of all anomalies recorded (66.2%). This finding complied with the results of Thilander et al[4] and Lauc.[26] There is a general consensus that treatment of crowding should start in the permanent dentition.[5] The National Health and Nutrition Survey III, undertaken in the United States between 1989 and 1994, showed a frequency of crowding ranging from 42.3% at ages 8-11 to 54.5% at ages 12-17, which was lower than the frequencies observed in this investigation.[29] Nevertheless, other studies have reported lower rates of crowding located in anterior/both segments.[3,6,7,24,25]

Thilander et al[4] found the prevalence of median diastema in their population to be 13.5% in the early mixed and 4% in the permanent dentition. Lauc[26] observed a high rate of midline diastema (45.1%). In contrast, in our study, this rate was 12.7%. Perillo et al[7] showed the prevalence of median diastema as equal to 9.9%. The frequency of diastema in Nigeria was 24%.[30]

Administrators of publicly funded programs need a valid screening method to determine priority for orthodontic treatment.[15] Priority of orthodontic care through national health care plans in European countries has been a prime factor behind the development of indexes, such as the IOTN.

The need for orthodontic treatment has been presented in the literature by means of different indexes. In the present study, the classification by the IOTN was used because the authors' are familiar with this index.

In Turkey, there are few epidemiologic surveys. Guray et al[19] used the Treatment Priority Index (TPI) and found that 72.26 % of 483 students required orthodontic treatment in a primary school with a low socioeconomic standard from Konya district (South Anatolia). Ugur et al[20] found a 37.77% orthodontic treatment need, by using the TPI in 572 6 to 10-year-old Turkish primary school children with a high socioeconomic standard in central Anatolia. Our study was carried out in a large adolescent sample with moderate socioeconomic status, and treatment need was lower than those two studies. These studies conducted in different regions show similar results in terms of the need for orthodontic treatment in individuals with different socio-cultural features in different locations. The results of this study were not in agreement with Ugur et al[20] who determined that orthodontic treatment needs increase with age. In our study, according to the DHC of the IOTN, 28.7% of the whole sample was classified as being in need of orthodontic treatment (grades 4 and 5). The results showed that the percentage was relatively greater than those reported by Souames et al[16] in France and Perillo et al[7] in Italy (21.3 and 27.3%, respectively). However, the British studies found a higher prevalence rate for untreated subjects: 32.7%,[10] 33% and, 35%.[14] Josefsson et al[13] found 39.5% of orthodontic treatment need in a Swedish sample. The findings of the present study, therefore, indicated that a substantial need for orthodontic intervention was present at a similar level to French and Italian children, but generally lower than northern European populations (United Kingdom and Sweden).

The AC for IOTN, in the present study, reduced orthodontic treatment need (16.7%). This has also been reported in other studies.[10,13,16] Tausche et al[5] claimed that the AC alone failed to identify any children needing orthodontic treatment. Because of the AC alone is an inappropriate method for screening treatment need, lack of agreement occurs between the normative component and the IOTN-AC. However, Josefsson et al[13] used the AC both by the examiner and the subject. This study also hunted up a difference between males and females for orthodontic treatment need. Treatment need did not differ significantly as a result of sex. AC alone is unsuitable for screening treatment need.

CONCLUSION

The results of this investigation demonstrated that Class II, Division 1 malocclusion was the most prevalent occlusal pattern among adolescents, and the high incidence of increased overjet and overbite are a reflection of the high prevalence of Class II malocclusion. Also, a high percentage of crowding is noteworthy.

Nearly one-third of the evaluated population would have a mandatory need for orthodontic treatment, if the DHC scores were used as the main criterion for such decisions. If the AC scores were used, the need would decrease to one-fifth of the sample. These results revealed the high percentage of need for orthodontic treatment in Turkey.

REFERENCES

1. Bentele MJ, Vig KW, Shanker S, Beck FM. Efficacy of training dental students in the index of orthodontic treatment need. Am J Orthod Dentofacial Orthop. 2002 Nov;122(5):456-62.

2. Brunelle JA, Bhat M, Lipton JA. Prevalence and distribution of selected occlusal characteristics in the US population, 1988-1991. J Dent Res. 1996 Feb;75 Spec No:706-13.

3. Tschill P, Bacon W, Sonko A. Malocclusion in the deciduous dentition of Caucasian children. Eur J Orthod. 1997 Aug;19(4):361-7.

4. Thilander B, Pena L, Infante C, Parada SS, de Mayorga C. Prevalence of malocclusion and orthodontic treatment need in children and adolescents in Bogota, Colombia. An epidemiological study related to different stages of dental development. Eur J Orthod. 2001 Apr;23(2):153-67.

5. Tausche E, Luck O, Harzer W. Prevalence of malocclusions in the early mixed dentition and orthodontic treatment need. Eur J Orthod. 2004 Jun;26(3):237-44.

6. Ciuffolo F, Manzoli L, D'Attilio M, Tecco S, Muratore F, Festa F, et al. Prevalence and distribution by gender of occlusal characteristics in a sample of Italian secondary school students: a cross-sectional study. Eur J Orthod. 2005 Dec;27(6):601-6. Epub 2005 Jul 11.

7. Perillo L, Masucci C, Ferro F, Apicella D, Baccetti T. Prevalence of orthodontic treatment need in southern Italian schoolchildren. Eur J Orthod. 2010 Feb;32(1):49-53.

8. Gelgör IE, Şişman Y, Malkoç S. Prevalence of congenital hypodontia in the permanent dentition. Turkiye Klinikleri J Dental Sci. 2005;11(2):43-8.

9. Evans R, Shaw W. Preliminary evaluation of an illustrated scale for rating dental attractiveness. Eur J Orthod. 1987 Nov;9(4):314-8.

10. Brook PH, Shaw WC. The development of an index of orthodontic treatment priority. Eur J Orthod. 1989 Aug;11(3):309-20.

11. Shaw WC, Richmond S, O'Brien KD, Brook P, Stephens CD. Quality control in orthodontics: indices of treatment need and treatment standards. Br Dent J. 1991 Feb 9;170(3):107-12.

12. Cooper S, Mandall NA, DiBiase D, Shaw WC. The reliability of the index of orthodontic treatment need over time. J Orthod. 2000 Mar;27(1):47-53.

13. Josefsson E, Bjerklin K, Lindsten R. Malocclusion frequency in Swedish and immigrant adolescents: influence of origin on orthodontic treatment need. Eur J Orthod. 2007 Feb;29(1):79-87.

14. Chestnutt IG, Burden DJ, Steele JG, Pitts NB, Nuttall NM, Morris AJ. The orthodontic condition of children in the United Kingdom, 2003. Br Dent J. 2006 Jun;200(11):609-12.

15. Krey KF, Hirsch C. Frequency of orthodontic treatment in German children and adolescents: influence of age, gender, and socio-economic status. Eur J Orthod. 2012 Apr;34(2):152-7.

16. Souames M, Bassigny F, Zenati N, Riordan PJ, Boy-Lefevre ML. Orthodontic treatment need in French schoolchildren: an epidemiological study using the Index of Orthodontic Treatment Need. Eur J Orthod. 2006 Dec;28(6):605-9.

17. Nobile CG, Pavia M, Fortunato L, Angelillo IF. Prevalence and factors related to malocclusion and orthodontic treatment need in children and adolescents in Italy. Eur J Public Health. 2007 Dec;17(6):637-41.

18. Gelgör IE, Karaman AI, Ercan E. Prevalence of malocclusion among adolescents in central Anatolia. Eur J Dent. 2007 Jul;1(3):125-31.

19. Güray E, Ertas E, Orhan M, Doruk C. An epidemiologic survey using "Treatment Priority Index" (TPI) on primary school children in Konya. Türk Ortodonti Derg. 1994 Nov;7(2):195-200.

20. Ugur T, Ciger S, Aksoy A, Telli A. An epidemiological survey using the Treatment Priority Index (TPI). Eur J Orthod. 1998 Apr;20(2):189-93.

21. World Health Organization. International collaboration study of oral health outcomes (ICS II), document 2: oral data collection and examination criteria. Geneva: WHO; 1989.

22. Silva RG, Kang DS. Prevalence of malocclusion among Latino adolescents. Am J Orthod Dentofacial Orthop. 2001 Mar;119(3):313-5.

23. Landis JR, Koch GG. The measurement of observer agreement for categorical data. Biometrics. 1977 Mar;33(1):159-74.

24. Haynes S. The prevalence of malocclusion in English children aged 11-12 years. Report of the congress. Eur Orthod Soc. 1970:89-98.

25. Foster TD, Day AJ. A survey of malocclusion and the need for orthodontic treatment in a Shropshire school population. Br J Orthod. 1974 Apr;1(3):73-8.

26. Lauc T. Orofacial analysis on the Adriatic islands: an epidemiological study of malocclusions on Hvar Island. Eur J Orthod. 2003 Jun;25(3):273-8.

27. McNamara JA Brudon WL. Orthodontics and dentofacial orthopedics. Ann Arbor: Needham Press; 2001.

28. Goose DH TD, Winter FC. Malocclusion in school children of the West Midlands. Br Dent J. 1957;102:174-8.

29. Proffit WR, Fields HW Jr, Moray LJ. Prevalence of malocclusion and orthodontic treatment need in the United States: estimates from the NHANES III survey. Int J Adult Orthodon Orthognath Surg. 1998;13(2):97-106.

30. Otuyemi OD, Ogunyinka A, Dosumu O, Cons NC, Jenny J. Malocclusion and orthodontic treatment need of secondary school students in Nigeria according to the dental aesthetic index (DAI). Int Dent J. 1999 Aug;49(4):203-10.

8

Assessment of first molars sagittal and rotational position in Class II, division 1 malocclusion

Paulo Estevão Scanavini[1], Renata Pilli Jóias[2], Maria Helena Ferreira Vasconcelos[3],
Marco Antonio Scanavini[4], Luiz Renato Paranhos[5]

Objective: This study assessed the anterior-posterior positioning of the upper and lower first molars, and the degree of rotation of the upper first molars in individuals with Class II, division 1, malocclusion. **Methods:** Asymmetry I, an accurate device, was used to assess sixty sets of dental casts from 27 females and 33 males, aged between 12 and 21 years old, with bilateral Class II, division 1. The sagittal position of the molars was determined by positioning the casts onto the device, considering the midpalatal suture as a symmetry reference, and then measuring the distance between the mesial marginal ridge of the most distal molar and the mesial marginal ridge of its counterpart. With regard to the degree of rotation of the upper molar, the distance between landmarks on the mesial marginal ridge was measured. Chi-square test with a 5% significance level was used to verify the variation in molars position. Student's t test at 5% significance was used for statistical analysis. **Results:** A great number of lower molars mesially positioned was registered, and the comparison between the right and left sides also demonstrated a higher number of mesially positioned molars on the right side of both arches. The average rotation of the molars was found to be 0.76 mm and 0.93 mm for the right and left sides, respectively. **Conclusion:** No statistically significant difference was detected between the mean values of molars mesialization regardless of the side and arch. Molars rotation, measured in millimeters, represented ¼ of Class II.

Keywords: Molar tooth. Angle Class II malocclusion. Orthodontics.

[1] MSc in Orthodontics, UMESP. Professor, Specialization Course in Orthodontics, APCD.
[2] PhD Student, Oral Biopathology, UNESP.
[3] PhD in Orthodontics, FOB/USP. Professor, UMESP.
[4] PhD in Orthodontics, USP. Professor, UMESP.
[5] Post-Doc in Dentistry, UNICAMP. Adjunct Professor, Federal University of Sergipe.

» The authors report no commercial, proprietary or financial interest in the products or companies described in this article.

Paulo Estevão Scanavini
Rua Antônio Pereira de Camargo, 129 – Centro
CEP: 13.170-030 – Sumaré/SP – E-mail: paranhos@ortodontista.com.br

INTRODUCTION

Dental arch symmetry and dimension are of great interest for orthodontists when making diagnosis and treatment planning.[1,2]

Molar positioning in the anterior-posterior direction determines the sagittal classification of malocclusion[3,4] and can be easily detected in cases of Class II subdivision. However, molar positioning should also be considered in cases of bilateral malocclusion, since a molar more mesially positioned on one side, even if not clinically[2] apparent, can influence diagnosis, treatment planning and,[5-8] especially occlusal stability.

The asymmetric position may determine important aspects regarding the orthodontic mechanics that will be used, such as the correction of rotations, or distalization methods.[9-12] These procedures may be applied with different intensities in each to obtain an arch with symmetrical positioning of the posterior teeth.[13] With the purpose of carrying out a detailed assessment of teeth positioning, the dental cast analysis is an important tool due to its practicality, reliability and reproducibility.[1,14-20]

Thus, this study aimed at assessing the positioning of contralateral molars in the maxillary and mandibular arches in the anterior-posterior direction, as well as to examine the degree of rotation of the upper molars in individuals with Class II, division 1 malocclusion.

MATERIAL AND METHODS

This research was previously approved by the Institutional Review Board of the Metodista University of São Paulo (UMESP), under protocol number 0210135. The sample of this study was obtained from the files of the Postgraduate Program of the aforementioned University. Sixty sets of plaster models from 27 females and 33 males, aged between 12 and 21 years, with Class II, division 1 malocclusion, were selected.

Measurements were made directly in the study models by using Asymmetry I, a device developed in the Postgraduate Program Department to enable the visualization of the sagittal positioning of molars as well as the existence of possible rotations. This device consists of a structure similar to a parallelometer, containing: A base for positioning the model, a transparent horizontal acrylic plate with a millimeter ruler, and a rod which enables the identification of the molars positioning (Figs 1A and B).

The midpalatal suture was used as a symmetry reference.[1,2] It was delimited in the maxillary arch by demarcating landmarks over the mid-palatal suture from the incisive papilla until the most posterior visible landmark.[19,20] The symmetry axis was obtained by connecting these landmarks. Then, it was extended anteriorly up to the incisal edge of the maxillary incisor to determine the landmark As (anterior-superior). Conversely, it was posteriorly extended up to the posterior surface of the maxillary model to determine Ps (posterior-superior) (Fig 2A).

The midline projection, obtained in the maxillary arch, was used when the midpalatal suture was transferred to the lower model.[15,16] The upper midline was transferred to the lower model by using the reference landmarks As and Ps.

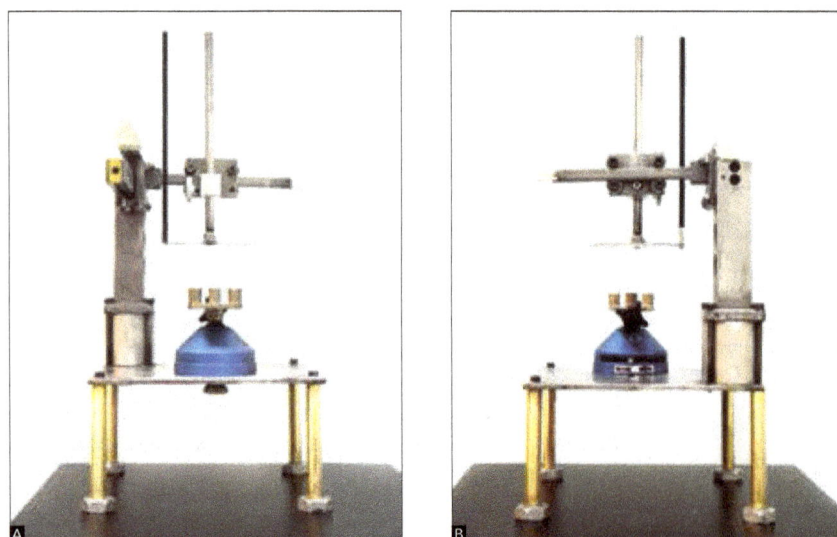

Figure 1 - Measuring device - Asymmetry I -, frontal view (**A**); posterior view (**B**).

The models, properly trimmed, were placed in occlusion, so that the posterior surfaces matched in the same plane. The landmark Ps of the upper model was transferred to the lower model by means of a set triangle ruler positioned perpendicularly to the base of the lower model, thereby determining the landmark Pi (posterior-inferior) on the lower model (Fig 2B).

With the models still in occlusion and with the set triangle ruler equally placed anteriorly to the models matching with the landmark As of the upper model, the landmark Ai (anterior-inferior) was demarcated in the mandibular model (Fig 2C).

Obtaining and connecting Ai and Pi landmarks enabled the lower midline to be determined (Fig 2D).

The models were then placed onto the base of the parallelometer which was fixed to the base of the Asymmetry I device (Figs 3A and B). When positioning the models, the occlusal surface of the teeth should be parallel to the horizontal plane, and the protractor pointer positioned over the midpalatal suture. The reference used for assessing the molar positioning was the mesial marginal ridge. Subsequently, the distance between the mesial marginal ridge positioned more distally and the mesial marginal ridge of the opposite molar was measured in the longitudinal direction, as shown in Figures 4 and 5.

In order to verify the possible association of variation in molar positioning, concerning the arch and side of the molars mesially positioned, chi-square test (c^2) was used. Student's t test was employed to compare these values. In all tests, a significance level of 5% was adopted.

In addition to assessing the position of the molars in the anterior-posterior direction, the degree of rotation of the upper molars was also assessed, as follows: the distance between the most mesial portion of the mesial marginal ridge toward the mesiodistal sulcus (point CM), and the apex of the mesiobuccal cusp, at its most mesial portion, was measured. One horizontal line was projected from the CM landmark, and another from the VM landmark, both parallel. Thus, the distance between these lines was measured, in millimeters, indicating the rotation of the molars in the mesiodistal direction (Fig 6).

RESULTS

Table 1 shows the distribution of the individuals comprising the sample, considering the side of the molar mesially positioned and the dental arch.

The variation in the mean value of molar mesialization was found to be 0.05 mm for the maxillary arch, with mean values of 1.55 mm and 1.50 mm for the left and right sides, respectively. For the mandibular arch, this

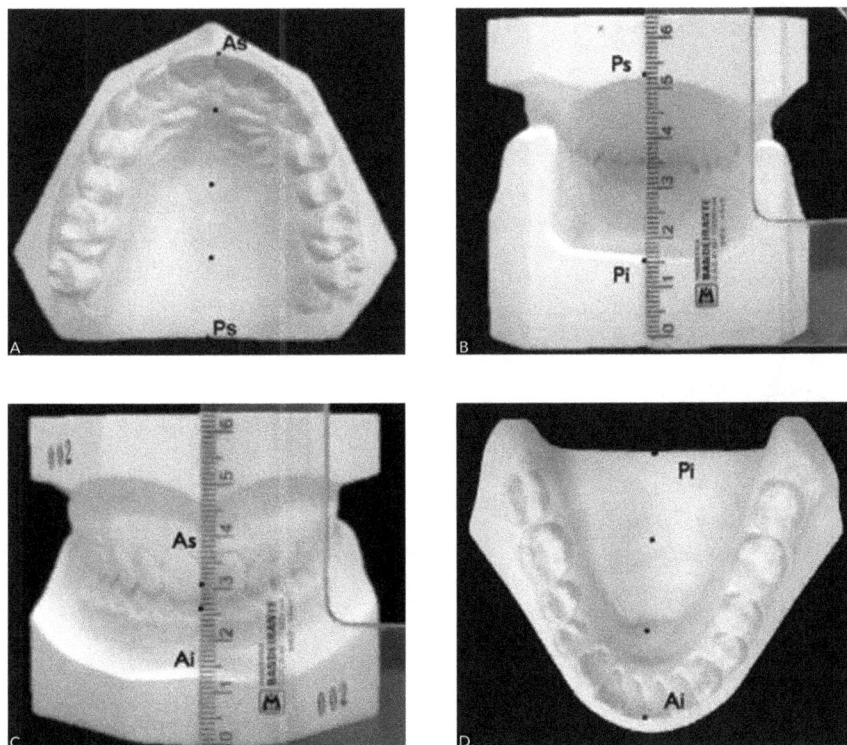

Figure 2 - A) determination of the upper midline (landmarks As and Ps); B) transference of the Ps to the lower model - obtaining Pi; C) transference of the As landmark to the lower model – obtaining Ai; D) determination of the lower midline (landmarks Ai and Pi).

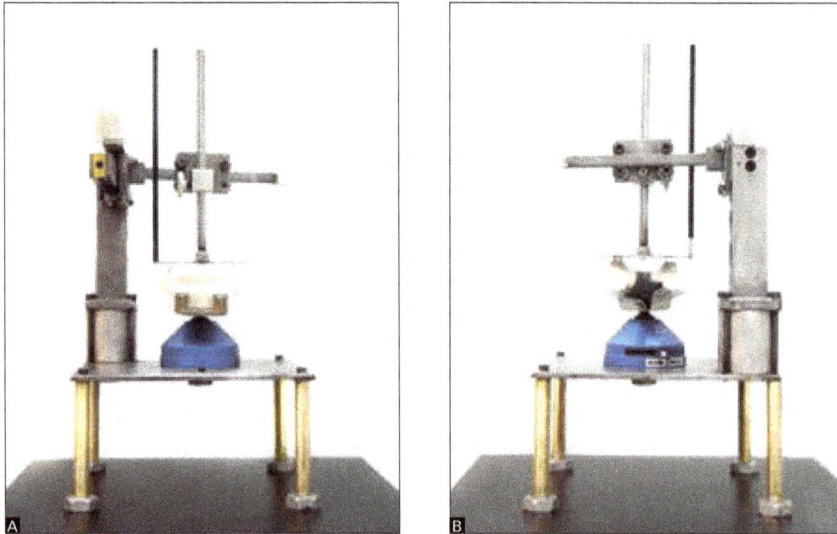

Figure 3 - Models positioned for measurement: **A)** front view, **B)** back view.

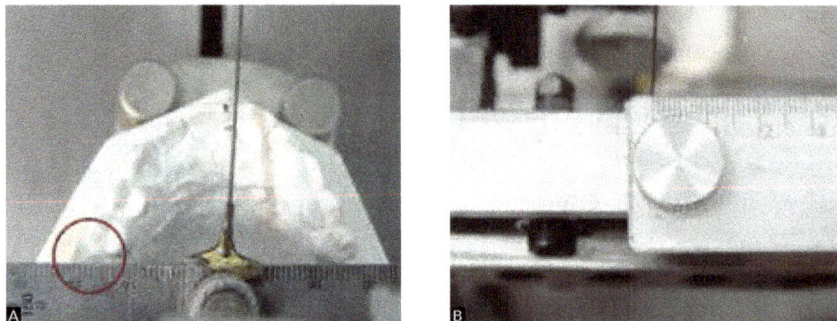

Figure 4 - **A)** Model positioned evidencing the more mesial position of the maxillary right first molar, in relation to left-side counterpart; **B)** ruler recording the position of the right maxillary first molar at zero position.

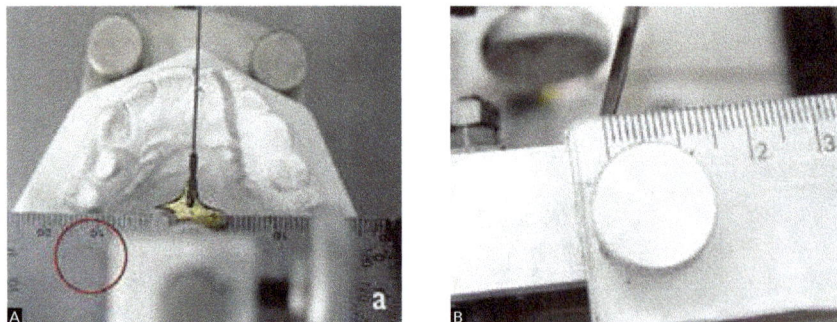

Figure 5 - **A)** Device positioned on the mesial marginal ridge of the right maxillary first molar **B)**; ruler registering the most mesial position of the right maxillary first molar by 1.5 mm, in relation to left-side counterpart.

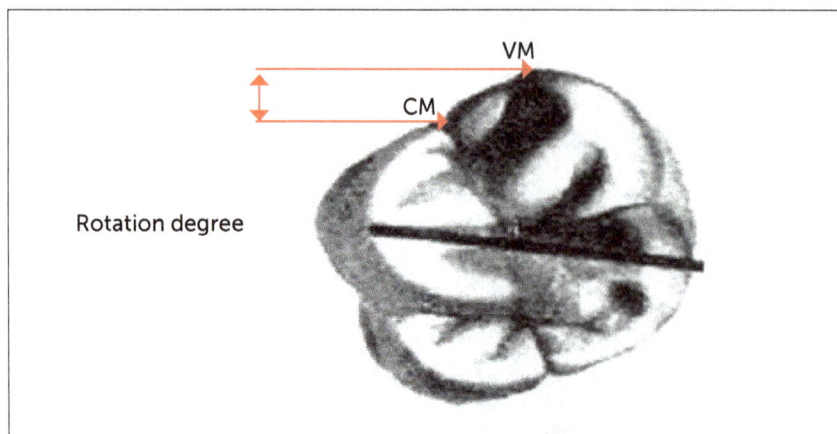

Figure 6 - method used to assess the rotation of the first maxillary molars.

variation was 0.45 mm, with mean values of 2.19 mm and 1.74 mm for the left and right sides, respectively. Table 2 shows the mean values and respective standard deviation of molar mesialization with regard to the arch and side. The t test indicated no significant difference in the respective comparisons.

With regard to the rotation of the upper molars, mean rotations of 0.76 ± 0.37 mm and 0.93 ± 0.53 mm were observed for the right and left molars, respectively, and a mean rotation of 0.85 ± 0.45 mm was observed between both sides.

DISCUSSION

The models used herein were assessed by a device exclusively developed for the dental arch asymmetry analyses. It was carefully designed not only to allow the models to be positioned on a flat surface, but also to observe the inclination of the occlusal plane. Additionally, it was used a small-caliber rod (0.5 mm) to avoid improper interferences on the measurements.[14-17]

In order to achieve more accurate and standardized measures, the models were placed onto a parallelometer base fixed to the base of the device, considering the midpalatal suture as a symmetry reference.[1,2] The occlusal surfaces of the teeth on the models were leveled to the horizontal plane by means of a leveling board. Two-millimeter rulers were adapted, one on

the protractor base, and the other on the upper part of the device as a way to measure the positioning and degree of rotation of the molars. The part of the device where the protractor with the pointer was fixed could move in transverse and longitudinal directions, through a set of rollers, causing the measurements to be easily and agilely obtained, thus, permitting higher reliability and standardization — once the models remained static after been positioned, and only the protractor with the pointers could move.

The analysis of the results demonstrated that the comparison between maxillary and mandibular arches showed a great number of lower molars more mesially positioned, corroborating the literature,[15,21,22] while the comparison between the sides showed a higher number of molars mesially positioned on the right side of both arches.

The mean values regarding variation in molar mesialization suggest that the sample of this study showed greater variation in molar positioning in the mandibular arch, which leads to a high incidence of asymmetry. This fact occurs because the mesialization of a molar in relation to its counterpart reveals an asymmetric positioning of these teeth, which can also indicate asymmetry in the respective dental arch. Although numerical differences were observed with regard to the sagittal positioning of these molars, our results pointed out that the mean values and standard deviation of molar mesialization have no significant difference when compared between the arches, neither when compared to the side of the molar mesially positioned. These findings are in disagreement with those of other authors[15,16,21] who assessed dental asymmetry in individuals with the same malocclusion and found significant differences between the maxillary and mandibular arches.

Asymmetric positioning of molars can be attributed to genetic, postural, chewing and harmful habits.[1,6,7,21] A correct diagnosis and adequate treatment planning are of paramount importance for obtain-

Table 1 - Distribution of the individuals comprising the sample considering the side of the molar mesially positioned and arch.

Mesialization	Arch			
	Maxillary		Mandibular	
	n	%	27	45.0
Right molar	21	35.0	27	45.0
Without mesialization	29	48.3	17	28.3
Left molar	10	16.7	16	26.7
Total	60	100.0	60	100.0

χ^2 = 5.27; p = 0.072 (non-significant difference).

Table 2 - Mean value and standard deviation of molar mesialization with regard to the arch and side, and t test values for the respective comparisons.

	Left	Right	Comparison between sides	
	Mean ± SD	Mean ± SD	t	p
Maxillary	1.55 ± 0.76	1.50 ± 0.50	0.219	0.828 (ns)
Mandibular	2.19 ± 1.12	1.74 ± 0.96	1.381	0.175 (ns)
Comparison between the arches	t = 1,576; p =0.128 (ns)	t = 1.039; p = 0.304 (ns)		

ns – non-significant difference.

ing a stable occlusion at retention and post-retention stages. In addition, achieving a symmetrical positioning of molars at an early stage of the orthodontic treatment favors the success of such a treatment.[6,7,8]

With regard to factors that possibly influence the asymmetric positioning of molars, the rotation of maxillary molars was assessed. This rotation may indicate an increased length of the maxillary dental arch, besides being responsible for the Class II relationship of molars. Accordingly, it is justified the need to assess the rotation of the first maxillary molars, once the degree of rotation may determine the level of Class II malocclusion. The correction of rotation of the first maxillary molars can even transform a Class II molar relationship into a Class I molar relationship, depending on the degree of rotation of the first maxillary molars.

This study aimed at assessing the rotation of molars in millimeters, i.e., foreseeing the space that would be gained in the dental arch so that the molars would be driven to the ideal position. The mean values of

rotation of the molars were found to be 0.76 mm and 0.93 mm for the right and left molars, respectively.

In general, the literature quantifies Class II into ¼ or ½ Class II, or full Class II. Taking into account that the average mesiodistal width of an upper molar is 10.41 mm[23] and that the average rotation of the molars was 0.84 mm, it was possible to understand that the molar rotation observed herein, when singly considered, would correspond to ¼ of Class II.

CONCLUSION

In conclusion, the results obtained by the methodology applied showed that:

» No significant difference was detected between the mean values and standard deviation of the molars mesialization when compared per side (right and left) and per arch (maxillary and mandibular);

» When singly observed, the molar rotation, quantified in millimeters, accounted for ¼ of Class II.

REFERENCES

1. Lundstrom A. Some asymmetries of dental arches, jaws, and skull, and their etiological significance. Am J Orthod. 1961;47(2):81-106.

2. Lear C. Symmetry analyses of the palate and maxillary dental arch. Angle Orthod. 1968;38(1):56-62.

3. Angle EH. Classification of malocclusion. Dent Cosmo. 1899;41(3):248-64.

4. Andrews LF. The six keys to normal occlusion. Am J Orthod. 1972; 62(3):296-309.

5. Nery PCB, Barbosa JA. Rotação de primeiros molares superiores na oclusão normal e má oclusão de Classe II divisão 1 de Angle. Rev Dental Press Ortod Ortop Facial. 2003;8(5):101-12.

6. Burstone CJ. Diagnosis and treatment planning of patients with asymmetries. Semin Orthod. 1998;4(3):153-64.

7. Shroff B, Siegel SM. Treatment of patients with asymmetries using asymmetric mechanics. Semin Orthod. 1998;4(3):165-79.

8. Paranhos LR, Andrews WA, Jóias RP, Bérzin F, Daruge Júnior E, Triviño T. Dental arch morphology in normal occlusions. Braz J Oral Sci. 2011; 10(1):65-8.

9. Moscardini MS. Estudo comparativo da eficiência do aparelho extrabucal e da barra transpalatina como meios de ancoragem durante a fase de retração. Rev Dental Press Ortod Ortop Facial. 2007;12(2):86-95.

10. Shimizu RH, Ambrosio RA, Shimizu IA, Godoy-Bezerra J, Ribeiro JS, Staszak KR. Princípios biomecânicos do aparelho extrabucal. Rev Dental Press Ortod Ortop Facial. 2004;9(6):122-56.

11. Dahlquist A. The effect of a transpalatal arch for the correction of first molar rotation. Eur J Orthod. 1996;18(3):257-67.

12. Choi YJ, Lee JS, Cha JY, Park YC. Total distalization of the maxillary arch in a patient with skeletal Class II malocclusion. Am J Orthod Dentofacial Orthop. 2011;139(6):823-33.

13. Quaglio LC, Freitas KMS, Freitas MR, Janson G, Henriques JFC. Stability and relapse of maxillary anterior crowding treatment in Class I and Class II division 1 malocclusions. Am J Orthod Dentofacial Orthop. 2011;139(6):768-74.

14. Wertz RA. Diagnosis and treatment planning of unilateral Class II malocclusions. Angle Orthod. 1975;45(2):85-94.

15. Araújo TM. Skeletal and dental arch asymmetries in individuals with normal dental occlusion. Int J Adult Orthod Orthog Surg. 1994;9(2):111-8.

16. Araújo TM. Skeletal and dental arch asymmetries in Class II division 1 malocclusion. J Clin Pediatr Dent. 1994;18(3):181-5.

17. Korkhaus G. A new orthodontic symmetrograph. Int J Orthod Oral Surg Radiol. 1930;16(6):665-8.

18. Mucha JN, Bolognese AM. Análise de modelos em Ortodontia. Rev Bras Odontol. 1985;42(1):28-44.

19. Maurice TJ, Kula K. Dental arch asymmetry in the mixed dentition. Angle Orthod. 1998;68(1):37-44.

20. Alavi DG. Facial and dental arch asymmetries in Class II subdivision malocclusion. Am J Orthod Dentofacial Orthop. 1988;93(1):38-46.

21. Janson GR. Assimetria dentária e suas complicações no tratamento ortodôntico: Apresentação de um caso clínico. Ortodontia. 1995;28(3):68-73.

22. Rose JM. Mandibular skeletal and dental asymmetry in Class II malocclusions. Am J Orthod Dentofacial Orthop. 1994;105(5):489-95.

23. Jóias RP, Velasco LG, Scanavini MA, Miranda ALR, Siqueira DF. Evaluation of the Bolton ratios on 3D dental casts of Brazilians with natural normal occlusions. World J Orthod. 2010;11(1):67-70.

9

Mandibular growth and dentoalveolar development in the treatment of Class II, division 1, malocclusion using Balters Bionator according to the skeletal maturation

Paulo Roberto dos Santos-Pinto[1], Lídia Parsekian Martins[2], Ary dos Santos-Pinto[3], Luiz Gonzaga Gandini Júnior[3]
Dirceu Barnabé Raveli[3], Cristiane Celli Matheus dos Santos-Pinto[4]

Objective: The purpose of the study was to evaluate the influence of the skeletal maturation in the mandibular and dentoalveolar growth and development during the Class II, division 1, malocclusion correction with Balters bionator. **Methods:** Three groups of children with Class II, division 1, malocclusion were evaluated. Two of them were treated for one year with the bionator of Balters appliance in different skeletal ages (Group 1: 6 children, 7 to 8 years old and Group 2: 10 children, 9 to 10 years old) and the other one was followed without treatment (Control Group: 7 children, 8 to 9 years old). Lateral 45 degree cephalometric radiographs were used for the evaluation of the mandibular growth and dentoalveolar development. Tantalum metallic implants were used as fixed and stable references for radiograph superimposition and data acquisition. Student's t test was used in the statistical analysis of the displacement of the points in the condyle, ramus, mandibular base and dental points. Analysis of variance one-fixed criteria was used to evaluate group differences (95% of level of significance). **Results:** The intragroup evaluation showed that all groups present significant skeletal growth for all points analyzed (1.2 to 3.7 mm), but in an intergroup comparison, the increment of the mandibular growth in the condyle, ramus and mandibular base were not statically different. For the dentoalveolar modifications, the less mature children showed greater labial inclination of the lower incisors (1.86 mm) and the most mature children showed greater first permanent molar extrusion (4.8 mm).

Keywords: Angle Class II malocclusion. Orthopedics. Growth and development.

[1] Professor, Barretos University - UNIFEB
[2] PhD in Orthodontics. Assistant Professor, Children's Clinic Department, School of Dentistry of Araraquara - UNESP.
[3] Full Professor, Children's Clinic Department, School of Dentistry of Araraquara - UNESP.
[4] MSc in Orthodontics, FOB-USP. Professor, Ribeirão Preto University - UNAERP.

» The authors report no commercial, proprietary or financial interest in the products or companies described in this article.

Prof. Paulo Roberto dos Santos-Pinto
Orthodontic Center – Rua Américo Brasiliense, 1702 – Sala 5,
CEP: 14015-050 – Ribeirão Preto/SP – Brazil
E-mail: dr-pauloroberto@hotmail.com

INTRODUCTION

The treatment of Class II malocclusion with functional appliances, studied for decades in experimental studies in animals and humans, prove that this therapy is able to rearrange the growth and normal development of the face,[26,28] with skeletal and dentoalveolar effects, important for the correction of malocclusion.[12,21,23] Regarding mandible, studies with different methodologies have proven that functional therapy in patients with Class II malocclusion, can alter condylar growth and promote mandibular bone remodeling.[26,28] However, the condylar growth is up to nowadays, a controversial and poorly defined fact.[22]

The importance of this study of Class II treatment with Balters bionator appliance lies in the use of 45° lateral teleradiographs, to allow an evaluation without overlapping anatomical structures,[16] by referential of metallic implants[24] and the distribution of these patients by bone age, which makes the results more reliable.

There are studies already that used similar methodologies[23] however, the clinician still has difficulty in defining the ideal stage to start intervention, because literature is often contradictory, with authors arguing that in young patients the mandibular length increase may occur with the use of these appliances,[5,24] challenged by authors who claim that this form of treatment does not grow the mandible, because puberty is where the child has more growth earnings.[22]

The objective of this study is to evaluate the influence of bone maturation, in mandibular and dentoalveolar growth and development, natural and induced by treatment of Class II malocclusion, division 1, with Balters bionator.

MATERIAL AND METHODS

This study used radiographs of a sample composed by 23 Caucasian patients being 09 males and 14 females, with bone ages between 7-10 years, Angle's Class II malocclusion, division 1, and mandibular deficiency. Oblique lateral radiographs, 45° (oblique teleradiography), of right and left hemimandibles, and hand and wrist radiographs were taken by the same technician on the same day, using X-ray machine (Funk Orbital X15), Lanex screens and TMG film with the factors: 82 kVp, 80 mA and 0.5 seconds exposure. These radiographs were collected prospectively in two stages with an interval of 1 year and archived in the Post-Graduation Course in Orthodontics, School of Dentistry - UNESP, in the city of Araraquara (SP).

Patients in the study were divided into 3 groups according to bone age obtained by the method of Eklöf and Ringertz using the program Radiocef Studio, Radiocef Studio version, based on measurements of 10 dimensions of the bones of the hand and wrist in radiographs images scanned. Control group (C),

Table 1 - Descriptive statistics of samples per treatment group.

| | | Values | | | Mean ± S.D. |
		n	Minimum	Maximum	
Control group	Chronological age - start	7	6.9	10.2	8.7 ± 1.05
	Chronological age - end	7	7.9	11.2	9.7 ± 1.07
	Treatment time	7	0.9	1	1 ± 0.06
	Skeletal maturity - start	7	8.5	9.4	9 ± 0.34
	Skeletal maturity - end	7	9.3	10.3	9.8 ± 0.41
Group 1	Chronological age - start	6	7.1	9.8	8.4 ± 1.11
	Chronological age - end	6	7.9	10.7	9.4 ± 1.16
	Treatment time	6	0.8	1.1	1 ± 0.09
	Skeletal maturity - start	6	7	8.5	8 ± 0.54
	Skeletal maturity - end	6	8.6	9.7	9.1 ± 0.36
Group 2	Chronological age - start	10	8.7	11.2	9.8 ± 0.78
	Chronological age - end	10	9.8	12.2	10.8 ± 0.78
	Treatment time	10	1	1.2	1.1 ± 0.07
	Skeletal maturity - start	10	9.3	10.7	10 ± 0.42
	Skeletal maturity - end*	9	9.9	11.5	10.6 ± 0.57

* It was not reported the skeletal maturity of a Group 2 patient.

with patients without treatment with 8.5 to 9.4 years of bone age and, treated Groups 1 and 2, with patients with initial bone age 7 to 8.5 years and 9.3 to 10.7 years, respectively (Table 1).

The appliance used in patients of treated groups was the bionator described by Balters,[4] with acrylic deep extension of the lower arch seeking greater mucosal support in the lingual region and always made by the same professional.[23]

All patients received three tantalum metal implants, measuring 0.5 mm in diameter and 1.5 mm length, positioned on the mandible cortical surface as the method developed by Björk.[8] The first positioned at the center of the symphysis, between the roots of the incisors and the other two positioned in the posterior region, between the roots of the lower first permanent molars, right and left.

Aiming to evaluate mandibular growth and tooth development, natural and induced by orthopedic treatment with Balters bionator, it was established 16 cephalometric points marked in visualized right and left oblique radiographs of the mandible: Condylar points (co, coa, cop, cla, and clp) points in the ramus region (ramp, rams, rma and rmi) and lower border (gop, go, goa, me, bora, borm and borp) (Table 1).

The points marked on the permanent teeth were icp, iip, cp, m1p, m2p, p1m and p2m and on deciduous teeth: cd, m1d and m2d, totaling 10 dental points, and 2 reference points of implant (Fig 1, Table 2).

For analysis of the displacements of cephalometric landmarks it was used a Cartesian coordinate system.

The X axis is represented by the horizontal line formed by the orbital plane determined in the initial radiographic (T_1) and transferred to subsequent radiographs through the superimposition of the images of metallic implants located at the anterior and posterior mandible (Ip and Ia). The Y axis is represented by the vertical line perpendicular to the orbital plane passing through a fiducial point located at the rear end of the orbit plane in a rearmost position to skeletal and dental structures of cephalometric tracing. The anteroposterior position of each cephalometric point was obtained by linear distance from point referred to the Y axis, parallel to the axis X. Similarly, the vertical position of each cephalometric point was obtained by linear distance from the point to the X axis parallel to the Y axis (Fig 1).

The horizontal displacement for each point was calculated as the difference between the linear horizontal distance of the points at two different instants (I_2-I_1) where I_1 represents the beginning of orthopedic treatment (treated group) or beginning of the observation period (control) and I_2, the displacement after 1 year of orthopedic therapy (treated group) or end of the observation period (Control group). The total displacement of each point was obtained using the rule of the right triangle (total displacement equal to the square root of the sum of squared horizontal displacement and vertical displacement squared).

This study was approved on May 4, 2009 by the research ethics committee of the Faculty of Dentistry of Araraquara under protocol 39/06, which is in accordance with resolution 196/96 of the National Health Council/MS.

STATISTICAL ANALYSES

The predetermined points in the radiographs were digitized twice by the same calibrated operator every 15 days, using the IBM compatible personal computer with the program Dentofacial Planner Plus version 2.02, on Numonics Accugrid digitizing tablet. Data were taken to the Excel Program in IBM micro-

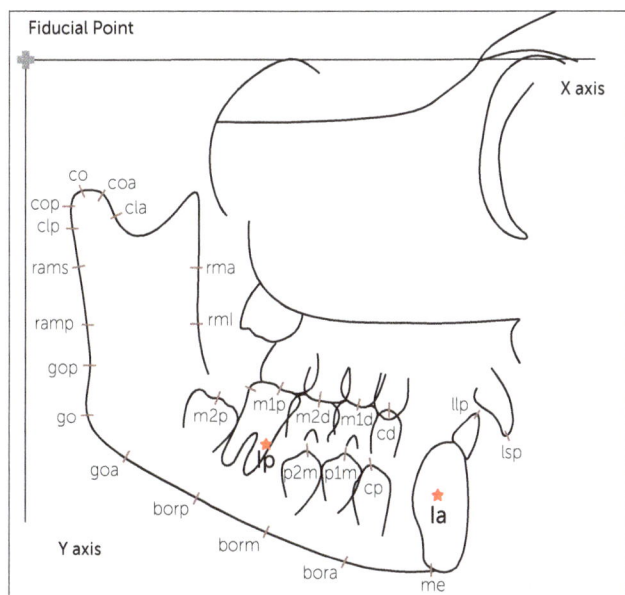

Figure 1 - X axis represented by the horizontal line formed by the orbital plane determined on the initial radiograph (T_1), transferred to the subsequent radiographs through the superposition of metallic implants. Y axis determined by a vertical line passing through the fiducial point located at the posterior end of the orbital plane with points on the mandibular body: Condylar (co, coa, cop, cla, and clp); mandibular ramus points (ramp, rams, rma and rmi); lower border (gop, go, goa, me, bora, borm, and borp); and dental points (isp, iip, cp, m1p, m2p, p1m, p2m, m1d, m2d and cd).

Table 2 - Skeletal and dental cephalometric measurements:

Point	Name	Definition
Condylion	co	Most superior point of the mandibular condyle
Anterior condylion	coa	Most anterior point of the mandibular condyle
Posterior condylion	cop	Most posterior point of the mandibular condyle
Anterior condylar neck	cla	Most anterior point of the mandibular condyle neck
Posterior condylar neck	clp	Most posterior point of the condylar neck
Posterior superior ramus	rams	Most posterior and superior point of the ramus of the mandible
Posterior median ramus	ramp	Most posterior and median point of the ramus of the mandible
Anterior superior ramus	rma	Located at the anterior and superior surface of the ramus of the mandible
Anterior median ramus	rmi	Located at the anterior and median surface of the ramus of the mandible
Superior gonion	gop	Most upper (superior) and posterior point of the gonial angle
Gonion	go	Most lower (inferior) and posterior point of the gonial angle
Antegonial notch	goa	Located at the antegonial notch region
Menton	me	Located at the base of the mandible. In the intersection with mandibular symphysis
The landmarks of the posterior, median and anterior base of the mandible	borp, borm and bora	Landmarks determined, respectively, from goa, by dividing the segment goa me in three equidistant points
Posterior implant	lp	Mandibular landmark which the implant is Located at the posterior surface of the mandibular body
Anterior implant	la	Mandibular landmark which the implant is Located at the anterior of the mandibular body
Upper permanent incisor	isp	Located at the incisal edge of the upper incisor
Lower permanent incisor	iip	Located at the incisal edge of the lower incisor
Lower permanent canine	cp	Located at the incisal edge of the lower canine
Lower deciduous canine	cd	Located at the incisal edge of the lower deciduous canine
Mandibular first premolar	p1m	Located at the incisal edge of the mandibular first premolar
Mandibular second premolar	p2m	Located at the incisal edge of the mandibular second premolar
Deciduous mandibular first molar	m1d	Located at the incisal edge of the deciduous mandibular first molar
Deciduous mandibular second molar	m2d	Located at the incisal edge of the deciduous mandibular second molar
Permanent mandibular first molar	m1p	Located at the middle portion of the occlusal surface of the permanent mandibular first molar
Permanent mandibular second molar	m2p	Located at the middle portion of the occlusal surface of the permanent mandibular second molar

computer and statistically analyzed using SPSS. This procedure was performed to evaluate the error of the method in the scanning process. It was applied Intraclass Correlation Coefficient (ICC) which showed variations from 0.893 to 0.996, with the smallest corresponding to the point m1d(v) and the highest to points oj, cop(v) coa(v) and rmd, demonstrating that the error method was not significant.

For comparison between groups, the data were annualized in order to balance the small difference in time for observation or treatment from 0.8 to 1.2 years (Table 1).

From each patient, at each study point, it was obtained two oblique teleradiographs one on the right side and another on the left side. The study of correlation of the displacements of the predetermined points on both sides employing the Pearson correlation coefficient showed that for 77 % of them

the correlation is zero or very weak and 16 % of the correlation is moderate showing that a promoted correction by the device or natural growth is not necessarily symmetric. Based on these results it was chosen to work with the measurements of both sides as independent measures.

For statistical analysis of the displacement of each point, it was employed Student's t test for the mean of a population. To assess whether the means of each measure in the three groups were equal, it was used analysis of variance with a criterion of classification (ANOVA) when the homogeneity test of variances was not significant, otherwise the statistical analysis was performed by the Brown-Forsythe test. It was conducted tests of multiple comparison of means for variables that showed statistically significant results in testing the hypothesis of equality of means. The significance level for all statistical tests was 95 % ($p < 0.05$).

Table 3 - Mean and standard deviation of mandibular growth, tooth eruption (total, horizontal and vertical) and significance of the Student's t test of the hypothesis that the mean is equal to zero - Control Group.

	Point	n	Total Mean ± SD	Horizontal Mean ± SD	Vertical Mean ± SD
Mandibular growth	me	14	1.20** ± 0.97	-0.35ns ± 1.12	0.74** ± 0.72
	bora	14	1.37** ± 1.12	-0.69ns ± 1.52	0.20ns ± 0.63
	borm	14	1.73** ± 1.42	-0.55ns ± 1.97	0.11ns ± 1.01
	borp	14	2.14** ± 1.40	-0.87ns ± 2.13	0.02ns ± 1.24
	goa	14	2.07** ± 1.01	-0.71ns ± 1.79	-0.20ns ± 1.37
	go	14	1.90** ± 1.29	-1.03** ± 1.00	-0.86ns ± 1.61
	gop	14	2.07** ± 1.25	-0.89** ± 0.80	-1.21* ± 1.77
	ramp	14	2.28** ± 1.11	-0.69* ± 0.90	-1.40* ± 1.84
	rams	14	2.10** ± 0.95	-0.78** ± 0.85	-1.42** ± 1.44
	clp	14	2.27** ± 1.41	-0.52* ± 0.83	-1.76** ± 1.79
	cop	14	2.18** ± 1.57	-0.68* ± 0.97	-1.51* ± 1.92
	co	14	2.29** ± 1.65	-0.69* ± 0.93	-1.68** ± 1.99
	coa	14	2.35** ± 1.71	-0.40ns ± 1.02	-1.83** ± 2.01
	cla	14	2.40** ± 1.52	-0.45* ± 0.76	-2.02** ± 1.82
	rma	14	1.83** ± 1.10	-0.55* ± 0.82	-1.11* ± 1.58
	rmi	14	2.94** ± 2.23	-0.30ns ± 3.20	-0.80ns ± 1.82
Tooth movement	m2p	14	2.18** ± 1.18	1.48** ± 1.31	-1.16** ± 1.00
	m1p	14	2.19** ± 1.14	0.49ns ± 1.07	-1.85** ± 1.16
	m2d	12	1.54** ± 0.58	0.48ns ± 1.03	-0.59ns ± 1.11
	p2m	14	2.79** ± 2.01	1.31** ± 1.24	-2.36** ± 1.75
	m1d	9	1.13** ± 0.88	0.08ns ± 1.23	-0.46ns ± 0.68
	p1m	14	2.67** ± 2.15	1.38* ± 2.28	-1.84** ± 1.16
	cp	13	4.96** ± 2.12	1.00* ± 1.36	-4.72** ± 2.01
	iip	14	1.52** ± 0.80	0.72** ± 0.84	0.58ns ± 1.22

* - the hypothesis that the mean is zero is rejected at a significance level of 0.05.
** - the hypothesis that the mean is zero is rejected at a significance level of 0.01.
ns - the hypothesis that the mean is zero is not rejected.

Table 4 - Mean and standard deviation of mandibular growth, tooth eruption (total, horizontal and vertical) and significance of the Student's t test of the hypothesis that the mean is equal to zero – Group 1.

	Point	n	Total Mean ± SD	Horizontal Mean ± SD	Vertical Mean ± SD
Mandibular growth	me	11	1.71** ± 0.73	0.58sn ± 1.31	0.69sn ± 1.07
	bora	11	1.39** ± 1.03	0.55sn ± 1.53	0.39sn ± 0.60
	borm	11	1.64** ± 1.79	0.36sn ± 2.06	0.19sn ± 1.32
	borp	11	1.67** ± 1.33	-0.55sn ± 1.65	-0.48sn ± 1.24
	goa	11	3.30** ± 2.68	-1.69sn ± 3.35	-0.78sn ± 2.03
	go	11	2.31** ± 1.45	-1.30** ± 0.74	-1.32** ± 1.92
	gop	11	2.63** ± 1.40	-1.31** ± 0.66	-1.79** ± 1.93
	ramp	11	2.65** ± 1.86	-0.95** ± 1.03	-2.01** ± 2.16
	rams	11	2.93** ± 1.77	-0.88** ± 1.07	-2.27** ± 2.22
	clp	11	2.64** ± 2.09	-0.73** ± 0.81	-2.22** ± 2.32
	cop	11	2.76** ± 1.67	-0.56sn ± 1.01	-2.39** ± 1.88
	co	11	2.75** ± 1.90	-0.58sn ± 1.13	-2.27** ± 2.16
	coa	11	2.94** ± 1.86	-0.45sn ± 1.18	-2.60** ± 1.98
	cla	11	2.65** ± 2.11	-0.27sn ± 0.60	-2.34** ± 2.39
	rma	11	2.25** ± 1.60	-0.38sn ± 1.48	-1.49** ± 1.84
	rmi	11	2.32** ± 1.26	-0.75sn ± 1.37	-1.59** ± 1.50
Tooth movement	m2p	11	2.55** ± 1.34	2.14** ± 1.32	-0.92** ± 1.12
	m1p	11	3.11** ± 1.93	0.84** ± 0.74	-2.66** ± 2.28
	m2d	8	1.30** ± 0.74	0.61** ± 0.67	-0.56ns ± 1.13
	p2m	11	2.73** ± 1.92	1.45** ± 1.23	-1.95** ± 1.97
	m1d	7	1.57** ± 1.11	0.79sn ± 1.56	-0.45ns ± 0.83
	p1m	11	3.21** ± 2.22	1.23** ± 1.25	-2.66** ± 2.28
	cp	11	4.14** ± 2.00	0.21sn ± 1.19	-3.90** ± 2.15
	iip	11	2.70** ± 1.31	1.86** ± 1.09	1.71** ± 1.26

* - the hypothesis that the mean is zero is rejected at a significance level of 0.05.
** - the hypothesis that the mean is zero is rejected at a significance level of 0.01.
ns - the hypothesis that the mean is zero is not rejected.

RESULTS

According to the analyzed sample and the measurements it is possible to say that, accompanied by one year without treatment, natural growth occurred promoting back horizontal changes at goa and go points and back and down at points gop, ramp, rams, clp, cop, co, coa, cla and rma and, only down at point me, with statistical significance (Table 3).

The results of the displacement of dental points of this Control group were significant for the overall tooth displacement. Horizontally it occurred labial migration of incisors, the m2p points, p2m, p1m and cp points moved to mesial and occlusal and m1p shifted toward occlusal significantly. The remaining evaluated teeth showed no significant changes in this group.

The data from Group 1 (Table 4), of patients with lower bone age or less mature, showed significant total displacement of all studied points, both for measures of skeletal origin as tooth measures.

The total tooth movements were all significant, with mesial movement of all teeth, except the first deciduous molars and canines, and significant extrusion of permanent teeth (m1p, m2p, p1m, p2m, cp).

Significant changes occurred in both horizontal and vertical at goa, go, gop, ramp, rams, clp, cop, co, coa, cla, rmi points, only horizontally at borp point, and vertically at me and rma points.

The dental changes in both horizontal and vertical occurred with significant mesial movement and extrusion of points m2p, p2m, and cp, only extrusion at m1p, p1m points.

Table 5 - Means and standard deviation of the mandibular growth and total dental eruption, horizontal and vertical, and t test significance of the hypothesis that the mean is equal to zero – Group 3.

	Point	n	Total Mean ± SD	Horizontal Mean ± SD	Vertical Mean ± SD
Mandibular growth	me	20	1.45** ± 0.75	-0.17[ns] ± 1.19	0.50* ± 1.04
	bora	20	1.95** ± 1.16	-0.73[ns] ± 1.95	0.29[ns] ± 0.94
	borm	20	1.77** ± 1.47	-0.89[ns] ± 1.93	0.01[ns] ± 0.94
	borp	20	2.18** ± 2.07	-1.31* ± 2.35	-0.48[ns] ± 1.30
	goa	20	2.68** ± 1.87	-1.61** ± 2.23	-1.13** ± 1.41
	go	20	2.42** ± 1.48	-1.26** ± 1.68	-1.27** ± 1.47
	gop	20	2.58** ± 1.69	-1.24** ± 1.52	-1.48** ± 1.91
	ramp	20	2.77** ± 1.64	-0.94** ± 1.18	-1.53* ± 2.45
	rams	20	3.05** ± 2.26	-0.83** ± 1.07	-2.22** ± 2.80
	clp	20	3.62** ± 3.12	-1.11** ± 1.51	-2.75** ± 3.47
	cop	20	3.53** ± 3.09	-1.04** ± 1.70	-2.70** ± 3.31
	co	20	3.57** ± 3.13	-1.23** ± 1.89	-2.68** ± 3.24
	coa	20	3.70** ± 3.27	-1.28** ± 1.70	-2.77** ± 3.52
	cla	20	3.54** ± 3.02	-1.08** ± 1.54	-2.62** ± 3.39
	rma	20	3.01** ± 1.79	-0.74[ns] ± 1.61	-1.67** ± 2.58
	rmi	20	3.05** ± 1.64	-1.01* ± 2.15	-1.55** ± 2.07
Tooth movement	m2p	20	3.14** ± 1.17	1.72** ± 0.95	-2.37** ± 1.35
	m1p	20	4.83** ± 2.52	0.40[ns] ± 0.94	-4.64** ± 2.68
	m2d	18	1.33** ± 0.73	0.14[ns] ± 1.18	-0.37[ns] ± 0.93
	p2m	20	2.21** ± 1.81	0.94** ± 1.42	-1.50** ± 1.76
	m1d	5	1.21* ± 0.87	0.95[ns] ± 1.10	-0.15[ns] ± 0.48
	p1m	20	5.35** ± 2.40	0.68[ns] ± 2.34	-4.64** ± 2.68
	cp	19	4.29** ± 2.22	1.08** ± 1.09	-3.97** ± 2.31
	iip	20	1.90** ± 1.12	0.40[ns] ± 1.55	0.59[ns] ± 1.46

* - the hypothesis that the mean is zero is rejected at a significance level of 0.05.
** - the hypothesis that the mean is zero is rejected at a significance level of 0.01.
ns - the hypothesis that the mean is zero is not rejected.

To evaluate whether the average of each measure in the three groups were equal it was used analysis of variance with one classification criterion (ANOVA) when the test for homogeneity of variance was not significant, otherwise the comparison of means was performed by Brown-Forsythe test. The results are shown in Tables 6 and 7, and in Table 8 the results of the multiple comparisons of means of variables that showed statistically significant results in test for difference of means.

The data in Table 6 show that, except for the measure iip, there are no statistical differences between the means of the horizontal measures of mandibular growth and tooth migration. The results of the multiple comparisons of means (Table 8) show that the

iip mean from Group 1 differs from means of Control group and Group 2. For measures of vertical growth, the results indicate that there is significant difference between the group's means only for some measures of tooth movement, m2p, m1p and p1m. Regarding to p1m it was also observed no significant difference between the variances of the three groups. The results of multiple comparisons of means show that, for the three measures cited above, the vertical growth in Group 2 was higher and significantly different from the other two groups.

DISCUSSION

This work was carried out at 45° oblique teleradiographs of patients who had metal implants inserted in the mandible, used as stable references, what allowed a more reliable evaluation of the results. This feature eliminates variables like the magnification of radiographic images[3] and incorrect positioning of the patients head in cephalostat. The images of implants as suggested by Bjork[8] were marked on the initial teleradiograph and transferred to the subsequent, providing an assessment of the real displacement of the points in evaluated time (for all groups), which otherwise would not be possible.[23]

Identifying whether the orthopedic device only changes the direction of condylar growth or the rate and amount of this growth has been the purpose of many authors. Bjork and Skieller[9] cite the importance, in longitudinal studies, the condylar growth in mandible length increase, being the growth direction of the condyle extremely variable and difficult to predict. The real role of the condyle in the mandibular growth is controversial in craniofacial growth studies. The cartilage of the condyle has a capacity of compensatory growth, generating enough growth to allow adaptation of the mandible to the skull base by articular fossa (mandibular fossa) and to maxillary complex.

In the Control group of our study, the growth of the condyle was significant in all its references, anterior and posterior condylar neck (cla and clp), posterior and superior portion (cop and co), up and back. The anterior condylar region (coa) was an exception and showed no backward growth.

With the use of the appliance in younger children (Group 1) the condyle showed no significant

Table 6 - Results of tests for homogeneity of variance (Levene's test) and to test the hypothesis that the mean of the 3 groups are equal (ANOVA or Brown Forsythe test) - points with vertical and horizontal movements.

Point	Horizontal movement						Vertical movement					
	Levene's test			ANOVA			Levene's test			ANOVA		
	F	gl1 / gl2	Sig.	F	gl1 / gl2	Sig.	F	gl1 / gl2	Sig.	F	gl1 / gl2	Sig.
me	0.24	2 /42	0.789	2.04	2 /42	0.142	0.47	2 /42	0.629	0.30	2 / 42	0.742
bora	1.29	2 /42	0.287	2.22	2 /42	0.121	1.10	2 /42	0.341	0.19	2 / 42	0.824
borm	0.02	2 /42	0.981	1.43	2 /42	0.252	0.02	2 /42	0.981	0.11	2 / 42	0.899
borp	0.73	2 /42	0.488	0.48	2 /42	0.619	0.10	2 /42	0.902	0.76	2 / 42	0.476
goa	1.90	2 /42	0.162	0.71	2 /42	0.496	0.62	2 /42	0.543	1.45	2 / 42	0.246
go	2.02	2 /42	0.146	0.17	2 /42	0.845	0.22	2 /42	0.807	0.33	2 / 42	0.719
gop	2.55	2 /42	0.090	0.51	2 /42	0.607	0.01	2 /42	0.989	0.29	2 / 42	0.746
ramp	0.40	2 /42	0.674	0.27	2 /42	0.765	0.75	2 /42	0.481	0.25	2 / 42	0.778
rams	0.03	2 /42	0.970	0.03	2 /42	0.971	1.77	2 /42	0.183	0.60	2 / 42	0.555
clp	1.72	2 /42	0.192	1.06	2 /42	0.357	3.02	2 /42	0.060	0.52	2 / 42	0.596
cop	1.55	2 /42	0.225	0.53	2 /42	0.592	2.22	2 /42	0.121	0.85	2 / 42	0.436
co	2.27	2 /42	0.116	0.91	2 /42	0.410	1.48	2 /42	0.239	0.58	2 / 42	0.566
coa	1.05	2 /42	0.359	2.09	2 /42	0.137	2.03	2 /42	0.144	0.50	2 / 42	0.612
cla	2.98	2 /42	0.062	2.20	2 /42	0.123	2.17	2 /42	0.127	0.20	2 / 42	0.823
rma	2.75	2 /42	0.076	0.25	2 /42	0.782	2.53	2 /42	0.091	0.28	2 / 42	0.754
rmi	1.15	2 /42	0.325	0.36	2 /42	0.700	0.93	2 /42	0.402	0.81	2 / 42	0.453
m2p	1.18	2 /42	0.317	1.01	2 /42	0.375	0.61	2 /42	0.550	6.82	2 / 42	**0.003**
m1p	1.08	2 /42	0.350	0.81	2 /42	0.452	5.63	2 /42	**0.007**	7.87[1]	2 / 32	**0.002**
m2d	0.61	2 /35	0.550	0.69	2 /35	0.508	0.58	2 /35	0.563	0.20	2 / 35	0.822
p2m	0.22	2 /42	0.803	0.60	2 /42	0.551	0.01	2 /42	0.988	0.96	2 / 42	0.392
m1d	1.45	2 /18	0.261	0.91	2 /18	0.421	0.46	2 /18	0.639	0.37	2 / 18	0.699
p1m	0.24	2 /42	0.787	0.52	2 /42	0.598	5.57	2 /42	**0.007**	7.93[1]	2 / 32	**0.002**
cp	0.06	2 /40	0.938	2.00	2 /40	0.149	0.48	2 /40	0.620	0.58	2 / 40	0.563
iip	1.50	2 /40	0.255	4.19	2 /40	**0.022**	0.20	2 /40	0.819	2.47	2 / 40	0.097

[1] The analysis of variance (ANOVA) was replaced by Brown and Forsythe statistical due to the heterogeneity of variances.

back growth and vertical growth similar to the Control group. In Group 2, with mature children, the condyle showed significant backwards and upwards growth, showing a modification of condylar growth more to posterior and superior as found by Araújo.[3] This pattern of condylar growth did not differ from that presented by the children in the Control group, but there was greater vertical growth in both treated groups (1 and 2) and horizontal in Group 2 being discordant from results of Bjork[8] who suggests that backward growth from treatment might have been statistically significant compared to the Control group and Huttgren et al,[15] who reported that activators caused a redirection of the condyle in posterior position. These results are consistent with Monini,[25] who found stability in the direction of condylar growth.

Our study showed that there were significant individual changes, but the comparison between groups, vidual changes, but the comparison between groups, changes in relation to the condyle were not significant, allowing us to reaffirm the hypothesis of several authors[3,20] who accepted the redirection of mandibular growth, however, nothing beyond the natural growth potential.

Regarding the mandibular ramus, it was found in the Control group a slip of the ramus to posterior represented by resorption of the anterior ramus (backward and upward) and apposition on the backward posterior. These data were observed both in the upper (rams and rma) and middle ramus (ramp and rmi).

The treated Groups 1 and 2 exhibited a displacement onto the upper anterior ramus and upward and backward in the lower ramus, similar to the Control group. These results are consistent with the process of ramus displacement relative to the mandibular body which occurs naturally during facial skeleton growth and development described by Gu and McNamara.[14]

Table 7 - Results of tests for homogeneity of variance (Levene's test) and to test the hypothesis that the mean of the 3 groups are equal (ANOVA or Brown Forsythe test) – landmarks with total movements.

Point	Total movement					
	Levene's test			ANOVA		
	F	gl1 / gl2	Sig.	F	gl1 / gl2	Sig.
me	0.05	2 /42	0.951	1.21	2 /42	0.309
bora	0.01	2 /42	0.991	1.45	2 /42	0.247
borm	0.08	2 /42	0.921	0.02	2 /42	0.977
borp	1.22	2 /42	0.307	0.34	2 /42	0.714
goa	2.18	2 /42	0.126	1.29	2 /42	0.286
go	0.20	2 /42	0.823	0.59	2 /42	0.562
gop	0.66	2 /42	0.524	0.59	2 /42	0.558
ramp	0.54	2 /42	0.586	0.42	2 /42	0.660
rams	1.83	2 /42	0.173	1.21	2 /42	0.307
clp	3.72	2 /42	**0.033**	1.64(1)	2 /36.6	0.207
cop	3.69	2 /42	**0.033**	1.68(1)	2 /38.7	0.199
co	3.06	2 /42	0.058	1.16	2 /42	0.323
coa	2.49	2 /42	0.095	1.16	2 /42	0.323
cla	1.55	2 /42	0.224	1.04	2 /42	0.364
rma	1.83	2 /42	0.173	2.51	2 /42	0.094
rmi	0.41	2 /42	0.663	0.64	2 /42	0.532
m2p	0.24	2 /42	0.789	2.66	2 /42	0.082
m1p	4.88	2 /42	**0.012**	8.44(1)	2 /34.7	**0.001**
m2d	0.09	2 /35	0.915	0.41	2 /35	0.669
p2m	0.23	2 /42	0.794	0.47	2 /42	0.627
m1d	0.50	2 /18	0.614	0.43	2 /18	0.655
p1m	0.45	2 /42	0.639	6.52	2 /42	**0.003**
cp	0.30	2 /40	0.745	0.54	2 /40	0.588
iip	1.02	2 /40	0.370	3.35	2 /40	**0.045**

(1) The analysis of variance (ANOVA) was replaced by Brown and Forsythe statistical due to the heterogeneity of variances.

Table 8 - Means and standard deviations of tooth eruption and results of multiple comparison tests of mean measures that showed a significant result in the ANOVA.

Point	Control Group	Group 1	Group 2
	Mean ± SD	Mean ± SD	Mean ± SD
	Total displacement		
m1p	2.19a ± 1.14	3.11a ± 1.93	4.83b ± 2.52
p1m	2.67a ± 2.15	3.21a ± 2.22	5.35b ± 2.40
iip	1.52a ± 0.80	2.70b ± 1.31	1.90ab ± 1.12
	Horizontal displacement		
iip	0.72a ± 0.84	1.86b ± 1.09	0.40a ± 1.55
	Vertical displacement		
m2p	-1.16a ± 1.00	-0.92a ± 1.12	-2.37b ± 1.35
m1p	-1.85a ± 1.16	-2.66a ± 2.28	-4.64b ± 2.68
p1m	-1.84a ± 1.16	-2.66a ± 2.28	-4.64b ± 2.68

Note: Different letters correspond to statistically different averages by Student–Newman–Keuls (SNK) test

The comparative results between the 3 groups analyzed show that the mandibular body showed growth in the vertical direction, without statistical significance, suggesting that Balters bionator did not influenced this growth. These results corroborate with Kessner and Faltin[18] because there is a joint remodeling that promotes mandibular adaptation more to anterior without changing mandibular length significantly. Schulhof and Engel,[29] disagree with these findings and emphasize that treatment with the bionator appliance promotes an increase in ascending ramus and mandibular body in relation to normal growth.

In the present study there was no significant increase in mandibular ramus because the condyle grew up to 1.68 mm (c), 2.27 mm (g1) and 2.68 mm (g2) and gonion grew in the same direction, from 0.86 mm (c), 1.32 mm (g1) and 1.27 mm (g2), resulting in a small increase in the co-go distance, respectively of 0.82 mm for the Control group, 0.95 mm for Group 1 and 1.41 mm for Group 2. The results found by Reis et al,[27] were similar to ours, where Balters bionator stimulated the growth of the mandibular body and ramus similarly in both age groups without modifying the tendency of individual growth. Moreover, Malta et al[19] showed that the difference in amount of mandibular growth occurs and is significant (3.3 mm) when comparing cases of Class II patients treated with Balters bionator appliance and untreated, demonstrating that this appliance is efficient.

The data show that the gonion region exhibited significant changes in all studied groups. The points goa, go and gop showed significant upward and backward displacement except for goa in Group 1. The displacement of these points in Group 2 was higher than in other groups, but without statistical significance. These results point to a pattern of remodeling gonion region, especially in mature children, compatible with the natural growth demonstrated by several authors,[8,9,10,14] who observed resorption in the mandible posterior border. So, part of the vertical growth seen in the condylar region is partially offset by reabsorption which occurs in the gonion region, resulting in small changes in mandibular ramus height. Bigliazzi, Kessner and Faltin Jr.,[7] found that in Class II, division 1, patients with mandibular retrognathia, the gonion angle remained unchanged during the treatment period with bionator.

Clinical observations have shown that the use of orthopedic devices can alter the growth of the mandible, however the exact nature of this change remains a topic of great controversy.[13] Our results showed that in the Control group there was a significantly downward movement of menton and that the mandibular border exhibited backward movement without statistical significance. These data are consistent with other studies,[14,30] which found bone apposition in the anterior portion of the mandibular border.

In Group 1 occurred forward and downward displacement of the mentum and anterior border, while the posterior border had a backward and upward movement, all insignificant. In Group 2, the mentum presented downward movement and the posterior border a significant backward movement and nothing significant of the anterior and middle border. These data indicate a relative stability of the mandibular lower border, mainly in young children.

The results observed for mature children were similar to the Control group, results that are in accordance with other studies.[20,21] On the other hand, Almeida,[1] who treated children aged 10.8 months observed an increase in mandibular protrusion and the effective length of the mandibular body, which according to Almeida-Pedrin,[2] promoted a significant improvement in the maxillomandibular relationship compared to the Control group, which agrees with the study of Basciftci et al,[5] in the same year, that the greatest amount of growth occurs during adolescence.

Opheij et al[26] did not find statistical significant skeletal changes in Class II malocclusion patients with mandibular retrognathia, treated with bionator, noticing the most significant effects on the dentoalveolar structures. For Janson[17] children treated in the pre-pubertal period exhibited dentoalveolar changes, notably a protrusion of the lower incisors and correction of molar relationship in distal-occlusion. It was observed[17] an overjet reduction of approximately 2 mm, similar to what was observed in our study (significant overjet decrease in 1.86 mm in Group 1, compared

with 0.72 mm in the Control group and 0.4 mm in Group 2). For Bastos and Mucha,[6] one of the bionator indications is when there is a possibility of backward projection of the lower incisors. For Martins[21] skeletal changes promoted by bionator occur in 32 % through increased lower facial height and 68 % dentoalveolar movement, higher of lower molars and upper incisors.

In the vertical direction occurred greater amount of eruption of posterior teeth, significant for Group 2 that showed nearly twice eruption of molars (2.37 mm of the first molars, 4.64 mm of second molars and 2.66 mm of the first premolars) when compared to the Control group and Group 1. These facts demonstrate that the bionator appliance with occlusal support allows the active eruption of permanent molars. With respect to premolars, these erupt in more mature individuals (Group 2), mainly due to more advanced stage of root formation that they are. For the authors[1,11] there was a significant increase in posterior facial height especially in the treated group with bionator by extrusion of posterior teeth, confirmed by our study when considering the results of the more mature group (Group 2) and the youngest (Group 1), which demonstrated the predominance of dentoalveolar adaptation in the horizontal direction.

CONCLUSION

Due to the methodology adopted in this study and the results, based on statistical analysis, we conclude that:

1 – When it was evaluated the skeletal and dental changes in groups individually, there was growth at all points analyzed.

2 – When the groups were compared with each other, skeletal mandibular changes were similar indicating that the mandibular growth pattern has not changed significantly with the established treatment and.

3 – When it was evaluated dental changes after using bionator, a greater extrusion of the first permanent molars and premolars in more mature group (Group 2) and the labial inclination of the lower incisors was higher in younger patients (Group 1).

REFERENCES

1. Almeida MR. Avaliação cefalométrica comparativa da interceptação da má-oclusão de Classe II, divisão 1, utilizando o aparelho de Frankel e o bionator de Balters [tese]. Bauru (SP): Universidade de São Paulo; 2000.

2. Almeida-Pedrin RR. Efeitos cefalométricos do aparelho extrabucal conjugado (Splint Maxilar) e do bionator, no tratamento de má oclusão de Classe II, divisão 1 [tese]. Bauru (SP): Universidade de São Paulo; 2003.

3. Araujo AM. Estudo cefalométrico com implantes metálicos dos efeitos do aparelho Bionator de Balters no desenvolvimento esquelético maxilomandibular durante o tratamento da má oclusão Classe II, divisão 1 [tese]. Araraquara (SP): Universidade Estadual Paulista; 2003.

4. Balters W. Guía de la técnica del Bionator. Buenos Aires: Editorial Mundi; 1969. 68p.

5. Basciftci FA, Uysal T, Büyükerkmen A, Sari Z. The effects of activator treatment on the craniofacial structures of Class II, division 1 patients. Eur J Orthod. 2003;25(1):83-7.

6. Bastos GK, Mucha JN. Aparelhos funcionais: uma revisão. Rev Bras Odontol. 2002;59(3):184-8.

7. Bigliazzi R, Kessner CA, Faltin Jr K. Estudo das alterações anatômicas e morfológicas em pacientes em Classe II, divisão 1, com retrognatismo mandibular, tratados com bionator de Balters, empregando-se a análise das contra-partes de Enlow. Rev Dental Press Ortod Ortop Facial. 2000;5(2):9-19.

8. Björk A. Facial growth in man, studied with aid of metallic implants. Acta Odontol Scand. 1955;13(1):9-34.

9. Björk A, Skieller V. Normal and abnormal growth of the mandible. A synthesis of longitudinal cephalometric implant studies over a period of 25 years. Eur J Orthod. 1983;5(1):1-46.

10. Buschang PH, Gandini Jr L. G. Mandibular skeletal growth and modelling between 10-15 years. Eur J Orthod. 2001;23:1-11.

11. Cavalcante CT. Alterações verticais decorrentes da interceptação da Classe II com o aparelho Bionator [tese]. Bauru (SP): Universidade de São Paulo; 2003.

12. Almeida MR, Henriques JF, Ursi W. Comparative study of the Frankel (FR- 2) and bionator appliances in the treatment of Class II malocclusion. Am J Orthod Dentofacial Orthop. 2002;121(5):458-66.

13. Graber TM, Neumann B. The Bionator removable orthodontic appliances. Philadelphia: Saunders Company; 1977.

14. Gu Y, McNamara JA Jr. Mandibular growth changes and cervical vertebral maturation. Angle Orthod. 2007;77(6):947-53.

15. Hultgren BW, Isaacson RJ, Erdman AG, Worms FW. Mechanics, growth, and class II corrections. Am J Orthod. 1978;74(4):338-95.

16. Iseri H, Solow B. Change in the width of the mandibular body from 6 to 23 years of age: an implant study. Eur J Orthod. 2000;22(3):229-38.

17. Janson I. A cephalometric study of the efficiency of the Bionator. Trans Eur Orthod. Soc. 1977;53:283-93.

18. Kessner CA, Faltin Jr K. Estudo cefalométrico radiográfico sobre a influência do Bionator de Balters no crescimento mandibular e o incremento vertical do ramo ascendente da mandíbula, nos tratamentos das más oclusões de Classe II, divisão I com retrognatismo mandibular. Rev Inst Ciênc Saúde. 1997;15(esp. issue):51-8.

19. Malta LA, Baccetti T, Franchi L, Faltin K, McNamara JA. Long-term dentoskeletal effects and facial profile changes induced by bionator therapy. Angle Orthod. 2010;80(1):10-7.

20. Maltagliati LA, Henriques JFC, Janson G, Almeida RR, Freitas MR. A influência do tratamento ortopédico nas estruturas faciais de indivíduos com má oclusão de Classe II, 1ª divisão. Um estudo comparativo. J Appl Oral Sci. 2004;12(2):164-70.

21. Martins RP, Rosa Martins JC, Martins LP, Buschang PH. Skeletal and dental components of Class II correction with the bionator and removable headgear splint appliances. Am J Orthod Dentofacial Orthop. 2008;134(6):732-41.

22. McNamara JA Jr, Carlson DS. Quantitative analysis of temporomandibular joint adaptations to protrusive function. Am J Orthod. 1979;76(6):593-61.

23. Melo ACM, Gandini Jr LG, Santos-Pinto A, Araújo AM, Gonçalves JR. Avaliação cefalométrica do efeito do tratamento da má oclusão Classe II, divisão 1, com o bionator de Balters: estudo com implantes metálicos Rev Dental Press Ortod Ortop Facial. 2006;11(3):18-31.

24. Melo ACM, Santos-Pinto A, Martins JCR, Martins LP, Sakima MT. Orthopedic and orthodontic component of Class II division 1 malocclusion correction with Balters bionator: a cephalometric study with metallic implants. World J Orthod. 2003;4:237-42.

25. Monini AC. Estudo cefalométrico com implantes metálicos das alterações esqueléticas, a longo prazo, após o uso do Bionator de Balters [tese]. Araraquara (SP): Universidade Estadual Paulista; 2008.

26. Opheij DG, Callaert H, Opdebeeck HM. The effect of the amount of protrusion built into the bionator on condylar growth and displacement: a clinical study. Am J Orthod Dentofacial Orthop. 1989;95(5):401-9.

27. Reis SAB, Moresca R, Goldenberg FC, Vigorito JW. Utilização da análise de Jarabak para a avaliação do tratamento da Classe II, divisão 1, com o Bionator de Balters. Ortodontia. 2000;33(2):42-52.

28. Ruf S, Pancherz H. Temporomandibular joint growth adaptation in Herbst treatment a prospective magnetic resonance imaging and cephalometric roentgenographic study. Eur J Orthod. 1998;20(4):375-88.

29. Schulhof RJ, Engel GA. Results of Class II to functional appliance treatment. J Clin Orthod. 1982;16(9):587-99.

30. Wang MK, Bushang PH, Behrents R. Mandibular rotation and remodeling changes during early childhood. Angle Orthod. 2009;79(2):271-5.

10

Changes in skeletal and dental relationship in Class II Division I malocclusion after rapid maxillary expansion

Carolina Baratieri[1], Matheus Alves Jr[2], Ana Maria Bolognese[3], Matilde C. G. Nojima[4], Lincoln I. Nojima[4]

Objective: To assess skeletal and dental changes immediately after rapid maxillary expansion (RME) in Class II Division 1 malocclusion patients and after a retention period, using cone beam computed tomography (CBCT) imaging. **Methods:** Seventeen children with Class II, Division 1 malocclusion and maxillary skeletal transverse deficiency underwent RME following the Haas protocol. CBCT were taken before treatment (T_1), at the end of the active expansion phase (T_2) and after a retention period of 6 months (T_3). The scanned images were measured anteroposteriorly (SNA, SNB, ANB, overjet and MR) and vertically (N-ANS, ANS-Me, N-Me and overbite). **Results:** Significant differences were identified immediately after RME as the maxilla moved forward, the mandible moved downward, overjet increased and overbite decreased. During the retention period, the maxilla relapsed backwards and the mandible was displaced forward, leaving patients with an overall increase in anterior facial height. **Conclusion:** RME treatment allowed more anterior than inferior positioning of the mandible during the retention period, thus significantly improving Class II dental relationship in 75% of the patients evaluated.

Keywords: Palatal expansion technique. Angle Class II malocclusion. Clinical trial. Orthodontics.

[1] Professor, Department of Orthodontics, Federal University of de Santa Catarina, UFSC.
[2] PhD resident inOrthodontics, Federal University of Rio de Janeiro.
[3] Full professor, Department of Orthodontics, Federal University of Rio de Janeiro.
[4] Professor, Department of Orthodontics, Federal University of Rio de Janeiro, UFRJ.

» The authors report no commercial, proprietary or financial interest in the products or companies described in this article.

Lincoln Issamu Nojima
Avenida Professor Rodolpho Paulo Rocco, 325 – Ilha do Fundão
Rio de Janeiro/RJ — Brazil — CEP: 21941-617 – E-mail: linojima@gmail.com

INTRODUCTION

Angle[1] defined Class II malocclusion as the distal relationship of the lower first molar in relation to the upper first molar. Studies have recently shown that in addition to the anteroposterior and vertical problems related to Class II malocclusions, posterior transverse discrepancy is also frequently associated with it.[2]

Diagnosis of posterior transverse discrepancy often passes unnoticed at clinical examination as this problem is camouflaged by the Class II skeletal pattern. The characteristics of Class II malocclusion, in all three spatial planes, pre-exist in deciduous dentition and persist into mixed dentition without correction.[3] As soon as transverse maxillary deficiency is diagnosed, rapid maxillary expansion (RME) should be implemented regardless of other skeletal alterations because transverse maxillary growth ends earlier than growth in other directions.[4]

The majority of studies assessing RME outcomes showed that the mandible rotated downward and backward,[5] which is usually an unwanted effect in Class II patients. Clinical observations and case reports reveal either an improvement or correction of the sagittal relationship in Class II patients during the retention period following RME.[6]

Cone beam computed tomography (CBCT) allows a complete scan of the face within a few seconds, with less ionizing irradiation than CT[7] or full-mouth radiographic survey for orthodontic diagnosis.[8] Recent technological advances in dental software allow cephalometric concepts and tools to be combined with CBCT advantages.

Despite a large number of studies reporting on the effects of RME, most of them failed to specify or distinguish the type of malocclusion (Class I, II or III) in the subjects evaluated. Accordingly, there is a lack of information surrounding Class II malocclusion patients who underwent RME as the only treatment intervention. Therefore, the aim of this study is to use CBCT imaging to assess changes in dental and skeletal relationships in Class II, Division 1 malocclusion patients immediately after RME as well as after a 6-month retention period.

MATERIAL AND METHODS

This prospective study was carried out in the Department of Orthodontics of the Federal University of Rio de Janeiro with the approval of the Institute of Collective Health Studies Research Ethics Committee (ref.128/2009-0052.0.239.000-09) and with an informed consent form signed by patients and parents.

Seventeen white Brazilian subjects (8 boys and 9 girls with mean age of 10.67 and 10.05 years old, respectively) presenting Class II Division 1 malocclusion and maxillary transverse skeletal deficiency were selected and diagnosed to receive RME therapy. In addition, patients were followed for the following six months.

In selecting the sample, the following inclusion criteria were applied: Chronological age ranging from 7 to 12 years old; overjet greater than 3 mm; Class II molar (unilateral or bilateral) and skeletal (ANB ≥ 4°) relationship; maxillary skeletal transverse deficiency (distance from J point to facial frontal line > 12 mm);[9] skeletal maturation CS1 through CS3 as evaluated by the Cervical Vertebral Maturation method.

All patients were submitted to RME following the Haas protocol.[4] The appliances were standardized with stainless steel wire, 0.047-in in diameter (Rocky Mountain Orthodontics) and expansion screw of 11 mm (Dentaurum, Magnum – 600.303.30). Upon insertion, the expansion screw was activated four turns (0.2 mm per turn) on the first day, and on the following days it was activated two turns per day, (0.4 mm daily). The active phase varied from 2 to 3 weeks, depending on the individual maxillary transverse deficiency originally diagnosed. Afterwards, the expander screw was stabilized with a 0.012-in double thread ligature and was passively kept in place for the following six months after which the appliance was removed.

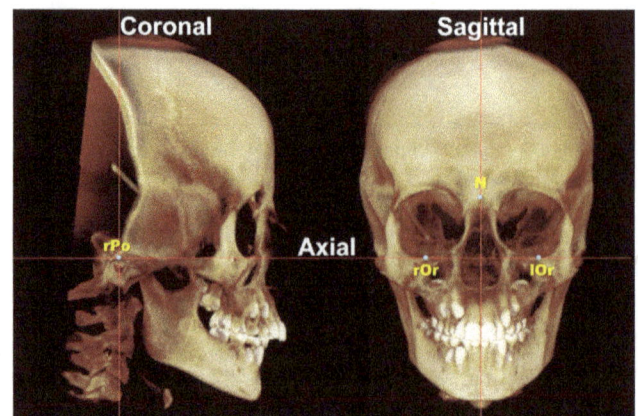

Figure 1 - 3D digital image of the head after orientation by axial, coronal and sagittal planes used as references.

CBTC scans were taken before treatment (T_1), immediately after stabilization of the expansion screw (T_2), and after removal of the expander (T3). The scans were performed with the same cone beam machine (i-CAT, Imaging Sciences International, Hatfield, Pennsylvania, USA), according to a standard protocol (120 KVp, 3 mA, FOV 13x17 cm and voxel 0.4 mm). Volume data at T_1, T_2, and T_3 were exported in DICOM (digital imaging and communication in medicine) format into Dolphin Imaging software® (Charsworth, Calif, USA).

Once imported by means of specific software tools, each 3D-volumetric data set was standardized using reference planes. The three planes are shown in Figure 1 and are defined by an axial plane passing through right and left infraorbitale points as well as right porion; a coronal plane passing through left and right porion perpendicular to the axial plane of choice; and a sagittal plane passing through the nasion point perpendicular to the axial and coronal planes of choice.

After standardization of head positioning, anatomical points (Sella, Nasion, A point, B point, Anterior Nasal Spine, and Menton) were analyzed through mid-sagittal slice images. Subsequently, landmarks 0.025 mm in diameter were identified (Table 1). The following measurements were performed (Fig 2): SNA (anteroposterior maxillary position), SNB (anteroposterior mandibular position), ANB (anteroposterior maxillo-mandibular relationship), N-ANS (upper anterior facial height), ANS-Me (lower anterior facial height), N-Me (anterior facial height), overjet, overbite, rMR (right molar relationship), and lMR (left molar relationship). Molar relationship

was determined as the perpendicular distance from the tip of mesiobuccal cusps of upper first permanent molar to the mesiobuccal sulcus of lower first permanent molar on the same side. Values of rMR and lMR could not be obtained at T_2 because of the artefacts caused by orthodontic bands in these CBCT images.

Measurements were performed separately at each time (T_1, T_2 and T_3) by the same examiner with a one-week interval in between. Intraexaminer reliability values were determined by means of intraclass correlation coefficient (ICC), with 95% confidence interval. Fifteen CBCT scans were randomly selected and remeasured by the same examiner (CB) within 2 weeks, under the same conditions, and compared

Table 1 - Definition of landmarks

Landmarks (abbreviation)	Definition
Orbitale (Or)*	Most inferior point on infraorbital rim
Porion (Po)*	Most superior point of anatomic external auditory meatus
Nasion (N)	Midsagittal point at junction of frontal and nasal bones at nasofrontal suture
Sella (S)	Midpoint of rim between anterior process at mid-sagittal plane
A point (A)	Deepest point of the maxillary alveolar bone concavity at mid-sagittal plane
B point (B)	Deepest point of the mandibular alveolar concavity at mid-sagittal plane
Anterior nasal spine (ANS)	Most anterior limit of floor of nose, at tip of ANS at mid-sagittal plane
Posterior nasal spine (PNS)	Most posterior point along palate at mid-sagittal plane
Menton (Me)	Most inferior point along curvature of chin at mid-sagittal plane

* Bilateral landmark

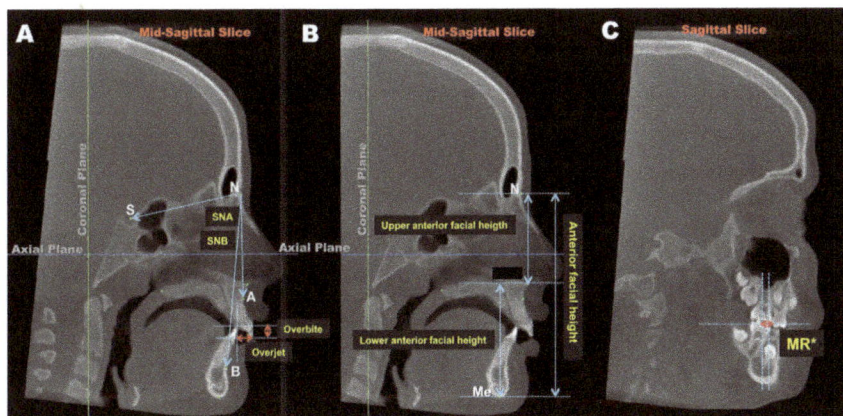

Figure 2 - Sagittal slice with landmarks and measurements. **A)** SNA, SNB, overbite and overjet; **B)** N-Me, N-ANS and ANS-Me; C. MR* (right molar relationship and left molar relationship).

with the first measurements. All measurement error coefficients were found to be close to 1.00 and within acceptable limits (higher than 0.95, except for MR measurement that was 0.91). The mean measurement difference obtained was less than 0.4 mm and 0.3°, which was considered not significant.

Means, standard deviations, minimum and maximum values were calculated for each measurement. After finding normal data distribution by means of the Kolmogorov-Smirnov non-parametric test, statistically significant differences were identified using paired Student's t-test (P < 0.05 - 95% interval confidence) between T_2 and T_1, T_3 and T_2, and T_3 and T_1. The percentage of patients who had the same qualitative mean changes during the interval T_1-T_3 was also calculated. Patients were considered to have increased measurement (mean difference ≥ 0.5 mm); no change

(-0.5 mm >and <0.5 mm); and decreased measurement (≤ −0.5 mm). Statistical analysis was carried out using the SPSS software version 16.0 (SPSS Inc., Chicago, IL, USA).

RESULTS

Separation of the mid-palatal suture was clinically confirmed in all patients with increased opening of inter-incisor diastema or within 3-5 days following expander activation. These data were confirmed on the CBCT image at T_2. During the retention period, one of the patients returned without the expander, thus, his data were not computed at T_3. Transverse deficiency was corrected in all patients. Data of RME transverse effects were previously published.[10]

Table 2 shows the descriptive analysis (minimum, maximum and standard deviation) of measurements

Table 2 - Descriptive analysis of measurements obtained in before treatment onset (T_1), immediately after expansion (T_2) and after retention (T_3).

	T_1 (n = 17)			T_2 (n = 17)			T_3 (n = 16)		
	Min.	Max.	Mean ± SD	Min.	Max.	Mean ± SD	Min.	Max.	Mean ± SD
SNA	74.38	86.20	79.71 ± 3.31	76.88	86.07	80.92 ± 2.99	76.53	86.07	80.09 ± 2.98
SNB	66.8	77.2	73.15 ± 3.41	67.71	76.6	72.92 ± 2.66	69.34	77.6	73.7 ± 2.72
ANB	4.00	9.49	6.61 ± 2.10	4.24	10.70	8.00 ± 2.25	2.50	10.03	6.39 ± 2.03
N-ENA	36.94	55.80	46.87 ± 4.54	36.84	56.52	47.27 ± 5.34	37.93	56.66	47.92 ± 4.76
ENA-Me	53.96	71.87	60.33 ± 4.16	56.59	74.23	61.30 ± 4.31	54.92	73.97	60.75 ± 4.41
N-Me	95.21	116.7	107.2 ± 6.06	94.96	117.57	108.6 ± 6.66	96.18	119.22	108.7 ± 6.51
Overjet	3.5	13.7	7.98 ± 3.56	3.51	14.67	9.38 ± 3.49	3.94	12.4	7.5 ± 2.78
Overbite	1.35	6.68	4.36 ± 1.61	0	5.5	2.59 ± 1.79	1.62	7.67	4.51 ± 1.78
RMd	0.5	9.09	3.18 ± 2.5	---	---	---	-2.68	6.83	1.84 ± 2.76
RMe	0.5	8.33	3.56 ± 2.27	---	---	---	-2.83	7.7	2.04 ± 2.59

n = number of patients; Min = minimum; Max = maximum; SD = standard deviation.

Table 3 - Results regarding skeletal and dental changes between pre-treatment and post-expansion (T_2 – T_1), post-retention and post-expansion (T_3 – T_2), and post-retention and initial (T_3 – T_1).

	T_2-T_1 (n = 17)	T_3-T_2 (n = 16)	T_3-T_1 (n = 16)
	Mean ± SD	Mean ± SD	Mean ± SD
SNA	1.21* ± 1.96	-0.83* ± 1.28	0.38 ± 1.32
SNB	-0.23 ± 2.05	0.78* ± 1.26	0.55 ± 1.76
ANB	1.39*** ± 1.09	-1.61*** ± 1.32	0.22 ± 0.84
N-ENA	0.40 ± 1.88	0.65 ± 1.31	1.06* ± 1.45
ENA-Me	0.97* ± 1.40	-0.55* ± 0.90	0.42 ± 1.40
N-Me	1.44*** ± 1.82	0.02 ± 1.18	1.46*** ± 1.42
Overjet	1.4* ± 1.96	-1.87*** ± 1.50	-0.47 ± 1.33
Overbite	-1.76*** ± 0.72	1.91*** ± 0.92	0.15 ± 0.56
RMd	---	---	-1.33** ± 1.23
RMe	---	---	-1.55** ± 1.55

n=number of patients; SD= Standard Deviation; Level of significance = * P < 0.05;**P < 0.01; ***P < 0.001.

obtained before treatment onset (T_1), immediately after expansion (T_2) and after retention (T_3). Table 3 shows Student's t-test results yielded between the following intervals: T_2-T_1, T_3-T_2 and T_3-T_1. Significant differences were identified immediately after RME $(T_2$-$T_1)$ as the maxilla moved forward (SNA mean increase was 1.21°), the mandible moved downward (ANS-Me mean increase was 0.97 mm and N-Me mean increase was 1.44 mm), overjet increased in 1.4 mm and overbite decreased in 1.76 mm. During the retention period $(T_3$-$T_2)$, the maxilla relapsed backward (SNA mean decrease was 0.83°) and the mandible was displaced forward (SNB mean increase was 0.78°), improving Class II ANB relationship (mean decrease of 1.61°), although patients were left with an overall increase in anterior facial height.

Table 4 shows a qualitative description of changes found within T_1-T_3. Class II dental relationship (rMR and lMR) improved in 75% of patients.

DISCUSSION

This study is part of a long-term prospective clinical investigation into the effects of RME on Class II malocclusions using CBCT imaging.[10,11] Understanding the effects of RME on Class II, Division 1 patients is of paramount importance, since transverse maxillary deficiency is often associated with this malocclusion.

Immediately after RME therapy, Class II relationship was worse in the anteroposterior and vertical dimensions. The maxilla significantly moved forward, whereas the mandible moved backward to a lesser degree. Skeletal changes were previously reported by Haas[12] and have been recently confirmed by meta-analysis[13] and systematic reviews.[14-16] Dental changes mirrored skeletal changes by showing significant increase in overjet and decrease in overbite. Changes in dental and skeletal relationships were more likely to be associated with premature contacts involving palatal cusps and dental-alveolar inclination caused by RME[17] than to inferior displacement of the maxilla. This effect was confirmed by the significant increase in buccal inclination (7.31°/6.46°)[10] found in upper first molars immediately after RME.

The 6-month retention period with the Haas expander did not only maintain the new skeletal, alveolar and dental transverse dimensions, (1.66 mm, 4.69 mm and 5.89 mm, respectively, $P < 0.001$),[10] but also resulted in significant decrease in dentoalveolar angulation of original levels. The wider maxilla allowed mandible to shift forward more than upward, therefore improving skeletal and dental relationships. This was revealed by overjet decrease, overbite increase and MR improvement.

By the end of the assessment period, sagittal skeletal changes were not significantly different when compared with initial data, except for patient's vertical dimension. However, Class II dental relationship significantly improved in 75% of patients. Studies assessing untreated Class II malocclusions determined that dental and skeletal patterns were not self-corrected,[3,18] but became even worse.[19] Wendling et al[20] observed

Table 4 - Number and percentage of patients with increased (≥ 0.5), no changes (- 0.5 > and < 0.5) or decreased (≤ - 0.5) measurements during the interval T_1-T_3.

	T_1-T_3		
	Increased n(%)	No changes n(%)	Decreased n(%)
SNA	6 (37.5)	9 (56.25)	1 (6.25)
SNB	8 (50)	5 (31.25)	3 (18.75)
ANB	5 (31.25)	3 (18.75)	8 (50)
N-ENA	13 (81.25)	3 (18.75)	----
ENA-Me	8 (50)	5 (31.25)	3 (18.75)
N-Me	13 (81.25)	2 (12.50)	1 (6.25)
Overjet	4 (25)	2 (12.5)	10 (62.5)
Overbite	3 (18.75)	11 (68.75)	1 (6.25)
RMd	1 (6.25)	3 (18.75)	12 (75)
RMe	1 (6.25)	3 (18.75)	12 (75)

n = number of patients.

that some patients had spontaneous Class II correction after RME during the retention period (6-12 months) in cases of moderate Class II malocclusions. McNamara et al[21] recently observed great improvement (1.8 mm) in MR after RME therapy in 81% of Class II patients when compared to non-treated controls (0.3 mm).

No statistically significant vertical changes were identified immediately after RME. This differs from previous studies that used cephalometric imaging[5,22-25] and reported downward displacement of the maxilla. However, after the retention period, a significant increase in the superior anterior facial height was observed in 81.25% of patients examined herein (N-ANS increased 1.06 mm). In contrast to RME active phase, the retention period was longer which could possibly explain the vertical growth of the maxilla over this period.[26,27] It is expected that untreated 9-year-old subjects would undergo vertical growth of 1.5 mm per year for boys and 1.2 mm for girls.[26] Mc Namara et al[21] observed a facial height increase of 3.4 mm in a RME group and 4.2 mm in the control group over a mean observation period of 3.7 years.

Despite the fact that the present study only assessed Class II Division 1 malocclusion patients, the severity of malocclusion was not considered (Table 2). The large variability of skeletal involvement may precipitate different responses to the same therapy. Vertical changes, resulting either from RME or growth, may limit horizontal mandibular changes and hinder forward positioning of the menton.[28] Vertical maxillary control during the active phase and the retention period would allow further anterior repositioning of the mandible.

The number of patients included in the present study, although sufficient to detect statistically significant changes, is likely insufficient to generalize the results to all Class II malocclusions. The lack of a control group was a limitation of the present study; however, a control group was unfeasible for the present study due to ethical reasons, since it is impossible not to intervene when a diagnosed transverse discrepancy is present.

The routine use of CBCT is not recommended for orthodontic procedures, given that conventional images emit lower radiation doses. However, some orthodontic patients require temporomandibular images, frontal and lateral cephalograms, panoramic, periapical, occlusal or bite-wing radiographs. It is worth noting that the effective dose related to a full-mouth radiographic survey, as reported by Gibbs,[8] and the sum of the effective doses for panoramic, lateral cephalometric and periapical images are similar, if not higher than that of CBCT without a 3D evaluation. This study used CBCT images because a 3D evaluation had also been carried out for other analyses and some data had already been previously reported.[10,11]

CONCLUSIONS

A 6-month retention period with the Haas expander after RME therapy in Class II Division 1 malocclusion patients allowed the mandible to be positioned significantly more forward and exhibit an improved anterior position rather than an inferior position. This improved Class II dental relationship in 75% of the patients evaluated.

REFERENCES

1.   Angle EH. Treatment of malocclusion of the teeth. Philadelphia: SS White; 1899.

2.   Tollaro I, Baccetti T, Franchi L, Tanasescu CD. Role of posterior transverse interarch discrepancy in Class II, Division 1 malocclusion during the mixed dentition phase. Am J Orthod Dentofacial Orthop. 1996;110(4):417-22.

3.   Baccetti T, Franchi L, McNamara JA Jr, Tollaro I. Early dentofacial features of Class II malocclusion: a longitudinal study from the deciduous through the mixed dentition. Am J Orthod Dentofacial Orthop. 1997;111(5):502-9.

4.   Haas AJ. Long-term posttreatment evaluation of rapid palatal expansion. Angle Orthod. 1980;50(3):189-217.

5.   Silva Filho OG, Boas CV, Capelozza LFO. Rapid maxillary expansion in the primary and mixed dentitions: a cephalometric evaluation. Am J Orthod Dentofacial Orthop. 1991;100(2):171-9.

6.   Lima Filho RMA, Lima AC, Ruellas ACO. Spontaneous correction of Class II malocclusion after rapid palatal expansion. Angle Orthod. 2003;73(6):745-52.

7.   Silva MAG, Wolf U, Heinicke F, Bumann A, Visser H, Hirsch E. Cone-beam computed tomography for routine orthodontic treatment planning: a radiation dose evaluation. Am J Orthod Dentofacial Orthop. 2008;133(5):640.e1-5.

8.   Gibbs SJ. Effective dose equivalent and effective dose: comparison for common projections in oral and maxillofacial radiology. Oral Surg Oral Med Oral Pathol Oral Radiol Endod. 2000;90(4):538-45.

9.   Ricketts RM. Perspectives in the clinical application of cephalometrics. Angle Orthod. 1981;51(2):115-50.

10. Baratieri C, Nojima LI, Alves Jr M, Souza MMGd, Nojima MG. Transverse effects of rapid maxillary expansion in Class II malocclusion patients: a cone-beam computed tomography study. Dental Press J Orthod. 2010;15(5):89-97.

11. Baratieri C, Alves Jr M, Sant'Anna EF, Nojima MdCG, Nojima LI. 3D Mandibular positioning after rapid maxillary expansion in Class II malocclusion Braz Dent J. 2011;22(5):428-34.

12. Haas AJ. The treatment of maxillary deficiency by opening the midpalatal suture. Angle Orthod. 1965;35(3):200-17.

13. Lagravére MO, Heo G, Major PW, Flores-Mir C. Meta-analysis of immediate changes with rapid maxxillary expansion treatment. J Am Dent Assoc. 2006;137(1):44-53.

14. Baratieri C, Alves Jr M, Souza MMG, Araújo MTS, Maia LC. Does rapid maxillary expansion have long-term effects on airway dimensions and breathing? Am J Orthod Dentofacial Orthop. 2011;140(2):146-56.

15. Lagravere MO, Major PW, Flores-Mir C. Long-term dental arch changes after rapid maxillary expansion treatment: a systematic review. Angle Orthod. 2005;75(2):155-61.

16. Lagravere MO, Major PW, Flores-Mir C. Long-term skeletal changes with rapid maxillary expansion: a systematic review. Angle Orthod. 2005;75(6):1046-52.

17. Wertz R. Skeletal and dental changes accompanying rapid midpalatal suture opening. Am J Orthod. 1970;58(1):41-66.

18. You Z-H, Fishman LS, Rosenblum RE, Subtelny JD. Dentoalveolar changes related to mandibular forward growth in untreated Class II persons. Am J Orthod Dentofacial Orthop. 2001;120(6):598-607.

19. Fröhlich FJ. Changes in untreated Class II type malocclusions. Angle Orthod. 1962;32(3):167-79.

20. Wendling LK, McNamara JA, Franchi L, Baccetti T. A prospective study of the short-term treatment effects of the acrylic-splint rapid maxillary expander combined with the lower Schwarz Appliance. Angle Orthod. 2004;75(1):7-14.

21. McNamara JA, Sigler LM, Franchi L, Guest SS, Baccetti T. Changes in Occlusal Relationships in mixed dentition patients treated with rapid maxillary expansion. Angle Orthod. 2010;80(2):230-8.

22. Haas AJ. Rapid expansion of the maxillary dental arch and nasal cavity by opening the midpalatal suture. Angle Orthod. 1961;31(2):73-90.

23. Akkaya S, Lorenzon S, Üçem TTA. A comparison of sagittal and vertical effects between bonded rapid and slow maxillary expansion procedures. Eur J Orthod. 1999;21(2):175-80.

24. Chung C-H, Font B. Skeletal and dental changes in the sagittal, vertical, and transverse dimensions after rapid palatal expansion. Am J Orthod Dentofacial Orthop. 2004;126(5):569-75.

25. Akkaya S, Lorenzon S, Üçem TTA. A comparison of sagittal and vertical effects between bonded rapid and slow maxillary expansion procedures. Eur J Orthod. 1999;21(2):175-80.

26. Riolo ML, Moyers RE, McNamara JA, Hunter W. An atlas of craniofacial growth -Cephalometric standards from the University School Growth Study. Michigan: University of Michigan-Monograph Craniofacial Series; 1974.

27. Wendling LK, McNamara JA, Franchi L, Baccetti T. A Prospective study of the short-term treatment effects of the acrylic-splint rapid maxillary expander combined with the lower Schwarz Appliance. Angle Orthod. 2005;75(1):7-14.

28. Schudy FF. Vertical growth versus anteroposterior growth as related to function and treatment. Angle Orthod. 1964;34(2):75-93.

11

Cephalometric effects of the Jones Jig appliance followed by fixed appliances in Class II malocclusion treatment

Mayara Paim Patel[1], José Fernando Castanha Henriques[2],
Karina Maria Salvatore de Freitas[3], Roberto Henrique da Costa Grec[4]

Objective: The aim of this study was to cephalometrically assess the skeletal and dentoalveolar effects of Class II malocclusion treatment performed with the Jones Jig appliance followed by fixed appliances. **Methods:** The sample comprised 25 patients with Class II malocclusion treated with the Jones Jig appliance followed by fixed appliances, at a mean initial age of 12.90 years old. The mean time of the entire orthodontic treatment was 3.89 years. The distalization phase lasted for 0.85 years, after which the fixed appliance was used for 3.04 years. Cephalograms were used at initial (T_1), post-distalization (T_2) and final phases of treatment (T_3). For intragroup comparison of the three phases evaluated, dependent ANOVA and Tukey tests were used. **Results:** Jones Jig appliance did not interfere in the maxillary and mandibular component and did not change maxillomandibular relationship. Jones Jig appliance promoted distalization of first molars with anchorage loss, mesialization and significant extrusion of first and second premolars, as well as a significant increase in anterior face height at the end of treatment. The majority of adverse effects that occur during intraoral distalization are subsequently corrected during corrective mechanics. Buccal inclination and protrusion of mandibular incisors were identified. By the end of treatment, correction of overjet and overbite was observed. **Conclusions:** Jones Jig appliance promoted distalization of first molars with anchorage loss represented by significant mesial movement and extrusion of first and second premolars, in addition to a significant increase in anterior face height.

Keywords: Malocclusion. Angle Class II. Corrective Orthodontics. Tooth movement.

[1] PhD in Orthodontics, School of Dentistry — University of São Paulo/Bauru.
[2] Full professor, University of São Paulo, USP.
[3] Adjunct professor, Masters program in Orthodontics, Ingá College, UNINGÁ.
[4] PhD resident in Orthodontics, School of Dentistry — University of São Paulo/Bauru.

» The authors report no commercial, proprietary or financial interest in the products or companies described in this article.

Karina Maria Salvatore de Freitas
Faculdade de Odontologia de Bauru, Universidade de São Paulo.
Rua Jamil Gebara 1-25, Apto 111 – CEP: 17017-150 — Brazil
E-mail: mayarapaim@hotmail.com

INTRODUCTION

Class II malocclusion is an anteroposterior discrepancy characterized by dentoalveolar or skeletal change or a combination of both, of which mandibular retrusion is the predominant etiologic factor.[1]

There are several methods used to treat this anteroposterior discrepancy, in which case treatment is certainly diversified by patients' etiologic factor, growth pattern, age, degrees of cooperation and, specially, their chief complaint. They may opt for a treatment with or without extractions, with the use of headgear, intermaxillary elastics, functional or mechanical orthopedics removable appliances, fixed intraoral appliances, and even surgical-orthodontic treatment.

Patient's cooperation is a determinant factor for successful orthodontic treatment, thus, protocols that require minimal collaboration are of great value in orthodontic practice. Intraoral distalizers fulfill this function, i.e., they correct Class II malocclusion without entirely depending on the patient to achieve satisfactory results by the end of treatment.[2-5]

Intraoral distalizers differ in the site of action, either buccal or palatal, and promote different results during distalization.[6] Another important factor is the type of anchorage which can be performed in deciduous molars or pre-molars, supported by two or four teeth.[7] Anchorage reinforcement can be currently accomplished by miniscrews fixed on the palate, thereby promoting skeletal anchorage and reducing adverse effects that are characteristic of intraoral distalizers.[8]

However, intraoral distalization through intraoral fixed appliances is only the first phase of treatment that will be finalized with fixed corrective mechanics. In the literature, there are only a few studies scientifically assessing the results of the two treatment phases;[9-12] most researches only assess the results of distalization.[2,4,7,13-17] Therefore, it is of paramount importance to conduct a study that assesses distalization phase and post-distalization fixed appliance phase, separately.

Thus, the aim of this study was to cephalometrically assess the skeletal and dentoalveolar changes of young subjects with Class II malocclusion treated with the Jones Jig appliance followed by corrective fixed appliances, comparing the changes caused by the distalization phase with the changes of the corrective fixed appliances phase.

MATERIAL AND METHODS

Material

This study was approved by Ingá College Institutional Review Board. The prospective sample comprised 75 lateral cephalograms of 25 subjects treated with the Jones Jig appliance followed by fixed appliances.

The criteria for sample selection were based on the following characteristics: Presence of Class II, division 1 malocclusion; mild to moderate crowding; absence of previous orthodontic treatment; absence of supernumerary teeth or agenesis.

Fourteen out of 25 patients were male, while 11 were female, all presenting Class II, division 1 malocclusion, 4 full-cusp Class II, 3 ¾-cusp Class II, 7 ½-cusp and 11 ¼-cusp Class II.

These patients were part of a prospective sample treated by a single student of Masters in Orthodontics at Ingá College. Class II molar relationship was initially corrected by means of the Jones Jig appliance and maintained as a result of the nightly use of headgear during the entire treatment. Fixed corrective appliances were also installed.

The mean initial age was 13.10 years (SD 1.40; minimum 10.83, maximum 16.24), the mean post-distalization age was 13.95 (SD 1.48; minimum 11.33, maximum 17.23), and the mean final age was 16.99 years (SD 1.87; minimum 15.03, maximum 23.15). The mean time of total orthodontic treatment was 3.89 years (SD 0.99). The distalization phase lasted for 0.85 years (SD 0.30; minimum 0.41, maximum 1.95) whereas the phase of fixed appliance after distalization lasted for 3.04 years (SD 0.97; minimum 1.73, maximum 5.93).

Methods

Orthodontic treatment with Jones Jig appliance

The Jones Jig appliance[5] was manufactured by Morelli®, and consisted of a 0.036-in steel body, a steel distal end of 0.016-in, a steel cursor on the mesial end and a stainless steel open spring which requires sequential activation. However, for this research, in order to dissipate light and continuous force, the steel spring was changed by a nickel-titanium spring of which mean size was 10 mm, GH manufacturer (Greenwood, USA & Canada). Distalizer installation started from the bandage of the maxillary second premolars in order to construct the modified Nance button. The compression spring corresponded to a distance of 5 mm, which promoted a dissipation of 120 grams (0.12N) of force, in average.

By the end of distalization and correction of molar relationship, an average overcorrection of 2 mm beyond normal molar relationship was endeavored. After removal of the Jones Jig, a modified Nance button was installed on the distalized molars in association with a headgear with middle-high traction (jeans helmet). This phase was followed by bonding of fixed orthodontic appliances (Morelli, Roth, slot 0.022 x 0.028-in). In the maxillary anterior retraction phase, the Nance button was removed and in addition to the night use of the headgear, (with a force of 250 grams, 0.25 N), 3/16-in Class II elastics were used, releasing an average force of 200 g/side (0.2 N), between 12 and 20 h/day. After the fixed orthodontic appliance was removed, a maxillary Hawley plate and a mandibular 3x3 were installed for retention.

Lateral cephalograms

Three lateral cephalograms of each patient were taken at three different times: T_1 (initial), T_2 (post-distalization) and T_3 (final).

Each radiograph was traced with landmarks set in a darkened room. Through a Numonics A-30TL digitizing table, attached to an AMD K-6 II 500MHz microcomputer, the location of the cephalometric landmarks was transferred to the Dentofacial Planner 7.02 software (Dentofacial Planner Software Inc., Toronto, Ontario, Canada) in which measurements involving planes and lines were processed. Magnification factors were set at 6% and 9.8%.

Error of the method

Intra-examiner error was assessed by retracing and obtaining new measurements of 20 randomly selected cephalometric radiographs. The first and second measurements were performed within a month interval. The formula proposed by Dahlberg[18] ($Se^2 = Sd^2/2n$) was applied to estimate the magnitude of casual errors, while systematic errors were analyzed by paired t-tests.[19]

Statistical analysis

Descriptive statistics was performed to obtain means and standard deviations of age and treatment times.

For intragroup comparisons of the three times evaluated, dependent ANOVA as well as Tukey tests were used whenever necessary.

STATISTICA for Windows (7.0 version, StatSoft. Inc.) software was used for analysis. Significance level was set at 5% (P < 0.05).

RESULTS

Two systematic errors were observed (PTVI-A and NAP). Casual error ranged from 0.26 mm of overjet to 1.75 degrees of NAP variable.

There were significant changes in almost all components of the three assessed phases (Table 1). The Jones Jig appliance did not affect the maxillary and mandibular component and did not change maxillomandibular relationship. There was distalization of first molars with loss of anchorage, extrusion and mesial movement of first and second premolars. Anterior face height was increased after treatment. Mandibular incisors were uprighted and protruded. By the end of treatment, overjet and overbite were corrected (Table 1).

DISCUSSION

The use of a control group could have added more data to this research by allowing the differentiation of changes produced by the Jones Jig and the fixed appliances from changes that occur with individuals' normal growth. However, the main objective of this study was to observe, separately, the changes in the period of use of the Jones Jig and in the period of use of fixed appliances, headgear and intermaxillary elastics. With this variation of time, there was no compatible control group that could have been used for comparison. Nevertheless, in no way, the lack of a control group invalidates the results obtained herein.

Maxillary component

Distalization with the Jones Jig followed by corrective fixed appliances did not produce statistically significant changes in the effective length of the maxilla (Fig 1, Table 1). This result was already expected, since intraoral distalizers do not promote skeletal changes, as reported in other studies.[9,14-16]

Nevertheless, there was significant maxillary retrusion.[9] This change is probably related to the use

Table 1 - Intragroup comparison of the three evaluated phases: Initial (T1), post-distalization (T2) and final (T3) (dependent ANOVA and Tukey tests).

Variables	T_1 Mean ± SD	T_2 Mean ± SD	T_3 Mean ± SD	P
Maxillary component				
SNA (degrees)	81.91 ± 3.96^AB	82.84 ± 4.20^A	81.72 ± 4.84^B	0.022*
Co-A (mm)	81.85 ± 5.21^A	82.97 ± 5.65^A	82.58 ± 5.48^A	0.216
PTVI-A (mm)	47.85 ± 4.51^A	48.06 ± 4.23^A	48.77 ± 4.72^A	0.148
Mandibular component				
SNB (degrees)	78.50 ± 3.00^A	79.31 ± 3.26^A	79.18 ± 4.37^A	0.210
Co-Gn (mm)	104.41 ± 5.02^A	106.30 ± 6.50^B	109.67 ± 6.90^C	0.000*
P-NB (mm)	1.40 ± 1.11^A	1.47 ± 1.17^A	1.66 ± 1.30^A	0.284
PTVI-B (mm)	47.28 ± 5.43^A	47.00 ± 5.11^A	49.36 ± 5.98^B	0.000*
Maxillomandibular relationship				
ANB (degrees)	3.42 ± 2.63^A	3.57 ± 2.41^A	2.54 ± 2.62^A	0.055
NAP (degrees)	5.44 ± 5.89^A	5.69 ± 5.77^A	3.34 ± 5.58^A	0.051
Vertical component				
FMA (degrees)	29.84 ± 4.17^A	31.99 ± 4.88^B	31.76 ± 4.04^B	0.005*
SN.PP (degrees)	6.40 ± 4.07^A	5.77 ± 3.70^A	6.84 ± 3.34^A	0.285
SN.GoGn (degrees)	31.80 ± 4.11^A	31.86 ± 4.98^A	32.25 ± 4.59^A	0.650
SN.GoMe (degrees)	34.95 ± 4.18^A	35.33 ± 4.46^A	35.40 ± 4.63^A	0.563
NS.Gn (degrees)	66.50 ± 3.58^A	66.32 ± 3.89^A	67.35 ± 4.34^A	0.059
SN.Ocl (degrees)	9.77 ± 4.05^A	10.04 ± 4.45^AB	11.85 ± 3.40^B	0.015*
LAFH (mm)	61.75 ± 5.54^A	63.77 ± 5.71^B	66.72 ± 6.95^C	0.000*
Maxillary dentoalveolar component				
SN.1 (degrees)	107.26 ± 5.52^A	111.77 ± 6.73^B	106.16 ± 6.29^A	0.000*
PTVI-1 (mm)	55.71 ± 5.23^A	56.82 ± 5.06^A	57.04 ± 5.35^A	0.086
PP-1 (mm)	26.90 ± 2.82^A	27.09 ± 2.95^A	28.58 ± 3.38^B	0.000*
1.NA (degrees)	25.33 ± 6.19^AB	28.73 ± 6.93^A	24.45 ± 6.95^B	0.015*
1-NA (mm)	5.05 ± 2.72 ^A	6.33 ± 2.67^A	5.48 + 3.36^A	0.087
SN 4 (degrees)	82.20 ± 4.57^A	94.60 ± 5.55^B	80.66 ± 5.61^A	0.000*
PTVI-4 (mm)	36.41 ± 3.87^A	38.87 ± 3.61^B	38.60 ± 4.21^B	0.000*
PP-4 (mm)	19.20 ± 2.47^A	20.61 ± 2.49^B	21.20 ± 2.81^C	0.000*
SN.5 (degrees)	78.24 ± 5.24^A	88.78 ± 5.53^B	79.80 ± 5.69^A	0.000*
PTVI-5 (mm)	29.99 ± 3.76^A	32.72 ± 3.73^B	32.14 ± 4.33^B	0.000*
PP-5 (mm)	18.69 ± 2.50^A	20.64 ± 2.44^B	20.69 ± 2.86^B	0.000*
SN.6 (degrees)	65.48 ± 4.82^A	55.30 ± 6.13^B	66.80 ± 5.21^A	0.000*
PTVI-6 (mm)	21.83 ± 3.61^A	19.66 ± 3.34^B	23.58 ± 4.23^C	0.000*
PP-6 (mm)	16.90 ± 2.29^A	16.46 ± 2.44^A	19.15 ± 3.04^B	0.000*
SN.7 (degrees)	50.26 ± 6.44^A	48.57 ± 6.08^A	55.42 ± 6.82^B	0.000*
PTVI-7 (mm)	12.14 ± 3.14^A	11.34 ± 3.36^A	13.53 ± 3.98^B	0.000*
PP-7 (mm)	11.48 ± 3.64^A	11.82 ± 3.24^A	15.68 ± 3.18^B	0.000*
Mandibular dentoalveolar component				
1.NB degrees)	25.79 ± 5.70^A	24.62 ± 5.75^A	28.48 ± 5.17^B	0.001*
1-NB (mm)	4.54 ± 2.21^A	4.73 ± 2.04^A	5.90 ± 1.93^B	0.000*
PTVI-6i (mm)	20.86 ± 4.51^A	21.04 ± 4.47^A	23.25 ± 4.34 ^B	0.000*
GoMe-6i (mm)	27.72 ± 2.78^A	28.29 ± 2.76^A	30.92 ± 3.62 ^B	0.000*
Dental relationships				
Molar relationship (mm)	-0.35 ± 1.09^A	-4.54 ± 1.07^B	-2.76 ± 0.58^C	0.000*
Overjet (mm)	4.59 ± 1.59^A	5.71 ± 1.98^B	2.80 ± 0.57^C	0.000*
Overbite (mm)	3.82 ± 1.52^A	3.40 ± 1.62^A	2.35 ± 0.51^B	0.000*

* statistically significant difference (p < 0.05)
- different letters mean statistically significant difference.

of an extraoral headgear, since after distalization performed by means of the Jones Jig the headgear was used as anchorage so as to maintain molars distalized as well as to verticalize their roots.[9,20]

Mandibular component

The effective length of the mandible was gradually and significantly increased, showing changes in the end of the distalization phase and at the end of corrective orthodontic treatment (Fig 1). Assessment of PTVI-B demonstrated statistically significant mandibular increase in the final phase of corrective treatment (Table 1). This change was probably related to craniofacial growth and development, which proves mandibular growth in the long-term.[21]

Maxillomandibular relationship

Maxillomandibular relationship was improved by the end of corrective orthodontic treatment; however, these changes were not statistically significant in all three stages (Table 1). This result was already expected, specially at the end of distalization of maxillary molars, since intraoral distalizers do not significantly interfere in changes of bone bases.[9,14-16]

Vertical component

The variables related to the vertical component showed a slight tendency towards angular increase in the phase of fixed corrective treatment; however, only FMA showed a statistically significant increase during distalization, a change that remained in the final stage. Likewise, the occlusal plane angle showed a statistically significant increase at the end of corrective treatment compared to the initial stage (Table 1). There was also a statistically significant increase in lower anterior face height in the post-distalization stage and at the end of corrective orthodontic treatment (Table 1).

Changes in cephalometric variables related to the vertical component certainly occurred due to clockwise rotation of the mandible probably caused by significant extrusion of first and second premolars during distalization.[9,16]

Changes in the occlusal plane and LAFH were also observed at the end of corrective orthodontic treatment and were related to extrusion of first premolars and first and second molars (Fig 2). However, in this

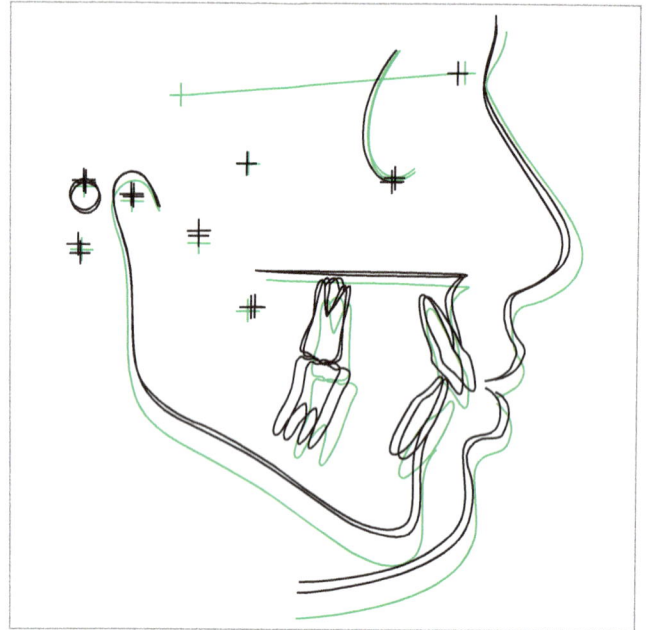

Figure 1 - Mean cephalometric landmarks in the three observation phases: (T_1, black; T_2, red; and T_3, green) (overlap on line SN).

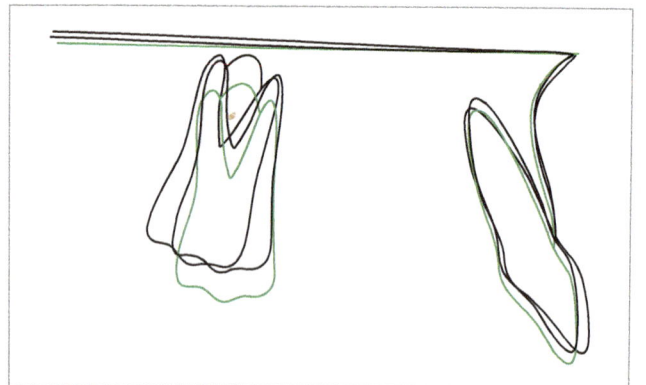

Figure 2 - Maxillary teeth alterations in the three observation phases (T1, black; T2, red; and T3, green) (overlap on palatal plane).

phase, vertical changes occurred to correct overbite, which decreased in 1.47 mm from the initial to the final stage.[9] Moreover, increased LAFH may also be credited to normal vertical facial growth.

Maxillary dentoalveolar component
Maxillary incisors

Maxillary incisors showed statistically significant buccal inclination in the post-distalization phase. This accentuated inclination is a characteristic of anchorage loss during intraoral distalization.[9,15-17] However, in the final phase of orthodontic treatment, maxillary incisors showed significant palatal inclination, thereby reversing anchorage loss. Protrusion of maxillary incisors was not statistically significant (Table 1).

In the final phase of corrective orthodontic treatment, maxillary incisors also showed significant extrusion related to correction of buccal inclination, vertical displacement of the maxilla due to the craniofacial growth[22] and the use of Class II elastics.

First and second maxillary premolars

In the post-distalization phase, first premolars demonstrated effects of anchorage loss related to distal movement through intraoral distalizers.[7,10-13,20] There was significant linear and angular mesial movement associated with extrusion in relation to the palatal plane. Mesial angulation was corrected at the end of orthodontic treatment; however, mesial positioning remained in the final stage (Table 1), probably due to anterior displacement of the maxilla in an attempt to accompany mandibular displacement.[10,20] First premolars showed significant extrusion at the end of distalization and orthodontic treatment.

Previous researches[9,16] also assessed the effects of the Jones Jig appliance, but focused only on second premolars, which are the anchorage teeth selected for placement of the Nance button during intraoral distalization.

Second premolars showed similar behavior to first premolars, also characterizing anchorage loss due to intraoral distalization.[2,4,7,9-13,15-17,20,23,24] There was statistically significant angular and linear mesial movement in the post-distalization phase. Conversely, in the final stage, mesial angulation was corrected, but mesial positioning also remained accompanying the displacement of the maxillary base in relation to the mandible.[10,20]

There was statistically significant extrusion during distalization in comparison to the initial position. This vertical change was related to mesial angulation and mesial movement, i.e., reflecting anchorage loss.[9,16]

Longitudinal observations show that extrusion, mesial angulation of premolars and anterior inclination of maxillary incisors are reversed effects that occur during active treatment with maxillary fixed appliances.[9,15] They may even occur spontaneously in the period of verticalization and stabilization with the Nance button positioned in distalized molars. However, the vertical positioning of second premolars remained at the end of corrective treatment, similarly to the post-distalization phase. In other words, it is probable that the accentuated curve of Spee

preserved extrusion of second premolars to correct overbite, which was greater at the beginning of treatment.

First and second maxillary molars

Maxillary first molars demonstrated significant distal angulation, as already anticipated in treatment of Class II with intraoral devices.[2-4,7,9,11-17,20]

Accentuated distal angulation is observed in all researches that assess distalization with the Jones Jig appliance,[5,9,14-17,25] including cases of absolute anchorage.[26] However, this angulation was reversed and, by the end of corrective orthodontic treatment, maxillary first molars showed a verticalized position in relation to the cranial base (Table 1 and Fig 2). This correction was already expected, since patients, by the end of the distalization process, used the extraoral headgear in order to anchor and verticalize distalized molars.[16,20]

Maxillary first molars were significantly distalized in the post-distalization phase; however, after corrective orthodontic treatment, significant angular and linear mesial movement was observed, probably due to correction of accentuated distal angulation and displacement of the maxilla of which goal is to maintain normal maxillomandibular relationship[10] (Fig 2).

By the end of corrective orthodontic treatment, molar extrusion was statistically significant, probably due to correction of overbite (Fig 2). Extrusion of maxillary first molars can also be related to appositional maxillary growth and vertical flotation process.[22] In this group, the use of headgear may not have promoted extrusion of first molars, since the headgear was used with medium-high traction (jeans helmet), thereby preventing tooth extrusion.

Maxillary second molars showed no statistically significant changes in the post-distalization phase; however, at the end of corrective orthodontic treatment, second molars showed mesial angulation in relation to the cranial base, as well as statistically significant mesialization. Statistically significant extrusion was also observed at the end of corrective orthodontic treatment. Changes caused to second molars were not only due to eruption, but also to movement of maxillary first molars in the corrective phase.[9]

In relation to maxillary first molars, second molars showed greater extrusion at the end of corrective treatment. This result can probably be attributed to the different stage of eruption of maxillary first and second molars.[9]

Mandibular dentoalveolar component
Mandibular incisors

With regard to mandibular incisors, there was statistically significant buccal inclination and protrusion at the end of corrective orthodontic treatment (Table 1 and Fig 3). This change was related to correction of overjet which was greater at the beginning of treatment. Therefore, changes observed in mandibular incisors occurred to decrease overjet and were due to the use of Class II elastics.

In the literature, only the study conducted by Brickman, Sinha and Nanda[9] assessed the effect of Class II treatment with the Jones Jig appliance followed by corrective fixed appliances. Nevertheless, the authors did not report the behavior of mandibular incisors. However, studies that assessed other distalizers observed buccal inclination during orthodontic treatment.[10,11,20] According to Angelieri et al,[20] mandibular incisors are buccally inclined due to anterior mandibular displacement and the use of Class II elastics.

Mandibular first molars

Mandibular molars showed statistically significant mesialization during corrective treatment when initial and post-distalization phases were compared (Table 1). Class II molar relationship was corrected not only by maxillary molars distalization, but also by mesial movement of mandibular molars.[10,20]

As for the vertical component, at the end of corrective treatment, mandibular molars showed significant extrusion when the initial and post-distalization phases were compared (Fig 3). Changes in mandibular molars are not reported by studies assessing distalization with the Jones Jig [5,15-17] followed by fixed appliances;[9] however, extrusion was observed in studies that use the Pendulum appliance.[10,11] Therefore, it is assumed that mandibular molars extrusion may be related to the use of Class II elastics, vertical displacement due to appositional growth of the lower base of the mandible and to vertical floating.[22]

Dental relationships

Molar relationship showed statistically significant changes in the three phases of assessment. In the initial phase, patients showed Class II relationship, whereas in the post-distalization phase, there was

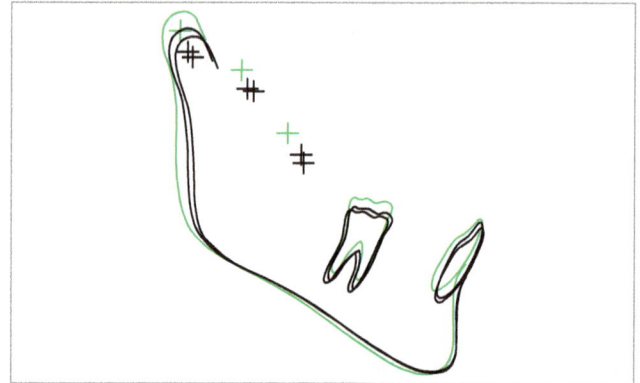

Figure 3 - Manibular teeth alterations in the three observation phases (T1, black; T2, red; and T3, green) (overlap on mandibular plane).

overcorrection with molars ending up in a "super" Class I relationship, as suggested by previous studies.[9,11,12] However, as expected, maxillary molars mesially moved during corrective treatment to establish normal molar relationship, (Table 1).

At the beginning of treatment, both overjet and overbite were increased. In the post-distalization phase, there was an increase in overjet due to buccal tipping of maxillary incisors, thereby characterizing anchorage loss related to distalization with the Jones Jig appliance.[16] By the end of corrective orthodontic treatment, both overjet and overbite were reduced, thus demonstrating that orthodontic treatment goals were achieved. Correction of overjet was related to uprighting of maxillary incisors and buccal tipping of mandibular incisors, as described above. Correction of overbite, on the other hand, was probably related to extrusion of first and second premolars and first and second molars, as previously reported.

Brickman, Sinha and Nanda[9] observed an increase of 0.45 mm in overjet and a decrease of 1.28 mm in overbite during distalization of maxillary molars. According to the authors, changes in overjet were related to mesial movement of maxillary premolars and buccal inclination of maxillary incisors, as reported by other studies assessing intraoral distalization.[12,13,16,20]

CONCLUSION

The Jones Jig appliance did not interfere in maxillary and mandibular components and did not change maxillomandibular relationship. The Jones Jig appliance promoted distalization of first molars with anchorage loss, significant mesialization and extrusion of first and second premolars, and a significant increase in anterior face height at the end of treatment. Most adverse effects occurred during the intraoral distalization phase and were subsequently corrected with corrective mechanics. There was buccal inclination and protrusion of mandibular incisors. At the end of treatment, overjet and overbite correction was observed.

REFERENCES

1. McNamara J. Components of class II malocclusion in children 8-10 years of age. Angle Orthod. 1981;51(3):177-202.

2. Fortini A, Lupoli M, Giuntoli F, Franchi L. Dentoskeletal effects induced by rapid molar distalization with the first class appliance. Am J Orthod Dentofacial Orthop. 2004;125(6):697-704.

3. Gianelly AA, Vaitas AS, Thomas WM. The use of magnets to move molars distally. Am J Orthod Dentofacial Orthop. 1989;96(2):161-7.

4. Hilgers J. The pendulum appliance for Class II non-compliance therapy. J Clin Orthod. 1992;26(11):706-14.

5. Jones RD, White JM. Rapid Class II molar correction with an open-coil jig. J Clin Orthod. 1992;26(10):661-4.

6. Antonarakis GS, Kiliaridis S. Maxillary molar distalization with noncompliance intramaxillary appliances in Class II malocclusion. A systematic review. Angle Orthod. 2008;78(6):1133-40.

7. Kinzinger GSM, Wehrbein H, Diedrich PR. Molar distalization with a modified pendulum appliance--in vitro analysis of the force systems and in vivo study in children and adolescents. Angle Orthod. 2005;75(4):558-67.

8. Oncag G, Seckin O, Dincer B, Arikan F. Osseointegrated implants with pendulum springs for maxillary molar distalization: a cephalometric study. Am J Orthod Dentofacial Orthop. 2007;131(1):16-26.

9. Brickman CD, Sinha PK, Nanda RS. Evaluation of the Jones jig appliance for distal molar movement. Am J Orthod Dentofacial Orthop. 2000;118(5):526-34.

10. Burkhardt DR, McNamara JA Jr, Baccetti T. Maxillary molar distalization or mandibular enhancement: a cephalometric comparison of comprehensive orthodontic treatment including the pendulum and the Herbst appliances. Am J Orthod Dentofacial Orthop. 2003;123(2):108-16.

11. Chiu PP, McNamara JA, Franchi L. A comparison of two intraoral molar distalization appliances: distal jet versus pendulum. Am J Orthod Dentofacial Orthop. 2005;128(3):353-65.

12. Ngantung V, Nanda RS, Bowman SJ. Posttreatment evaluation of the distal jet appliance. Am J Orthod Dentofacial Orthop. 2001;120(2):178-85.

13. Ghosh J, Nanda RS. Evaluation of an intraoral maxillary molar distalization technique. Am J Orthod Dentofacial Orthop. 1996;110(6):639-46.

14. Gulati S, Kharbanda OP, Parkash H. Dental and skeletal changes after intraoral molar distalization with sectional jig assembly. Am J Orthod Dentofacial Orthop. 1998;114(3):319-27.

15. Haydar S, Uner O. Comparison of Jones jig molar distalization appliance with extraoral traction. Am J Orthod Dentofacial Orthop. 2000;117(1):49-53.

16. Patel MP, Janson G, Henriques JF, Almeida RR, Freitas MR, Pinzan A, et al. Comparative distalization effects of Jones jig and pendulum appliances. Am J Orthod Dentofacial Orthop. 2009;135(3):336-42.

17. Runge ME, Martin JT, Bukai F. Analysis of rapid maxillary molar distal movement without patient cooperation. Am J Orthod Dentofacial Orthop. 1999;115(2):153-7.

18. Dahlberg G. Statistical methods for medical and biological students. New York: Interscience; 1940.

19. Houston WJ. The analysis of errors in orthodontic measurements. Am J Orthod. 1983;83(5):382-90.

20. Angelieri F, Almeida RR, Almeida MR, Fuziy A. Dentoalveolar and skeletal changes associated with the pendulum appliance followed by fixed orthodontic treatment. Am J Orthod Dentofacial Orthop. 2006;129(4):520-7.

21. Martins DR, Janson G, Almeida RR, Pinzan A, Henriques JFC, Freitas MR. Atlas de crescimento craniofacial. São Paulo: Ed. Santos; 1998.

22. Enlow DH, Kuroda T, Lewis AB. The morphological and morphogenetic basis for craniofacial form and pattern. Angle Orthod. 1971;41(3):161-88.

23. Bolla E, Muratore F, Carano A, Bowman SJ. Evaluation of maxillary molar distalization with the distal jet: a comparison with other contemporary methods. Angle Orthod. 2002;72(5):481-94.

24. Bussick T, McNamara J Jr. Dentoalveolar and skeletal changes associated with the pendulum appliance. Am J Orthod Dentofacial Orthop. 2000;117(3):333-43.

25. Mavropoulos A, Karamouzos A, Kiliaridis S, Papadopoulos MA. Efficiency of noncompliance simultaneous first and second upper molar distalization: a three-dimensional tooth movement analysis. Angle Orthod. 2005;75(4):532-9.

26. Papadopoulos MA. Orthodontic treatment of Class II malocclusion with miniscrew implants. Am J Orthod Dentofacial Orthop. 2008;134(5):604.e1-16.

12

Retention period after treatment of posterior crossbite with maxillary expansion

Julia Garcia Costa[1], Thaís Magalhães Galindo[1], Claudia Trindade Mattos[2], Adriana de Alcantara Cury-Saramago[2]

Objective: The aim of this systematic review was to evaluate the duration of the retention period in growing patients undergoing maxillary expansion and its relation with posterior crossbite stability. **Methods:** Search strategies were executed for electronic databases Cochrane Library, Web of Science, PubMed and Scopus, which were completed on January 15, 2016. The inclusion criteria included randomized, prospective or retrospective controlled trials in growing subjects with posterior crossbite; treated with maxillary expanders; retention phase after expansion; post-retention phase of at least 6 months. The exclusion criteria were anterior crossbite, craniofacial anomalies, surgery or another orthodontic intervention; case reports; author's opinions articles, thesis, literature reviews and systematic reviews. The risk of bias of selected articles was assessed with Cochrane risk of bias tool for RCTs and Downs and Black checklist for non-RCTs. **Results:** A total of 156 titles/abstracts was retrieved, 44 full-texts were examined, and 6 articles were selected and assessed for their methodological quality. The retention period after maxillary expansion ranged between 4 weeks and 16 months. Fixed (acrylic plate, Haas, Hyrax and quad-helix) or removable (Hawley and Hawley expander) appliances were used for retention. **Conclusions:** Six months of retention with either fixed or removable appliances seem to be enough to avoid relapse or to guarantee minimal changes in a short-term follow-up.

Keywords: Crossbite. Maxillary expansion. Retainer.

[1] Orthodontics department, Universidade Federal Fluminense, Niterói, Brazil.
[2] Professor of Orthodontics, Dental Clinic department, Universidade Federal Fluminense, Niterói, Brazil.

Adriana de Alcantara Cury-Saramago
Rua Mário Santos Braga, 30, 2º andar, sl. 214 – Campus do Valonguinho
Centro – Niterói/RJ – Brazil – CEP: 24.020-140
E-mail: adrianacury@id.uff.br

» The authors report no commercial, proprietary or financial interest in the products or companies described in this article.

INTRODUCTION

Posterior crossbite is a common malocclusion in the deciduous and mixed dentitions, with prevalence rates of 7.5%[1] to 22%,[2] and in the permanent dentition with rates of 10.2% to 14.4%.[3]

The etiology of this malocclusion may be dental, skeletal and/or functional.[4] Few studies have reported the self-correction of posterior crossbite in the deciduous dentition, related to the discontinuation of sucking habits and chronic respiratory childhood diseases.[5,6] However, this condition is usually not self-corrected.[4,7,8]

Studies with adolescents and adults have revealed that patients presenting posterior crossbite have an increased risk to develop craniomandibular disorders, showing more signs and symptoms of these conditions.[2,5] Several authors suggest the early treatment of crossbites to prevent mandibular dysfunction as well as craniofacial asymmetry.[7-10]

Adults can be submitted to maxillary expansion, although there are controversies regarding the nonsurgical treatment.[11,12]

Various methods have been suggested for correction and retention after treatment of posterior crossbite in growing patients: Haas,[8,13-16] Hyrax,[14,15,17,18] quad-helix appliance (QDH),[4,7,14,15,19-21] removable plates,[4,7,9,20-22] grinding[7,10] and edgewise fixed appliances.[23]

The successful treatment of a posterior crossbite is frequently reached not only by the expansion of the maxilla. In growing subjects, the treatment must also achieve the reestablishment of the normal growth rate on a longitudinal basis,[24] as well as improve the oral and general health.[25]

No consensus among authors exists regarding the optimal retention period after maxillary expansion. Some authors recommend that the retention phase should last for 6 weeks,[19] while others advocate 6[4,21] or 8 months.[8] Thus, a systematic review of the literature was deemed appropriate.

The aim of this systematic review was to evaluate the duration of the retention period in growing patients undergoing maxillary expansion and its relation with posterior crossbite stability. The PICOS is shown in Table 1.

MATERIAL AND METHODS

This systematic review was registered on the National Institute of Health Research Database:

www.crd.york.ac.uk/prospero.

The inclusion criteria were randomized controlled trials (RTCs) and controlled trials in human growing subjects; experimental group presenting posterior crossbite; treatment with maxillary expanders; retention phase after expansion; and a minimum 6-month post-retention phase.

The exclusion criteria were subjects presenting anterior crossbite, craniofacial anomalies, previous surgery or another orthodontic intervention; case reports; author's opinions articles, thesis, literature reviews and systematic reviews.

To identify the studies, detailed search strategies were developed and executed in the following electronic databases: Cochrane Library, Web of Science, PubMed and Scopus (Table 2). All electronic searches were conducted between May 28, 2015 and January 15, 2016. No restrictions for language or publication date were used.

The results were compiled into a reference manager (EndNote X5, Thomson Reuters), and duplicate records were excluded.

Two authors independently reviewed titles and abstracts according to the inclusion and exclusion criteria. Any disagreement was solved by consultation with two others authors until mutual agreement was reached and initial selection was completed.

Full texts of articles where it was not possible to decide for inclusion or exclusion only by reading the title and abstract were also screened to confirm their eligibility. Two authors independently read the full texts of the articles previously selected.

After electronic searches and the initial selection process, a supplementary hand search was implemented by checking the references of each selected study. Afterwards, two authors independently performed a structured quality assessment of the selected articles based on risk of bias. The Cochrane risk of bias tools[26] was used for randomized studies, and the Downs and Black checklist[27] for non-randomized studies. Any disagreement on the risk of bias assessment was resolved after consulting other two authors.

The following data from the included articles were extracted and independently compiled by two researchers: author/year; sample description; crossbite type; expander/activation time; activation rate; retainer appliance and retention time; measurements; follow-up time; overcorrection; experimental group *versus* control group (*p* value);

Table 1 - PICOS.

PICOS	Description
Population	Growing subjects presenting posterior crossbite
Intervention	Treated with maxillary expansion
Comparison	Another maxillary expansion procedure, untreated crossbite subjects or untreated subjects without posterior crossbite
Outcomes	Duration of the retention period after maxillary expansion and its relation with posterior crossbite stability
Study design	Randomized controlled trials (RTCs) and controlled trials in human growing subjects

Table 2 - Search strategy in databases.

Database	Search strategy
Cochrane Library	"palatal expansion technic" or "maxillary expansion" in Title, Abstract, Keywords and "retention" or "retainer" or "stability" or "relapse" in Title, Abstract, Keywords and "crossbite" in Title, Abstract, Keywords not "case report" in Title, Abstract, Keywords (Word variations have been searched)
Web of Science (Database=SCI-EXPANDED, SSCI, A&HCI, CPCI-S, CPCI-SSH, BKCI-S, BKCI-SSH)	1) TS=(palatal expansion technic OR maxillary expansion OR maxillary disjunction OR palatal disjunction OR expansion appliance OR maxillary expander OR palatal expander OR maxillary expander) 2) TS=(retention* OR retainer* OR relapse* OR stability*) 3) TS=(crossbite*) 4) #1 AND #2 AND #3 5) TI=(case report OR case series OR adult*) 6) #4 AND NOT #5
PubMed	(palatal expansion technique[MeSH Terms]) OR "maxillary expansion"[Title/Abstract]) OR "maxillary disjunction"[Title/Abstract]) OR "palatal disjunction"[Title/Abstract]) AND "retention"[Title/Abstract]) OR orthodontic retainer[MeSH Terms]) OR "stability"[Title/Abstract]) OR "relapse"[Title/Abstract]) AND "crossbite"[Title/Abstract]) NOT "case report"[Title]) NOT "case series"[Title]) NOT adult[Title]
Scopus	TITLE-ABS-KEY(palatal expansion technique) OR TITLE-ABS-KEY("maxillary expansion") OR TITLE-ABS-KEY("maxillary disjunction") OR TITLE-ABS-KEY("palatal disjunction") AND TITLE-ABS-KEY("retention") OR TITLE-ABS-KEY("retainers") OR TITLE-ABS-KEY("relapse") OR TITLE-ABS-KEY("post retention") OR TITLE-ABS-KEY("stability") OR TITLE-ABS-KEY("changes") AND TITLE-ABS-KEY(crossbite) AND NOT TITLE-ABS-KEY("case report") AND NOT TITLE-ABS-KEY("case series") AND NOT TITLE-ABS-KEY(adult)

relapse after follow-up time; crossbite correction stability after follow-up; conclusion.

In order to verify the percentage of relapse for each transversal measure given by the authors, the difference between the measure immediately after expansion (AE) and the measure after 6-month follow-up (FU) was calculated following the equation: $[(AE-FU) \times 100 / AE]$.

RESULTS

In the databases search, 281 articles were found. After duplicates were excluded, we screened 156 titles and abstracts; and 112 studies were excluded from this review; 44 full texts were screened, and 6 articles were selected according to the eligibility criteria. The search process is shown in the Prisma flow diagram (Fig 1).

Two articles included, which are randomized controlled trials, were assessed with the Cochrane tool and the corresponding graphs are shown in Figures 2 and 3. The non-randomized studies were classified according to their risk of bias, using the Downs and Black checklist, as: low risk,[4] medium[16] and high risk[8,22] (Table 3).

Data extracted from the included articles are displayed in Tables 4A and 4B. The retention period after maxillary expansion ranged from five[22] to sixteen months,[16] and the appliances used were: fixed (acrylic plate expander,[22] Haas,[8,16] Hyrax[17] and quad-helix[4,21]) or removable (hawley[4,22] and Hawley expander[4,21,22]).

The follow-up of these patients ranged from 6 months[4] to 60[16] months, and the relapses of the measurements described reached 0%[4] to 27%[17].

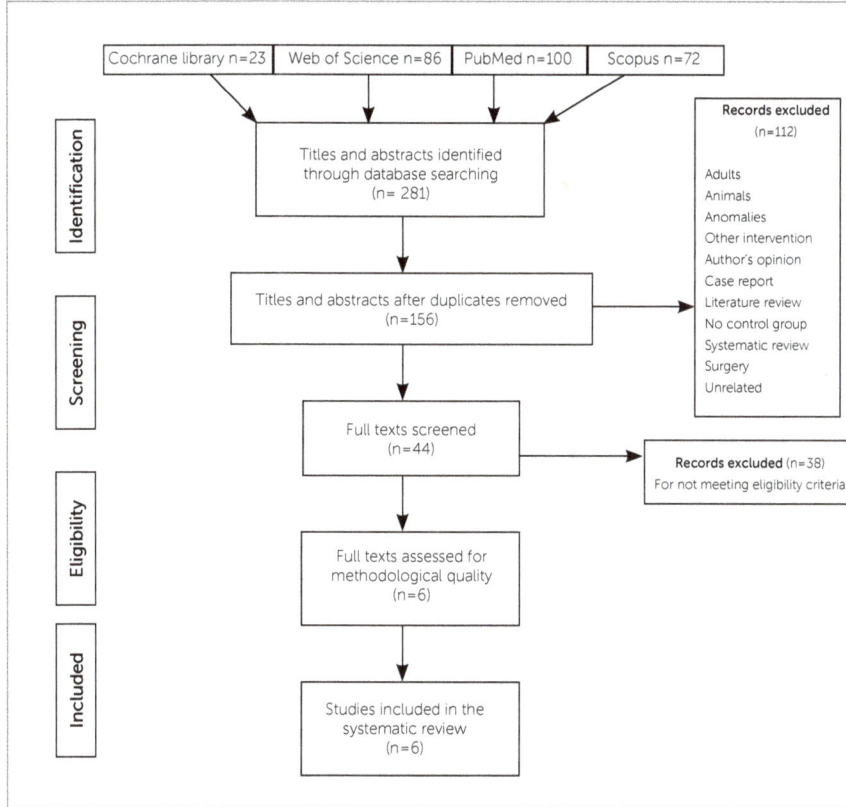

Figure 1 - Prisma flow diagram.

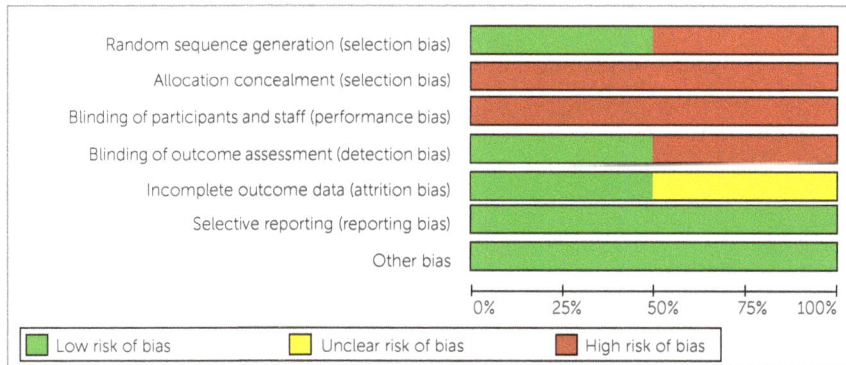

Figure 2 - Risk of bias graph for RCTs studies.

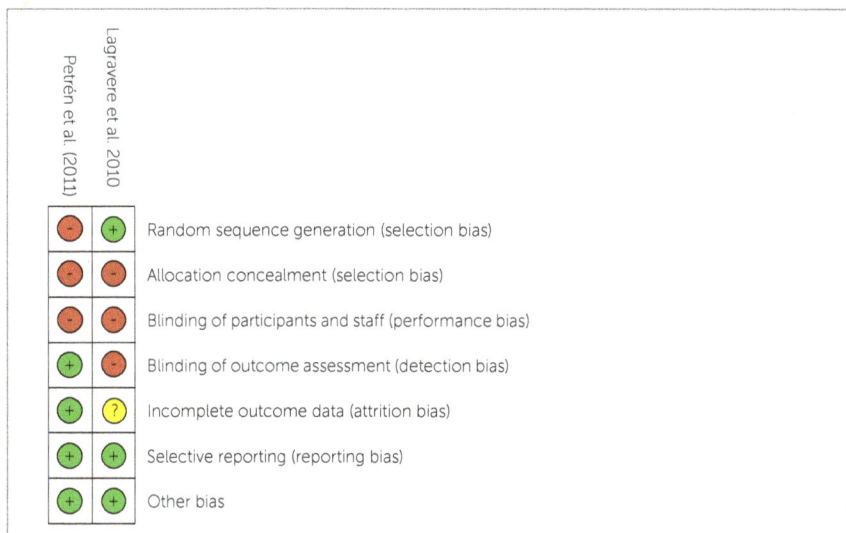

Figure 3 - Risk of bias summary for RCTs studies.

Table 3 - Downs and Black checklist for non-randomized studies.

ALL CRITERIA	DESCRIPTION OF CRITERIA (with additional explanation as required, determined by consensus of raters)	POSSIBLE ANSWERS	Cozzani et al[8]	Godoy et al[4]	Mutinelli et al[16]	Primožič et al[22]
1	Is the hypothesis/aim/objective of the study clearly described? Must be explicit	0/1	1	1	1	1
2	Are the main outcomes to be measured clearly described in the Introduction or Methods sections?	0/1	1	1	1	1
3	Are the characteristics of the patients included in the study clearly described?	0/1	1	1	1	1
4	Are the interventions of interest clearly described?	0/1	1	1	1	1
5	Are the distributions of principal confounders in each group of subjects to be compared clearly described?	0/1/2	0	2	2	0
6	Are the main findings of the study clearly described?	0/1	1	1	1	1
7	Does the study provide estimates of the random variability in the data for the main outcomes?	0/1	1	1	1	1
8	Have all important adverse events that may be a consequence of the intervention been reported?	0/1	1	1	0	1
9	Have the characteristics of patients lost to follow-up been described?	0/1	0	0	0	0
10	Have actual probability values been reported (e.g. 0.035 rather than <0.05) for the main outcomes except where the probability value is less than 0.001?	0/1	0	1	1	0
11	Were the subjects asked to participate in the study representative of the entire population from which they were recruited?	0/0/1	0	1	0	0
12	Were those subjects who were prepared to participate representative of the entire population from which they were recruited?	0/0/1	0	1	0	0
13	Were the staff, places, and facilities where the patients were treated, representative of the treatment the majority of patients receive?	0/0/1	0	1	0	0
14	Was an attempt made to blind study subjects to the intervention they have received?	0/0/1	0	0	0	0
15	Was an attempt made to blind those measuring the main outcomes of the intervention?	0/0/1	0	1	0	0
16	If any of the results of the study were based on "data dredging", was this made clear?	0/0/1	1	1	1	1
17	In trials and cohort studies, do the analyses adjust for different lengths of follow-up of patients, or in case control studies, is the time period between the intervention and outcome the same for cases and controls?	0/0/1	1	0	0	1
18	Were the statistical tests used to assess the main outcomes appropriate?	0/0/1	1	1	1	1
19	Was compliance with the intervention/s reliable?	0/0/1	1	0	1	1
20	Were the main outcome measures used accurate (valid and reliable)?	0/0/1	1	1	1	1
21	Were the patients in different intervention groups (trials and cohort studies) or were the cases and controls (case-control studies) recruited from the same population?	0/0/1	0	1	0	0
22	Were study subjects in different intervention groups (trials and cohort studies) or were the cases and controls (case-control studies) recruited over the same time?	0/0/1	1	1	0	0
23	Were study subjects randomized to intervention groups?	0/0/1	0	1	0	0
24	Was the randomized intervention assignment concealed from both patients and health care staff until recruitment was complete and irrevocable?	0/0/1	0	0	0	0
25	Was there adequate adjustment for confounding in the analyses from which the main findings were drawn?	0/0/1	0	0	1	1
26	Were losses of patients to follow-up taken into account?	0/0/1	0	1	0	1
27	Did the study have sufficient power to detect a clinically important effect where the probability value for a difference being due to chance <5%	1 - 5	0	4	4	0
TOTAL		Max. 32	13	25	18	14

0/1= No/Yes; 0/1/2= No/Partially/Yes; 0/0/1= Unable to determine/No/Yes.

Table 4A - Characteristics and data of included studies.

Author/ Year	Sample description	Type of crossbite	Expander/ Activation time	Activation rate	Retainer appliance/ Retention time
Cozzani et al[8] (2007)	» Group A (TG) = 31 (20 F/11M) CB experimental 7.3±1y » Group B (CG) = 30 (13F/17M) CB untreated 8.4y » Group C (CG) = 30 (13F/17M) CB untreated 10.8y	unilateral or bilateral posterior crossbite	Haas Group A (primary second molars and canines) mean 20 days (until permanent first molars correction)	RME once or twice/day 0.25 mm-0.5 mm/day	Haas at least 8m mean 1.1y
Lagravère et al[17] (2010)	» Group TG= 20 (15F/5M) CB experimental 14.05±1.35y » Group CG= 21 (15F/6M) CB untreated 12.86± 1.19y	posterior crossbite	Hyrax (until posterior CB overcorrection)	RME twice/day 0.5 mm	Hyrax/ 6 months
Godoy et al[4] (2011)	» Group QDH= 33 (26F/7M) CB-experimental 8.00±0.79y » Group EP= 33 (18F/15M) CB-experimental 7.82±0.85y » Group CG= 33 (14F/19M) CB-untreated 8.09±0.81y	unilateral posterior crossbite	QDH adjusted for buccal root torque mean 4.24±2.05m EP acrylic covering mean 6.12±3.25m (until CB correction) evaluated every 4 weeks	SME once a month QDH expanded 1 side to pass central fossa; and the other to the molar-band EP-0.25 mm/ week	Plate placed/ To be used 24 hours/ day for 3 months and for 3 more months just at night
Petrén et al[21] (2011)	» Group QDH= 20 (11F/9M) CB-experimental 9.00±1.19y » Group EP= 15 (10F/5M) 5M noncompliance excluded CB-experimental 8.5± 1.02y » Group CG= 20 (9F/11M) NCB- 8.8± 0.5y	unilateral posterior crossbite	QDH adjusted for buccal root torque QDH and EP (until CB correction) CG untreated	SME QDH activated 10 mm, reactivated every 6 weeks/ recemented EP 0.2 mm/week	QDH 6 months EP / 6 months 24 hours/day
Primožič et al[22] (2013)	» Group TG= 30 (17F/13M) CB experimental - 5.3± 0.7 y » Group CG= 30 (17F/13)M NCB- 5.3± 0.7 y	unilateral posterior crossbite, mandibular lateral shift	Acrylic plate expander cemented/ 4 weeks	SSME 0.25 mm/ every 2 days	Acrylic plate expander inactive/ 4 weeks Acrylic removable plate/ 4 months
Mutinelli et al[16] (2015)	» Group TG= 18 (10F/8M) CB experimental- 7.6±1.0y dental Class II » Group CG= 18 (10F/8M) CB-untreated- 13.1±1.6y dental Class II	unilateral or bilateral posterior crossbite	Haas/(primary second molars and canines) mean 28 days (until permanent first molars correction)	RME once or twice/ day 0.2 mm-0.4 mm/day	Haas/ 7 months 1.4y

TG= Treatment group; CG = Control group; F= female; M= male; PFM= Permanent first molar; PSM= Primary second molar; IC= Intercuspid canines; y= years; m= months; RME= Rapid maxillary expansion; QDH= Quad-Helix appliance;
EP= Expansion plate; NCB= Non crossbite group; CB= Crossbite; UPC= Unilateral posterior crossbite.

Table 4B - Characteristics and data of included studies.

Author/ Year	Measurements	Follow-up time	Overcorrec-tion	Experimental group x Control group (P value)	Relapse measurements after follow-up	Crossbite corrected after follow-up	Conclusion
Cozzaniet al[8] (2007)	» Maxillary arch width: » PFM- center of the fossa » PSM-center of the fossa » IC-cusp tip » DC	minimum 1y after appliance removal 2.4±1.7y	yes - primary teeth no - permanent first molar	PFM: ≤0.01 PSM: ≤0.01 IC: ≤0.05	PFM = 0.9% PSM = 6.0% IC = 5.5%	yes	Relapse: PFM < PSM Overexpand PSM PFM was stable for 2y 4m after treatment
Lagravere et al[17] (2010)	» PC- center of pulp chamber in molars and tip of premolars buccal pulp horn » MBA-mesiobuccal root apex of molars » BA-buccal root apex of premolars » AIB-outer cortex of alveolar bone at the vertical level of the root apex » mm » CBCT	Before fixed bonding (12m) long-term post-relapse	yes	all groups P<.001	PC16-PC26 = 27% PC14-PC24 = 39% MBA16-MBA26= 28% BA14-BA24 = 18% AIB16-AIB26 = 51% AIB14-AIB24 = 20%	yes	aprox 4mm (70%) expansion - at T4 at molars Dental expansion> skeletal expansion Midpalatal suture separation on TG. No significant changes at the level of the pterigoid plates TG=CG
Godoy et al[4] (2011)	Maxillary arch width: PSM-center of the fossa IC- cusp tip DC	6m after appliance removal	no	IMD: P<0.001 (QDH=EP; QDH≠ CG; EP≠ CG) ICD: P= 0.354	PSF QDH= 2.2% EP = 1.7% IC QDH = 0.3% EP = 0%	yes 9.1% of the each sample showed relapse	QDH=EP for correct posterior crossbite QDH> breakage EP> lost appliances QDH< treatment time Treatment may be performed in 1y for posterior CB correction and 6m for retention
Petrén et al[21] (2011)	Maxillary arch width: PSM-gingival margin (GM) PSM-mesiobuccal cusp tip (MCT) IC-gingival margin (GM) IC-buccal cusp tip (BCT) DC	QDH and EP group 4y after correction	no	IMD (MCT): P=NR (CG>QDH,EP) ICD (BCT): P=NR (CG>QDH)	PSM QDH = 1.6% EP = 5.6% IC (GM) QDH = 4.9% EP = 5.6% IC (BCT) QDH = 1.2% EP = 0.6%	yes	The long-term stability of crossbite correction in the mixed dentition is favorable. Results: QDH=EP
Primozic et al[22] (2013)	Palatal surface area (mm²) 3D digital DC	12 months later 18 months later 30 months later	yes	Surface(mm²): P= NR NS (TG=CG)	Palatal surface area (TG) = - 0.5%	26.7% of the TG showed relapse	Treatment of unilateral CB in the deciduous dentition also create conditions for normal occlusal and craniofacial development. Improves facial symmetry and increase palatal area and volume
Mutinelli et al[16] (2015)	Maxillary arch width: PSM and IC (mm); 3D digital DC	In the permanent dentition 5.3±0.8y	yes - primary teeth no - permanent first molar	IC P= 0.02 PSM P= 0.001	PSM = 1% IC = 5.1%	yes	In patients in canine Class II, early treatment of lateral CB with a modified Haas expander anchored to deciduous teeth is effective and presented stable results until the stage of permanent dentition

TG= Treatment group; CG = Control group; PFM= Permanent first molar; PSM= Primary second molar; IC= Intercuspid canines; DC= Dental cast; y= years; m= months; RME= Rapid maxillary expansion; QDH= Quad-Helix appliance; EP= Expansion plate; IMD= Intermolar distance; ICD= intercanine distance; GM = Gingival margin; MCT= Mesiobuccal cusp tips; BCT= Gingival margin and buccal cusp tips; NCB= Non crossbite group; CB= Crossbite; NS= Not significant; NR= Not reported.

DISCUSSION

The duration of the steady retention after maxillary expansion that guarantees the correction of posterior crossbite is not well established in the literature and this was the main reason that led to this systematic review.

The evidence collected in this systematic review combined low, medium and high risk of bias studies. The main drawback in RCTs and non-RCTs was blinding, which is unfeasible in the assessed type of intervention. In non-RCTs, another main problem was the description of the characteristics of subjects lost to follow-up.

However, the heterogeneity among the studies made the comparison difficult. Dental and skeletal measures varied widely, as follows: intermolar distance measured between the center of the fossae of maxillary permanent first molars,[4,8,16] measured between the mesiobuccal cusp tips and gingival margin,[21] distance between the center of the fossae of maxillary primary second molars,[8] intercanine distance measured between cusp tips,[4,8,21] gingival margin,[21] palatal surface area,[22] and distance of center of pulp chamber in molars and tip of premolar buccal pulp horn, mesial buccal root apex of molars, buccal root apex of premolars, outer cortex of alveolar bone at the vertical level of the root apex.[17]

The appliances used for maxillary expansion in the studies included were Haas,[8,16] Hyrax,[17] QDH,[4,21] removable acrylic expansion plate,[4,21] and cemented acrylic plate.[22] All authors used the same expander appliance for retention of the maxillary expansion,[4,8,16,17,21,22] except the quad-helix group in the study from Godoy et al,[4] who used a removable Hawley retainer for retention.

The control group also differed among the studies. In some studies, subjects presenting posterior crossbite were included in the control group,[4,8,16,17] while other authors selected only patients with no posterior crossbite (normal occlusion or a different malocclusion with no transverse discrepancies) for the control group.[21,22] When these studies featured more than one control group, it was taken into account only the group of subjects with similar occlusion.[17]

Four studies[4,8,16,17] where the control group comprised subjects with posterior crossbite were approved by ethics committees and the authors followed their guidelines. Lagravere et al[17] benefited from a treatment control group with delay of 12 months, and there were no negative consequences for the treatment of patients.

However, that may be an ethical issue, since delaying the correction of a problem, which is known to be better solved as early as possible may be considered unethical. This was the reason why Petrén et al[21] did not include a control group of crossbite untreated subjects as their follow-up reached three years after treatment.

Overcorrection of the posterior crossbite is recommended by some authors[4,19,28,29] due to the tooth crown buccal inclination, which is usually a consequence of tooth-supported expanders.[21] The physiology of the relapse demonstrate that molars tend to return to their original buccolingual inclination after retention is discontinued, that would not allow relapse of the posterior crossbite if overexpansion was performed.[11] Four of the included studies[8,16,17,22] expanded the maxilla until the crossbite was overcorrected in all groups, particularly it was performed only in primary teeth for Cozzani et al[8] and Mutinelli et al.[16] In two articles[4,21] however, no overexpansion was produced.

Petrén et al[21] claims that overcorrection might be unnecessary, since their results without overexpansion were found to be stable in a long-term, the rate of relapse was 1.6% in the intermolar cusp distance, even so to avoid buccal tipping of the molars, the appliance was adjusted for buccal root torque.

Authors that used Haas as retainers for at least 7 months[16] and 8 months[8] presented a relapse of 1.0% and 0.9% respectively, in the intermolar distance. These results may suggest that a longer time of retention after maxillary expansion — that is, more than 7 months — would favor stability and less relapse. Moreover, the difference of the mean relapse was only 0.1 mm, which may be clinically irrelevant.

Lagravere et al[17] who used Hyrax as a retainer, observed the highest relapse of measurements, 27% in the molar distance, probably related to patient age, since their sample of the treated group was 14 years. All others authors[4,8,16,21,22] presented younger samples, between 5.1 a 9.7 years old, in the mixed dentition.

When removable appliances were used as retainers for 6 months, a relapse of 3.2%[4] and 1.2%[21] was found in the intermolar distance. Godoy et al[4] instructed the patients to use the removable plate 24 hours a day for 3 months and just at night for 3 more months, while Petrén et al[21] recommended a 24-hour/day use for 6 months. That may have influenced on the first authors' higher rates of relapse.

The overall comparison among fixed and removable retainers when a six-month retention was used, showed a very small range of variation, between 1.2%[21] and 3.2%[4] in the intermolar distance. When comparing treatment groups which had as their expander/retainer the QDH and EP, Petrén et al[21] observed similar results. According to Godoy et al,[4] the greatest disadvantage of EP was lost appliances and subsequent laboratory costs, and QDH's frequent breakage. In spite of this, one of the most cited disadvantages of removable appliances in the literature is the need for patients' compliance.[4,30]

Primozic et al[22] assessed skeletal measures through the palatal surface area. Considering a 30-month follow-up, there was no relapse in this skeletal measure. On the contrary, there was an increment of 6.38%. They found that increase in the experimental group to be similar to or greater than the increase observed in the control group of normal occlusion. According to the authors, that indicates the reestablishment of a normal growth rate and the condition for normal occlusion and craniofacial development.

However, relapse in dental and skeletal measures does not necessarily represent a relapse in the posterior crossbite. Four authors have reported recurrence of posterior crossbite. That relapse is expressed in percentage of patients as reported by authors or calculated according to their data: 0%[16,21] (Haas group for at least 7 months; removable plate group, 6 months of retention), 5%[21] (QDH group, 6 months of retention), 9.1%[4] (QDH and removable plate, 6 months of retention), 26.7%[22]

(acrylic cemented plate group, cemented as retention for 1 month and removable for 4 months). Relapse is not a rare event after correction of posterior crossbite.[21,22,30]

Primozic et al[22] showed the biggest recurrence of posterior crossbite after the treatment, amounting of 8 participants, they suggest that part of this relapse could be explained because the subjects expressed a Class III growth trend, inverse overjet and facial asymmetries.

Limitations of this review are: not enough RCTs were found that were able to answer our question; additionally, no study specifically aimed at answering this question, nor did any study assessed or compared different periods of retention in patients wearing the same kind of appliance. Our systematic review clearly shows the need for randomized controlled trials that specifically assess different periods of retention with the same appliances and the stability of correction of the posterior crossbite, so that a protocol may be created for successful treatment maintenance.

The clinical implication of this systematic review is that six months of retention of crossbite correction used 24 hours a day should be able to maintain the results obtained. However, the evidence for this conclusion is moderate.

CONCLUSION

Based on the results from this systematic review, there is moderate evidence to assert that six months of retention with either fixed or removable appliances seem to be enough to avoid relapse or to guarantee minimal changes in a short-term follow-up.

REFERENCES

1. Keski-Nisula K, Lehto R, Lusa V, Keski-Nisula L, Varrela J. Occurrence of malocclusion and need of orthodontic treatment in early mixed dentition. Am J Orthod Dentofacial Orthop. 2003 Dec;124(6):631-8.

2. Tausche E, Luck O, Harzer W. Prevalence of malocclusions in the early mixed dentition and orthodontic treatment need. Eur J Orthod. 2004 June;26(3):237-44.

3. Jonsson T, Arnlaugsson S, Karlsson KO, Ragnarsson B, Arnarson EO, Magnusson TE. Orthodontic treatment experience and prevalence of malocclusion traits in an Icelandic adult population. Am J Orthod Dentofacial Orthop. 2007 Jan;131(1):8.e11-8.

4. Godoy F, Godoy-Bezerra J, Rosenblatt A. Treatment of posterior crossbite comparing 2 appliances: a community-based trial. Am J Orthod Dentofacial Orthop. 2011 Jan;139(1):e45-52.

5. Egermark-Eriksson I, Carlsson GE, Magnusson T, Thilander B. A longitudinal study on malocclusion in relation to signs and symptoms of craniomandibular disorders in children and adolescents. Eur J Orthod. 1990 Nov;12(4):399-407.

6. Thilander B, Wahlund S, Lennartsson B. The effect of early interceptive treatment in children with posterior cross-bite. Eur J Orthod. 1984 Feb;6(1):25-34.

7. Petrén S, Bondemark L, Söderfeldt B. A systematic review concerning early orthodontic treatment of unilateral posterior crossbite. Angle Orthod. 2003 Oct;73(5):588-96.

8. Cozzani M, Guiducci A, Mirenghi S, Mutinelli S, Siciliani G. Arch width changes with a rapid maxillary expansion appliance anchored to the primary teeth. Angle Orthod. 2007 Mar;77(2):296-302.

9. Defraia E, Marinelli A, Baroni G, Tollaro I. Dentoalveolar effects induced by a removable expansion plate. Prog Orthod. 2007;8(2):260-7.

10. Flores-Mir C. Grinding is effective in early orthodontic treatment of unilateral posterior crossbite. Evid Based Dent. 2005;6(1):24.

11. Handelman CS, Wang L, BeGole EA, Haas AJ. Nonsurgical rapid maxillary expansion in adults: report on 47 cases using the Haas expander. Angle Orthod. 2000 Apr;70(2):129-44.

12. Lee KJ, Park YC, Park JY, Hwang WS. Miniscrew-assisted nonsurgical palatal expansion before orthognathic surgery for a patient with severe mandibular prognathism. Am J Orthod Dentofacial Orthop. 2010 June;137(6):830-9.

13. Haas AJ. Long-term posttreatment evaluation of rapid palatal expansion. Angle Orthod. 1980 July;50(3):189-217.

14. Huynh T, Kennedy DB, Joondeph DR, Bollen AM. Treatment response and stability of slow maxillary expansion using Haas, hyrax, and quad-helix appliances: a retrospective study. Am J Orthod Dentofacial Orthop. 2009 Sept;136(3):331-9.

15. Wong CA, Sinclair PM, Keim RG, Kennedy DB. Arch dimension changes from successful slow maxillary expansion of unilateral posterior crossbite. Angle Orthod. 2011 July;81(4):616-23

16. Mutinelli S, Cozzani M. Rapid maxillary expansion in early-mixed dentition: effectiveness of increasing arch dimension with anchorage on deciduous teeth. Eur J Paediatr Dent. 2015 June;16(2):115-22.

17. Lagravère MO, Carey J, Heo G, Toogood RW, Major PW. Transverse, vertical, and anteroposterior changes from bone-anchored maxillary expansion vs traditional rapid maxillary expansion: a randomized clinical trial. Am J Orthod Dentofacial Orthop. 2010 Mar;137(3):304.e1-12; discussion 304-5.

18. Wangsrimongkol T, Manosudprasit M, Pisek P, Leelasinjaroen P. Correction of complete maxillary crossbite with severe crowding using Hyrax expansion and fixed appliance. J Med Assoc Thai. 2013 Sept;96 Suppl 4:S149-56.

19. Bell RA, Le Compte EJ. The effects of maxillary expansion using a quad-helix appliance during the deciduous and mixed dentitions. Am J Orthod. 1981 Feb;79(2):152-61.

20. Bjerklin K. Follow-up control of patients with unilateral posterior cross-bite treated with expansion plates or the quad-helix appliance. J Orofac Orthop. 2000;61(2):112-24.

21. Petrén S, Bjerklin K, Bondemark L. Stability of unilateral posterior crossbite correction in the mixed dentition: a randomized clinical trial with a 3-year follow-up. Am J Orthod Dentofacial Orthop. 2011 Jan;139(1):e73-81.

22. Primožič J, Richmond S, Kau CH, Zhurov A, Ovsenik M. Three-dimensional evaluation of early crossbite correction: a longitudinal study. Eur J Orthod. 2013 Feb;35(1):7-13.

23. Gurel HG, Memili B, Erkan M, Sukurica Y. Long-term effects of rapid maxillary expansion followed by fixed appliances. Angle Orthod. 2010 Jan;80(1):5-9.

24. Kau CH, Zhurov A, Scheer R, Bouwman S, Richmond S. The feasibility of measuring three-dimensional facial morphology in children. Orthod Craniofac Res. 2004 Nov;7(4):198-204.

25. McNamara JA Jr, Lione R, Franchi L, Angelieri F, Cevidanes LH, Darendeliler MA, et al. The role of rapid maxillary expansion in the promotion of oral and general health. Prog Orthod. 2015;16:33.

26. Higgins JPT, Green S, editors. Cochrane handbook for systematic reviews of interventions. 2009. version 5.1.0, updated March 2011.

27. Downs SH, Black N. The feasibility of creating a checklist for the assessment of the methodological quality both of randomised and non-randomised studies of health care interventions. J Epidemiol Community Health. 1998 June;52(6):377-84.

28. Mew J. Relapse following maxillary expansion. A study of twenty-five consecutive cases. Am J Orthod. 1983 Jan;83(1):56-61.

29. Sandikçioğlu M, Hazar S. Skeletal and dental changes after maxillary expansion in the mixed dentition. Am J Orthod Dentofacial Orthop. 1997 Mar;111(3):321-7.

30. Agostino P, Ugolini A, Signori A, Silvestrini-Biavati A, Harrison JE, Riley P. Orthodontic treatment for posterior crossbites. Cochrane Database Syst Rev. 2014 Aug 8;(8):CD000979.

13

Dental and skeletal effects of combined headgear used alone or in association with rapid maxillary expansion

Milton Meri Benitez Farret[1], Eduardo Martinelli de Lima[2], Marcel M. Farret[3], Laura Lutz de Araújo[4]

Objective: The aim of this study was to assess the effects of combined headgear used alone or in association with rapid maxillary expansion, as the first step for Class II malocclusion treatment. **Methods:** The sample comprised 61 patients divided into three groups: Group 1, combined headgear (CH); Group 2, CH + rapid maxillary expansion (CH + RME); and Group 3, control (CG). In Group 1, patients were treated with combined headgear until Class I molar relationship was achieved. In Group 2, the protocol for headgear was the same; however, patients were previously subject to rapid maxillary expansion. **Results:** Results showed distal displacement of maxillary molars for both experimental groups ($p < 0.001$), with distal tipping only in Group 1 (CH) ($p < 0.001$). There was restriction of forward maxillary growth in Group 2 (CH + RME) ($p < 0.05$) and clockwise rotation of the maxilla in Group 1 (CH) ($p < 0.05$). **Conclusion:** Based on the results, it is possible to suggest that treatment with both protocols was efficient; however, results were more significant for Group 2 (CH + RME) with less side effects.

Keywords: Cephalometry. Extraoral traction appliance. Angle Class II malocclusion.

[1] Professor of Orthodontics, Undergraduate Program, Universidade Federal de Santa Maria, Santa Maria, Rio Grande do Sul, Brazil.

[2] Adjunct professor of Orthodontics, Pontifícia Universidade Católica do Rio Grande do Sul (PUC/RS), Porto Alegre, Rio Grande do Sul, Brazil.

[3] PhD in Orthodontics, Pontifícia Universidade Católica do Rio Grande do Sul (PUCRS), Porto Alegre, Rio Grande do Sul, Brazil.

[4] MSc in Orthodontics, Pontifícia Universidade Católica do Rio Grande do Sul (PUC/RS), Porto Alegre, Rio Grande do Sul, Brazil.

» The authors report no commercial, proprietary or financial interest in the products or companies described in this article.

Milton Meri Benitez Farret
Rua Floriano Peixoto 1000/113, Santa Maria, RS, Brazil
E-mail: milton@farretodontologia.com.br

INTRODUCTION

Class II malocclusion can result from multiple combinations of dental and/or skeletal relationships established between the maxilla and mandible.[1] Headgear followed by the use of full fixed orthodontic appliance can be considered the gold standard treatment for children and adolescents with skeletal Class II malocclusion.[2] Extraoral forces hold maxillary forward displacement while the mandible grows forward naturally. Since the 1950s, orthodontists have used headgears successfully and produced favorable dental and orthopedic effects proved by cephalometric analysis.[3] There is scientific evidence that headgear can reduce facial convexity and improve the sagittal relationship between upper and lower dental arches.[4-7]

The morphological characteristics of Class II malocclusions usually include transverse maxillary deficiency.[8,9,10] In those cases, patients should undergo rapid maxillary expansion.[9,10,11] According to Haas[10] and Lima Filho et al,[9] there is marked upper arch constriction in the region between canines in individuals with Class II, Division 1 malocclusion. Maxillary constriction should be corrected by rapid maxillary expansion, followed by the use of headgear whenever necessary. Headgear appliances provide different force systems according to the direction of traction.[12] Cervical headgear is generally indicated for patients with hypodivergent facial types, while high-pull headgear is more commonly used in hyperdivergent faces.[13-16] Nevertheless, combined headgear has been used in a wide variety of cranial-facial architetures.[17]

From the clinical orthodontist's standpoint, the question is whether the benefits of rapid maxillary expansion before combined traction headgear is used are really worth it when treating Class II malocclusion. Therefore, the aim of this study was to assess maxillary dental and skeletal effects caused by combined headgear used alone or in association with rapid maxillary expansion in adolescents with Class II, Division 1 malocclusion.

MATERIAL AND METHODS

The experimental sample comprised 41 individuals (18 boys and 23 girls) with Class II, Division 1 malocclusion, aged between 9 and 13 years old and treated by combined headgear (CH) as the first step of orthodontic treatment. A total of 20 individuals (8 boys and 12 girls) with Class I malocclusion were assessed during the development of dentition and served as controls.

Research subjects were selected from the records of 400 individuals available in the files of the Clinic of Orthodontics, School of Dentistry, Pontifícia Universidade Católica do Rio Grande do Sul, Brazil. All treated and control individuals had good general and oral health conditions, were in the pubertal growth period, and had less than 3 mm of crowding in the lower arch. The research was approved by the university Institutional Review Board (10/05127).

Initial records (T_1) included patient's medical and dental history, dental casts, and Lateral cephalograms. Dental casts determined the diagnosis of Class II malocclusion associated or not with transverse maxillary deficiency. In Class II, first molars should at least present a cusp-to-cusp relationship. Transverse maxillary deficiency was determined when the distance between maxillary molars was 4 mm less than the distance between mandibular molars, as described previously.[16] Based on anteroposterior and transversal first molar relationship, subjects were allocated into Group 1 (Class II, normal transverse maxilla) or Group 2 (Class II, transverse maxillary deficiency). Group 3 comprised control individuals with Class I molar relationship and normal transverse maxilla.

Subjects in Group 1 (n = 20, 8 boys and 12 girls) had Class II malocclusion with normal transverse maxilla and were treated with combined headgear (CH), 12 to 14 hours per day, during six months. The headgear outer bow was parallel to the inner bow and had hooks in the region of first molars. The inner bow was expanded 2 mm before being inserted into the molar tubes. Forces of 300 g/f were applied in both parietal and cervical direction on each side. The equation $V_r = \sqrt{V_c^2 + V_p^2}$, in which V_r is the resultant vector, V_c the cervical vector, and V_p is the parietal vector, established that the resultant vector was equal to 424 f/g. Subjects allocated in Group 2 (n = 21, 10 boys and 11 girls) had Class II malocclusion associated with transverse maxillary deficiency. Thus, before headgear therapy, patients underwent rapid maxillary expansion (RME + CH) during 14 days. A modified Haas expander, banded to first molars and bonded up to first premolars or first deciduous molars, was activated four times a day on the first day and twice a day thereafter, until transverse overcorrection was achieved. On the seventh day of expansion, patients started the 6-month therapy with combined headgear, following the same protocol applied for Group 1 (CH). In Group 3, control subjects (n = 20, 8 boys and 12 girls) had Class I malocclusion with normal transverse maxilla. During the 6-month period of the study, they underwent space supervision procedures only, including space maintenance or wearing of deciduous teeth.

At baseline, cephalometric measurements showed that all groups were representative of slightly hyperdivergent individuals. Mandibular plane angle (SN.GoGn) was $36.9 \pm 3.9°$ in Group 1 (CH), $36.4 \pm 6.3°$ in Group 2 (RME+CH) and $36.9 \pm 4.1°$ in Group 3 (control). On the other hand, ANB angle highlighted a Class II skeletal pattern in the treated groups (CH = $5 \pm 1.9°$, RME+CH = $5.9 \pm 1.8°$) and a Class I skeletal pattern in the control group ($3.7 \pm 2.2°$).

Follow-up records (T_2) of experimental groups (Group 1 [CH], Group 2 [RME+CH]) included lateral cephalograms taken when Class I molar relationship was achieved, on average, six months after headgear therapy onset. The follow-up records of Group 3 (control) were taken six months later, on average; similar to the experimental groups when Class I molar relationship was achieved. Cephalograms were manually taken in random order. Afterwards, the cephalometric landmarks were digitized with the aid of Dentofacial Planner Plus (DFP 2.0) software by an operator blind to subject and group. Cephalometric measurements were selected to assess dental and skeletal effects of treatment on the maxilla (Fig 1). Statistical analysis was performed by Student's t-test for comparison between T_1 and T_2 in each group. One-way analysis of variance (ANOVA) and Tukey's multiple comparison tests were applied to compare differences ($T_2 - T_1$) between groups.

RESULTS
Molars

Distal movement of maxillary molars occurred in both experimental groups during the study period ($p < 0.001$), but distal tipping occurred only in Group 1 (CH) ($p < 0.001$) (Tables 1 and 2). However, the amount of distal tipping of maxillary molars did not differ whether the headgear was used alone or in association with maxillary expansion ($p > 0.05$) (Table 4). There was no extrusion of maxillary molars in either one of the experimental groups ($p > 0.05$).

Maxilla

Clockwise rotation of the maxilla occurred between T_1 and T_2 only in Group 1 (CH) ($p < 0.05$) (Table 1). Nevertheless, the values of maxillary clockwise rotation did not differ whether the headgear was used alone or in association with maxillary expansion ($p > 0.05$) (Table 4). There was restriction of forward maxillary growth between T_1 and T_2 only in Group 2 (CH + RME) ($p < 0.05$) (Table 2). However, the variation occurring in Group 2 did not differ from that found in Groups 1 and 3 ($p > 0.05$) (Table 4).

Class I molar relationship was achieved in 6.5 ± 1 months in Group 1 and 5.5 ± 1.1 months in Group 2.

DISCUSSION

The combined headgear is well indicated to treat patients with Class II malocclusion and mesodivergent or hyperdivergent facial patterns.[12,14,15] On the other hand,

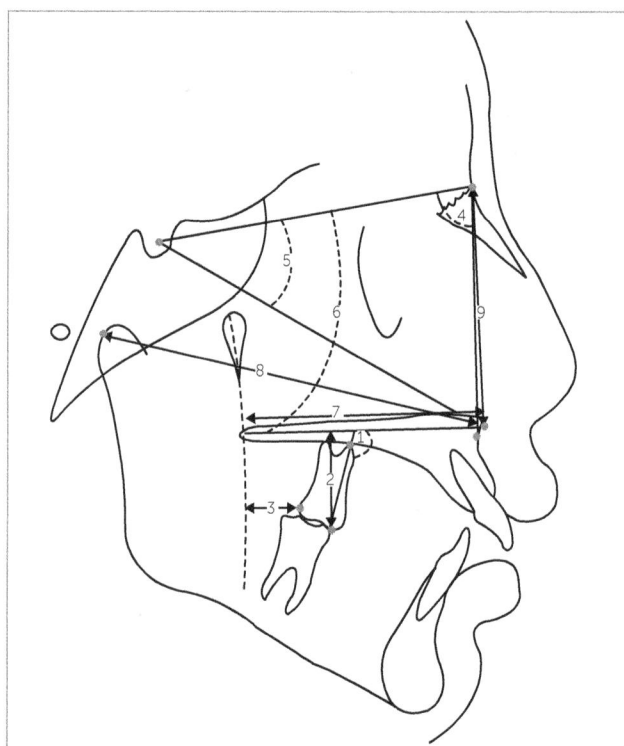

Figure 1 - Anatomical tracing and cephalometric measurements. Dental measurements: molar inclination (1), molar height (2) and anteroposterior molar (3). Maxillary measurements: SNA (4), SN.Ptm-Sn (5), SN.PP(6), Ptm-Sn (7), Co-Sn (8) and N-Sn (9).

Table 1 - Means, standard deviation, mean difference and Student's t-test comparing initial (T_1) and control (T_2) values in Group 1 (CH) (n = 20).

Measurements	T_1		T_2		Mean difference	P-value
	Mean	SD	Mean	SD		
Molars						
Molar inclination (degrees)	101.9	3.8	108.3	6.3	6.4	0.000***
Molar height (mm)	19.1	2.2	19.0	2.4	-0.1	0.66
Anteroposterior molar (mm)	-8.7	2.4	-6.4	2.3	2.3	0.000***
Maxilla						
SNA (degrees)	81.4	3.8	80.7	3.3	-0.3	0.24
SN.SSn (degrees)	23.4	1.6	24.0	1.6	0.5	0.02*
SN.PP (degrees)	10.5	2.1	11.7	2.3	1.2	0.001**
Ptm-Sn (mm)	51.1	3.4	50.7	2.9	-0.4	0.14
Co-Sn (mm)	88.4	5.1	89.7	5.2	1.2	0.01*
N-Sn (mm)	54.5	4.1	56.2	3.7	1.6	0.000***

* $p < 0.05$; ** $p < 0.01$; *** $p < 0.001$.

Table 2 - Means, standard deviation, mean difference and Student's t-test comparing initial (T_1) and control (T_2) values in Group 2 (CH + RME) (n = 21).

Measurements	T_1		T_2		Mean difference	P-value
	Mean	SD	Mean	SD		
Molars						
Molar inclination (degrees)	102.8	3.2	104.3	4.4	1.4	0.18
Molar height (mm)	21.0	2.3	21.5	2.2	0.4	0.07
Anteroposterior molar (mm)	-8.0	3.1	-6.5	2.9	1.4	0.001**
Maxilla						
SNA (degrees)	81.3	3.5	80.7		-0.6	0.02*
SN.SSn (degrees)	23.5	2.2	23.8	2.3	0.3	0.15
SN.PP (degrees)	9.7	2.8	10.3	2.8	0.5	0.06
Ptm-Sn (mm)	52.1	3.6	52.1	3.3	0.0	0.77
Co-Sn (mm)	89.7	4.6	89.8	4.7	0.1	0.75
N-Sn (mm)	54.0	2.5	55.2	2.8	1.1	0.001**

* $p < 0.05$; ** $p < 0.01$; *** $p < 0.001$.

Table 3 - Means, standard deviation, mean difference and Student's t-test comparing initial (T_1) and control (T_2) values in Group 3 (C) (n = 20).

Measurements	T_1		T_2		Mean difference	P-value
	Mean	SD	Mean	SD		
Molars						
Molar inclination (degrees)	102.2	3.6	102.8	5.9	0.6	0.62
Molar height (mm)	20.7	2.1	21.1	2.6	0.4	0.14
Anteroposterior molar (mm)	-8.4	2.8	-8.7	3.5	-0.2	0.60
Maxilla						
SNA (degrees)	80.0	3.5	79.9	2.9	-0.3	0.91
SN.SSn (degrees)	23.8	2.6	23.2	2.4	-0.5	0.18
SN.PP (degrees)	9.6	3.0	9.1	3.0	-0.4	0.25
Ptm-Sn (mm)	50.3	2.1	51.0	2.8	0.6	0.06
Co-Sn (mm)	86.4	4.0	87.2	4.1	0.8	0.01*
N-Sn (mm)	51.2	2.7	51.9	2.9	0.7	0.04*

* $p < 0.05$; ** $p < 0.01$; *** $p < 0.001$.

Table 4 - Minimum and maximum differences, means, standard deviation and one-way analysis of variance supplemented by Tuke's multiple comparisons test comparing groups at two intervals.

Measurements	Groups	Difference ($T_2 - T_1$)			SD	P-value
		Minimum	Maximum	Mean		
Molars						
Molar inclination (degrees)	Group 1 (CH)	-1.0	18.6	6.4^B	5.2	
	Group 2 (CH + RME)	-11.9	8.0	1.4^{AB}	5.0	0.002**
	Group 3 (Control)	-8.4	14.0	0.6^A	5.7	
Molar height (mm)	Group 1 (CH)	-1.7	2.4	-0.1	1.1	
	Group 2 (CH + RME)	-1.7	3.4	0.4	1.1	0.22
	Group 3 (Control)	-1.6	2.8	0.4	1.1	
Anteriorposterior molar (mm)	Group 1 (CH)	-0.5	6.1	2.3^B	1.6	
	Group 2 (CH + RME)	-2.2	3.7	1.4^B	1.6	0.000***
	Group 3 (Control)	-3.3	6.6	-0.2^A	2.4	
Maxilla						
SNA (degrees)	Group 1 (CH)	-2.3	1.5	-0.0	1.1	
	Group 2 (CH + RME)	-2.6	1.4	-0.6	1.1	0.33
	Group 3 (Control)	-1.7	4.2	-0.3	1.3	
SN.SSn (degrees)	Group 1 (CH)	-1.0	3.0	0.5^B	0.9	
	Group 2 (CH + RME)	-2.0	3.0	0.3^{AB}	1.1	0.02*
	Group 3 (Control)	-4.1	2.7	-0.5^A	1.8	
SN.PP (degrees)	Group 1 (CH)	-1.0	4.0	1.2^B	1.4	
	Group 2 (CH + RME)	-2.4	2.7	0.5^{AB}	1.3	0.004**
	Group 3 (Control)	-3.4	2.8	-0.4^A	1.6	
Ptm-Sn (mm)	Group 1 (CH)	-3.8	1.3	-0.4	1.3	
	Group 2 (CH + RME)	-2.7	4.4	0.1	1.4	0.5
	Group 3 (Control)	-1.9	4.0	0.6	1.5	
Co-Sn (mm)	Group 1 (CH)	-3.6	5.1	1.2	2.2	
	Group 2 (CH + RME)	-3.3	5.0	0.1	1.9	0.15
	Group 3 (Control)	-1.3	3.9	0.8	1.3	
N-Sn (mm)	Group 1 (CH)	-1.1	4.8	1.6	1.3	
	Group 2 (CH + RME)	-1.2	4.4	1.1	1.3	0.11
	Group 3 (Control)	-2.5	3.4	0.7	1.4	

* $p < 0.05$; ** $p < 0.01$; *** $p < 0.001$. Means followed by the same letter do not differ.

cervical headgear is more suitable in cases of hypodivergent or mesodivergent facial patterns in which extrusion of maxillary molars would not hinder facial esthetics.[14,18,20] Molar extrusion can cause clockwise rotation of the mandible and increase anterior facial height.[17] High-pull headgear is usually recommended for cases of marked hyperdivergent facial pattern associated or not with anterior open bite.[15,20,22]

Transverse maxillary deficiency is often associated with Class II malocclusion, especially Class II, Division 1.[9,11,16] Upper arch constriction in the region of canines may lead to mandibular retrognathism, which impairs natural anteroposterior growth of the mandible.[9,11] Should transverse maxillary deficiency be diagnosed, rapid maxillary expansion should be carried out to maximize the benefits of orthodontic treatment for Class II patients.[8,10]

Mesodivergent and hyperdivergent facial patterns are predominant in cases of Class II, Division 1 malocclusion. However, the literature lacks evidence on the effects of combined headgear, associated or not with rapid maxillary expansion, over dentofacial structures. The present study analyzed the primary effects of combined headgear associated or not with rapid maxillary expansion, as the first step of comprehensive treatment of Class II malocclusions.

Follow-up records were taken when maxillary and mandibular first molars achieved Class I relationship. Despite the importance of assessment presented herein, further studies should include the final results of treatment. Cephalometric measurements were selected based on their potential to analyze the behavior of dental and skeletal maxillary structures.

The design of the appliance followed standards adopted in a previous study,[16] with the outer bow parallel to the inner bow and ending in the region of first permanent molars. The design of the headgear is strongly associated with its effects on maxillary molars. In combined headgears, longer and/or downward angled outer bows produce resultant forces that maximize vertical upward vectors, avoiding molar extrusion, but increasing distal tipping.[11] On the other hand, cervical headgears with shorter outer bows would maximize the horizontal vectors, producing a resultant force in distal direction, which can reduce the tendency towards molar inclination, but still prevent extrusion.[16] Although outer bows angled upward can eliminate molar inclination, this design may lead to undesirable extrusion of molars usually associated with clockwise rotation of the mandible, which jeopardizes Class II malocclusion treatment.[12,16,22]

Distal movement of maxillary molars was found occur in both Class II malocclusion treatment approaches. It was clear that combined headgear was effective in producing distal dental movement whether associated or not with maxillary expansion. Distal tipping of maxillary molars was found only in Group 1, which included individuals treated by headgear alone. In the present study, mean maxillary molars distal tipping was of 6.4 degrees in Group 1 (CH), very close to the value of 6.9 degrees found by Üçem and Yüksel.[22] In Group 2 (CH+RME), molar distal tipping decreased to 1.4 degrees. Despite no statistical significant differences being found between groups, it seems that maxillary expansion was useful in preventing molar inclination. The connection of maxillary molars with the expander's acrylic plate and premolars would increase anchorage against distal tipping.[16] There was no extrusion of maxillary molars either if the headgear was used alone or in association with the maxillary expander. Üçem and Yüksel have already showed that combined headgear avoided extrusion of maxillary molars.[22] This is a positive result, since molar extrusion would be an undesirable effect in the treatment of Class II malocclusion.

Restriction of forward maxillary growth is one of the objectives of the headgear used to treat Class II malocclusions.[5,6,16] In the present study, there was a reduction in the SNA angle between T_1 and T_2 only in Group 2 (CH + RME). However, comparison between groups did not show significant differences. Likewise, Üçem and Yüksel did not report effects over the SNA angle when combined headgear was used alone.[22] One can consider that the greater restriction in forward maxillary growth observed in subjects treated by rapid maxillary expansion is related to the distribution of forces over the maxilla provided by the connection of maxillary molars and premolars to the expander's acrylic plate and due to marked mobility caused by sutures separation.[10]

Clockwise rotation of the maxilla was observed between T_1 and T_2 in Group 1 (CH), but without significant difference from that found in Group 2 (CH+RME). The clockwise rotation of the maxilla is related to the direction of forces applied over maxillary molars. As molars are located in the posterior region of the arch, they can rotate the palatal plane and tilt the occlusal plane.[14] This effect is undesirable, especially in patients with excessive exposure of gingival tissues and deep bite.[14] According to O'Reilly et al,[17] clockwise rotation of the maxilla also happens in Class II patients treated with cervical headgear; and according to Üçem and Yüksel,[22] clockwise rotation may also be observed in patients treated with combined headgear. Therefore, it seems that only high-pull headgears would prevent or at least reduce maxillary clockwise rotation, based on a system of forces in which the resultant force passes through or above the center of resistance of the maxilla.[14]

Treatment effect can be considered equivalent to changes in the treated group minus changes in the control group. Comparison of mean differences (T_2 - T_1) between groups, as disclosed in Table 4, depict the main results of our study.

There was distal movement of maxillary molars in both treated groups when compared to the control group. On the other hand, distal tipping of molars was found only in Group 1 (CH). This finding is in agreement with those reported by Üçem and Yüksel.[22] Clockwise rotation of the maxilla was also considered a treatment effect of combined headgear used alone, based on the significant difference with the control group. This undesirable behavior could be expected, since it was previously found by O'Reilly et al[17] and by Gautam et al.[14]

Based on these results, we consider that combined headgear, used alone or in association with rapid maxillary expansion, is an effective strategy as the first step of Class II malocclusion treatment. Additionally, rapid maxillary expansion seems to reduce initial treatment time, probably due to anterior accommodation of the mandible and favorable environment to anteriorposterior mandibular growth after expansion.[8,9,11] Furthermore, deciduous molars and premolars are distally tipped together by their connection with the Haas expander, which reduces time and prevents a second phase of treatment. The clinical findings provided by this study allow the authors to recommend maxillary expansion before headgear appliance used to treat Class II associated with transverse maxillary deficiency. Further investigation, including final records (T_3), should be carried out to provide better information about this treatment strategy.

CONCLUSION

Combination headgear used as the first step of Class II malocclusion treatment results in the following:

» Distal movement of maxillary molars whether the headgear is used alone or in association with RME.

» Distal tipping of maxillary molars when the headgear is used alone: Group 1 (CH).

» Clockwise rotation of the maxilla when used alone: Group 1 (CH).

REFERENCES

1. Johnston LE, Answers in search of questioners. Am J Orthod Dentofacial Orthop. 2002;121(6):552-3.

2. Garbui IU, Nouer PR, Nouer DF, Magnani MB, Pereira Neto JS. Cephalometric assessment of vertical control in the treatment of class II malocclusion with a combined maxillary splint. Braz Oral Res. 2010;24(1):34-9.

3. Baumrind S, Molthen R, West EE, Miller DM. Distal displacement of the maxilla and the upper first molar. Am J Orthod. 1979;75(6):630-40.

4. Gandini MRS, Gandini LG Jr, Martins JCR, Del Santo M Jr. Effects of cervical headgear and edgewise appliances on growing patients. Am J Orthod Dentofacial Orthop. 2001;119(5):531-8.

5. Jacob HB, Buschang PH, Santos-Pinto A. Class II malocclusion treatment using high-pull headgear with a splint: a systematic review. Dental Press J Orthod. 2013;18(2):21.e1-e7.

6. Ramos DS, Lima EM. A longitudinal evaluation of the skeletal profile of treated and untreated skeletal Class II individuals. Angle Orthod. 2005;75(1):47-53.

7. Tollaro I, Baccetti T, Franchi L, Tanasescu CD. Role of posterior transverse interarch discrepancy in Class II, Division 1 malocclusion during the mixed dentition phase. Am J Orthod Dentofacial Orthop. 1996;110(4):417-22.

8. Lima Filho RM, Lima AC, Ruellas ACO. Spontaneous correction of Class II malocclusion after rapid palatal expansion. Angle Orthod. 2003;73(6):745-52.

9. Haas AJ. Palatal expansion: just the beginning of dentofacial orthopedics. Am J Orthod. 1970;57(3):219-55.

10. Lima Filho RM, Ruellas ACO. Long-term maxillary changes in patients with skeletal Class II malocclusion treated with slow and rapid palatal expansion. Am J Orthod Dentofacial Orthop. 2008;134(3):383-8.

11. Armstrong MM. Controlling the magnitude, direction, and duration of extraoral force. Am J Orthod. 1971;59(3):217-43.

12. Freeman CS, McNamara JA Jr, Baccetti T, Franchi L, Graff TW. Treatment effects of the bionator and high-pull facebow combination followed by fixed appliances in patients with increased vertical dimensions. Am J Orthod Dentofacial Orthop. 2007;131(2):184-95.

13. Gautam P, Valiathan A, Adhikari R. Craniofacial displacement in response to varying headgear forces evaluated biomechanically with finite element analysis. Am J Orthod Dentofacial Orthop. 2009;135(4):507-15.

14. Gkantidis N, Halazonetis DJ, Alexandropoulos E, Haralabakis NB. Treatment strategies for patients with hyperdivergent Class II Division 1 malocclusion: is vertical dimension affected? Am J Orthod Dentofacial Orthop. 2011;140(3):346-55.

15. O'Reilly MT, Nanda SK, Close J. Cervical and oblique headgear: a comparison of treatment effects. Am J Orthod Dentofacial Orthop. 1993;103(6):504-9.

16. Tortop T, Yuksel S. Treatment and posttreatment changes with combined headgear therapy. Angle Orthod. 2007;77(5):857-63.

17. Farret MM, Lima EMS, Araujo VP, Rizzatto SMD, Menezes LM, Grossi ML. Molar changes with cervical headgear alone or in combination with rapid maxillary expansion. Angle Orthod. 2008;78(5):847-51.

18. Casaccia GR, Gomes JC, Squeff LR, Penedo ND, Elias CN, Gouvêa JP, et al. Analysis of initial movement of maxillary molars submitted to extraoral forces: a 3D study. Dental Press J Orthod. 2010;15(5):37.e1-e8.

19. Tamburus VS, Neto JSP, Siqueira VCV, Tamburus WL. Treatment effects on Class II division 1 high angle patients treated according to the Bioprogressive therapy (cervical headgear and lower utility arch), with emphasis on vertical control. Dental Press J Orthod. 2011;16(3):70-8.

20. Ibitayo AO, Pangrazio-Kulbersh V, Berger J, Bayirli B. Dentoskeletal effects of functional appliances vs bimaxillary surgery in hyperdivergent Class II patients. Angle Orthod. 2011;81(2):304-11.

21. Marsan G. Effects of activator and high-pull headgear combination therapy: skeletal, dentoalveolar, and soft tissue profile changes. Eur J Orthod. 2007;29(2):140-8.

22. Ucem TT, Yuksel S. Effects of different vectors of forces applied by combined headgear. Am J Orthod Dentofacial Orthop. 1998;113(3):316-23.

14

Comparative evaluation of soft tissue changes in Class I borderline patients treated with extraction and nonextraction modalities

Aniruddh Yashwant V.[1], Ravi K.[2], Edeinton Arumugam[3]

Objective: To compare soft tissue changes in Class I borderline cases treated with extraction and nonextraction modalities. **Methods:** A parent sample of 150 patients with Class I dental and skeletal malocclusion (89 patients treated with premolar extraction and 61 patients without extraction) was randomly selected and subjected to discriminant analysis which identified the borderline sample of 44 patients (22 extraction and 22 nonextraction patients). Pretreatment and post-treatment cephalograms of the borderline subsample were analyzed using 22 soft tissue parameters. **Results:** Upper and lower lips were more retracted and thickness of the upper lip increased more in the borderline extraction cases ($p < 0.01$). The nasolabial angle became more obtuse and the interlabial gap was reduced in the borderline extraction cases ($p < 0.01$). Lower lip, interlabial gap and nasolabial angle showed no changes in the borderline nonextraction cases. **Conclusion:** The soft tissue parameters which can be used as guideline in decision making to choose either extraction or nonextraction in Class I borderline cases are upper and lower lip protrusion in relation to the E-plane and Sn-Pg' line, lower lip protrusion in relation to the true vertical line (TVL), upper lip thickness, nasolabial angle and interlabial gap.

Keywords: Angle Class I malocclusion. Borderline cases. Discriminant analysis. Soft tissue changes.

[1] Senior lecturer, Department of Orthodontics and Dentofacial Orthopedics, Indira Gandhi Institute of Dental Sciences, MGMCRI campus, SBV University, Pillayarkuppam, Pondicherry, India.
[2] Professor and Head of Department, Department of Orthodontics and Dentofacial Orthopedics, SRM Dental College, Ramapuram, Chennai, India.
[3] Associate professor, Department of Orthodontics and Dentofacial Orthopedics, SRM Dental College, Ramapuram, Chennai, India.

» The authors report no commercial, proprietary or financial interest in the products or companies described in this article.

Aniruddh Yashwant V.
E-mail: aniruddhyashwant@yahoo.com

INTRODUCTION

Orthodontics is the branch of Dentistry which mainly deals with malocclusion and dentofacial deformities and their correction for optimal function and esthetics. Orthodontic treatment should not focus only on occlusal relations, but also on facial esthetics, in particular profile esthetics, as they are the primary motive that encourages most patients to seek orthodontic treatment.[1] In the present era, several treatment modalities emphasize soft tissue paradigm.[2,3] Wuerpel E.H [4] discussed the changes in soft tissue that must be considered during orthodontic treatment, instead of moving teeth without anticipating soft tissue outcomes after treatment.

In treating a Class I malocclusion, there are two main approaches in comprehensive Orthodontics: extraction and nonextraction. Extractions are routinely used to correct dental crowding and protrusion of teeth and the overlying soft tissue. The nonextraction approach requires expansion of the arches, molar distalization or proximal stripping. The common demerits of extraction treatment were hypothesized to be "dished-in profiles," narrower dental arches, increased width of the buccal corridor; while those of nonextraction treatment were hypothesized to be poor stability and protrusive profile in borderline cases.[5]

There have been numerous studies about posttreatment soft tissue changes in Class II malocclusions, but the impact of facial esthetics in Class I cases has seldom been given importance.[6,7,8] This study was undertaken to compare the soft tissue changes seen in extraction and nonextraction treatment modalities in Class I borderline malocclusions.

MATERIAL AND METHODS

The treatment records of 150 patients with dental and skeletal Class I malocclusion were randomly selected from the record archive of patients treated over the past five years in the Department of Orthodontics and Dentofacial Orthopedics, SRM Dental College, Ramapuram, Chennai, India. Only patients whose treatment was finished with bilateral Class I canine and molar relationship were included in the study. Pretreatment and post-treatment cephalograms, which were taken from the same cephalostat with teeth occluding in centric occlusion and lips relaxed, were gathered. The study design was approved by the institutional Ethics Committee.

It is difficult to segregate borderline Class I malocclusions based only on specific parameters, especially when a large sample of patients is to be studied. Discriminant analysis is a multivariate statistical method wherein many parameters that influence treatment modality can be assessed. It can also help in identifying the predictors of treatment modality and also to identify borderline patients.[6,8]

Hence, in this study, a stepwise discriminant analysis was performed to segregate the borderline subsample of patients who could have been treated with either extraction or nonextraction treatment modalities. A total of 15 cephalometric variables, 4 model measurements, besides age and sex (demographic variables) were used for the discriminant analysis (Table 1). The values of the 21 variables were noted for all the 150 cases of the parent sample and data were subjected to discriminant analysis using Statistica software (StatSoft, Inc. USA). At each step of the discriminant analysis, all the 21 variables were reviewed and evaluated to determine which variable would contribute most to the discrimination between groups. That variable was then included in the discriminant

Table 1 - Variables for discriminant analysis.

No	PARAMETERS	CHARACTERISTIC
1.	SNA	Maxillary position
2.	SNB	Mandibular position
3.	ANB	Maxillomandibular relationship
4.	FMA	Facial height/orientation of mandible
5.	U1-SN	Maxillary incisor protrusion
6.	U1-NA (linear)	Maxillary incisor protrusion
7.	U1-NA (angular)	Maxillary incisor inclination
8.	L1-NB (linear)	Mandibular incisor protrusion
9.	L1-NB (angular)	Mandibular incisor inclination
10.	Wits appraisal	Maxillomandibular relationship
11.	N-S-Ar	Mandibular position
12.	Z angle	Profile convexity
13.	L lip-E-plane	Lower lip protrusion
14.	L1-APog	Mandibular incisor position
15.	Jarabak ratio	Growth pattern/facial height
16.	Overbite	
17.	Overjet	
18.	Maxillary tooth material- arch discrepancy	
19.	Mandibular tooth material- arch discrepancy	
20.	Age	Demographic variable
21.	Sex	Demographic variable

model, and analysis was restarted. Thereby, the variables entered the discriminant function individually based on their discriminating power.

Based on the data incorporated for the parent sample, only the variables that were significant were deemed eligible to be included in the discriminant analysis. From the inferential statistics, the discriminant function used three significant variables in descending order of importance, which were (p <0.01):

1. Maxillary tooth material – arch length discrepancy;

2. Mandibular tooth material – arch length discrepancy;

3. Mandibular incisor to NB (linear).

By means of the discriminant analysis, a standardized discriminate score (Dz) was achieved for each of the 150 patients. The univariate representation of the scores is shown in Graph 1. The mean of the discriminate scores (group centroid score) was calculated for each group. The group centroid score was -0.7170 for the extraction group and 1.046 for the nonextraction group.

Using the formula below for calculating critical cutting score value for unequal group sizes, the optimal cutting score was obtained.[9]

$$ZCS = \frac{NAZB + NBZA}{NA + NB}$$

In which:

» Group A: Extraction.

» Group B: Nonextraction.

» ZCS: Critical cutting score between Group A and Group B.

» NA: Number of observations in Group A.

» NB: Number of observations in Group B.

» ZA: Centroid score for Group A.

» ZB: Centroid score for Group B.

The borderline subsample of patients was inferred to be those scores which were closest to the critical cutting score. Soft tissue landmarks were identified for soft tissue analysis of the 22 extraction and 22 nonextraction borderline cases, using the 22 parameters enlisted in Table 2 (Figs 1 to 13).

Ten random cephalometric radiographs were taken and assessed for the second time to test for the standard deviation of error in repeated measures for each soft tissue cephalometric measurement by means of Dahlberg's formula ($\sqrt{(\Sigma d)^2/2N}$).

Mean and standard deviation of the 22 soft tissue parameters were calculated for the extraction and nonextraction borderline samples before and after treatment. The mean and standard deviation for the differences that each treatment group experienced from pretreatment to post-treatment were also obtained.

Independent sample t-tests were used to test the significance of differences between treatment change values of the two different treatment groups. The null hypothesis stating that no difference exists in the cephalometric variables in each treatment group before and after treatment was tested using paired t-tests (p < 0.05 was considered statistically significant). The standard deviation of error of the repeated measures for soft tissue cephalometric measurements was calculated by means of Dahlberg's formula.

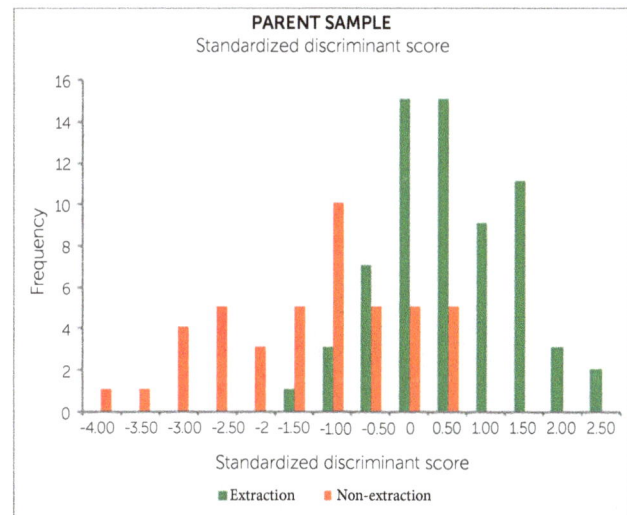

Graph 1 - Standardized discriminant scores for parent sample.
*p < 0.05 (significant at 5% level).

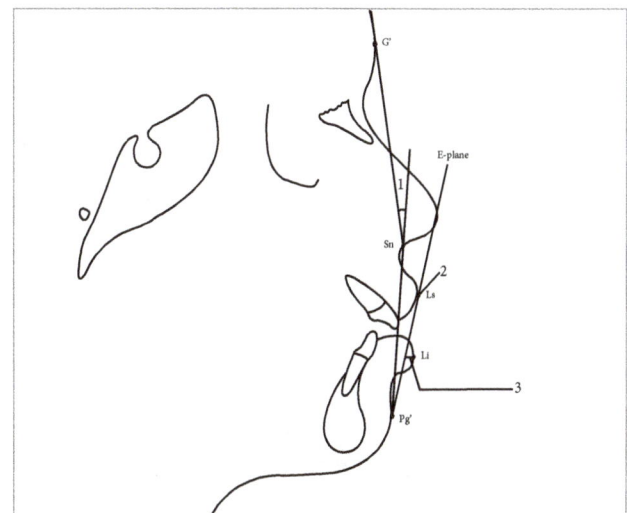

Figure 1 - 1 = Angle of facial convexity (G'-Sn-Pg'). 2 = Protrusion of upper lip (Ls to E-plane). 3 = Protrusion of lower lip (Li to E-plane).

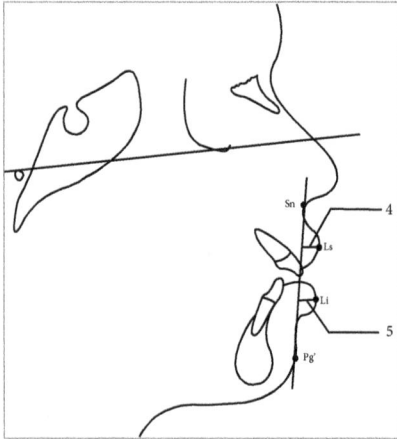

Figure 2 - **4** = Protrusion of upper lip (Ls–Sn-Pg' line). **5** = Protrusion of lower lip (Li–Sn-Pg' line).

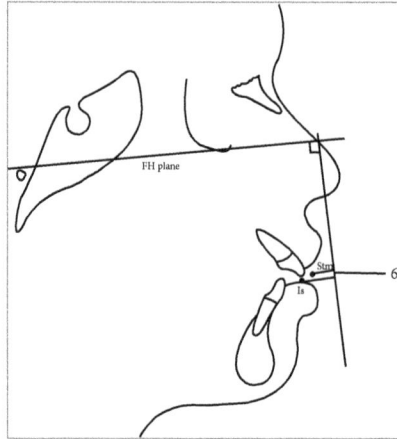

Figure 3 - **6** = Maxillary incisor exposure (Is-Stm).

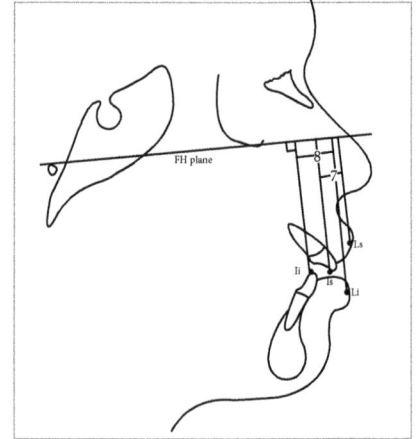

Figure 4 - **7** = Thickness of upper lip (Is-Ls). **8** = Thickness of lower lip (Ii-Li).

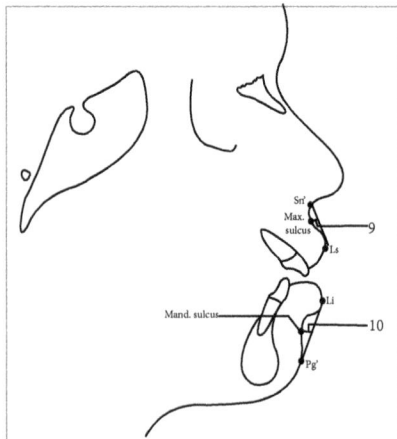

Figure 5 - **9** = Max. sulcus (Sn'-Ls). **10** = Mand. sulcus (Li-Pg').

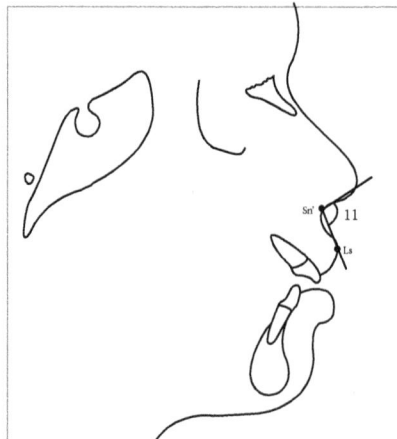

Figure 6 - **11** = Nasolabial angle.

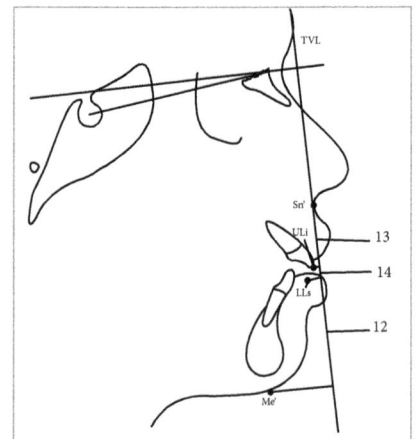

Figure 7 - **12** = Lower lip length (LLs - Me'). **13** = Upper lip length (Sn'-ULi). **14** = Interlabial gap (ULi-LLs).

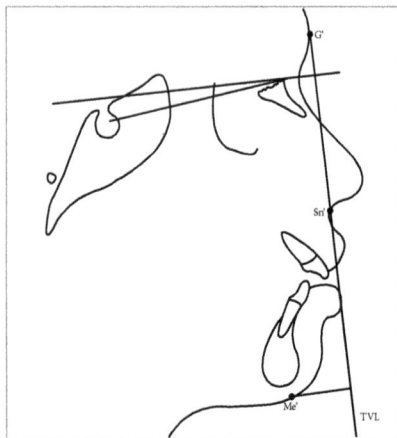

Figure 8 - **15** = Vertical height ratio (G'-Sn':Sn'-Me').

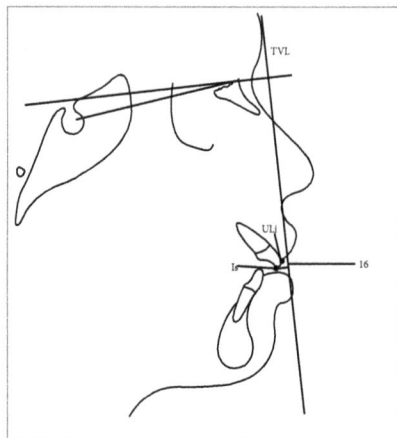

Figure 9 - **16** = Incisal exposure [ULi-Is (on TVL)].

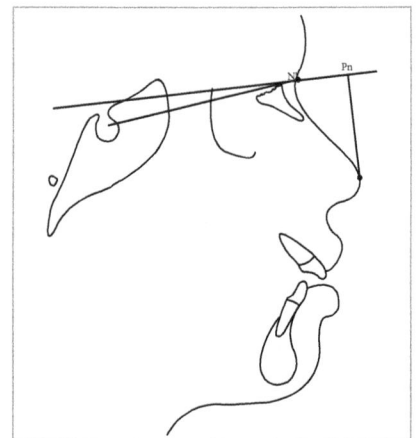

Figure 10 - **17** = N'-Pn (perpendicular to TVL).

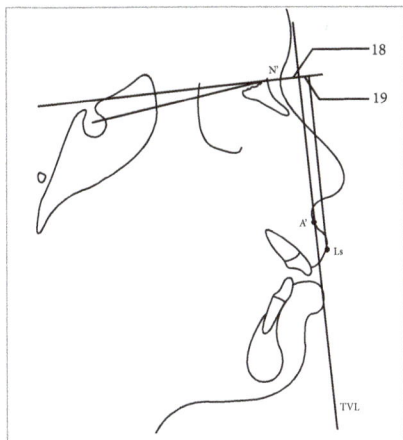

Figure 11 - **18** = N'-A' (perpendicular to TVL).
19 = N'-Ls (perpendicular to TVL).

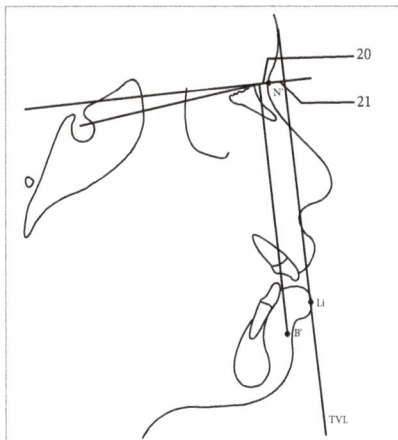

Figure 12 - **20** = N'-B' (perpendicular to TVL),
21 = N'-Li (perpendicular to TVL).

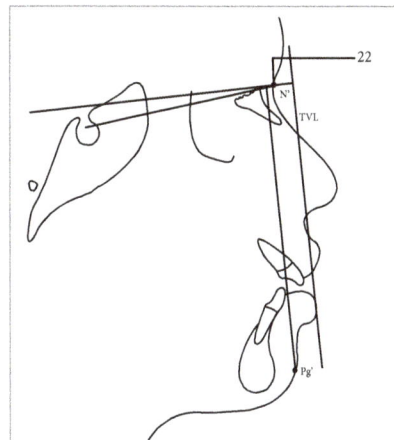

Figure 13 - **22** = N'-Pg' (perpendicular to TVL).

Table 2 - Soft tissue analysis.

No	MEASUREMENT	DESCRIPTION
1.	G'–Sn-Pg' (Fig 1)	Angle of facial convexity
2.	Ls–E-plane (Fig 1)	Protrusion of the upper lip in relation to E-plane
3.	LL–E-plane (Fig 1)	Protrusion of the lower lip in relation to E-plane
4.	Ls–Sn-Pg' line (Fig 2)	Protrusion of the upper lip in relation to Sn-Pg' line
5.	LL–Sn-Pg' line (Fig 2)	Protrusion of the lower lip in relation to Sn-Pq' line
6.	Is-Stm [perpendicular to FH plane] (Fig 3)	Maxillary incisor exposure
7.	Is-Ls [on FH plane] (Fig 4)	Thickness of the upper lip
8.	Ii-LL [on FH plane] (Fig 4)	Thickness of the lower lip
9.	Max. Sulcus - Sn'-Ls (Fig 5)	Maxillary sulcus depth
10.	Mand. Sulcus - LL-Pg' (Fig 5)	Mandibular sulcus depth
11.	Nasolabial angle (Fig 6)	Formed by the intersection of labrale superius and columella at subnasale
12.	LLs - Me' (Fig 7)	Lower lip length
13.	Sn'- ULi (Fig 7)	Upper lip length
14.	ULi-LLs (Fig 7)	Interlabial gap
15.	G'-Sn' : Sn'-Me' (Fig 8)	Vertical height ratio
16.	ULi-Is (on TVL) (Fig 9)	Incisal exposure
17.	N' – Pn (perpendicular to True Vertical Line [TVL]) (Fig 10)	Projection of the nose
18.	N' – A' (perpendicular to TVL) (Fig 11)	Thickness of the upper lip
19.	N'- Ls (perpendicular to TVL) (Fig 11)	Protrusion of the upper lip
20.	N'- B' (perpendicular to TVL) (Fig 12)	Thickness of the lower lip
21.	N'-Li (perpendicular to TVL) (Fig 12)	Protrusion of the lower lip
22.	N'- Pg' (perpendicular to TVL) (Fig 13)	Soft tissue thickness at chin

RESULTS

The descriptive and inferential statistics of all the 150 Class I cases using discriminant analysis are tabulated (Table 3). A total of 89 cases were treated by extraction of either first or second premolars and 61 cases by the nonextraction modality. Descriptive statistics of the parent sample of 150 cases showed that the sample consisted of patients with skeletal and dental Class I malocclusion.

Out of ten significant parameters in the discriminant analysis, maxillary tooth material-arch length discrepancy (Max tooth-arch length) is the most important in differentiating extraction and nonextraction groups, followed by mandibular tooth material-arch length discrepancy (Mand tooth-arch length) and linear relationship of mandibular incisor to NB [L1-NB(L)], as shown in Table 4.

Comparative statistics of the borderline extraction sample and borderline nonextraction sample is listed in Tables 5 and 6, respectively. Upper lip thickness increased significantly from 12.09 mm at treatment onset to 14.02 mm at the end of treatment in the borderline nonextraction sample. The other parameters did not show statistically significant changes.

Comparative statistics of mean differences between extraction and nonextraction borderline samples are listed in Table 7. In relation to the E-plane, the upper lip was retracted by 2.23 mm in the extraction and by 0.55 mm in the nonextraction group; whereas the lower lip was retracted by 2.59 mm in the extraction and by 0.05 mm in the nonextraction group. The mean soft tissue change values for the upper lip in relation to the Sn-Pg' line were -1.66 mm for the extraction and -0.36 mm for the nonextraction group; whereas for the lower lip in relation to the Sn-Pg' line, the mean change values were -2.09 mm for the extraction and 0.09 mm for the nonextraction group. The mean soft tissue change values for the lower lip in relation to true vertical line (TVL) were -2.50 mm for the extraction and -0.39 mm for the nonextraction group. Upper lip thickness increased by 3.41 mm in the extraction and 1.93 mm in the nonextraction group. The increases in nasolabial angle were 9.410° in the extraction group and 20° in the nonextraction group. Interlabial gap decreased by 2.77 mm in the extraction group and by 0.39 mm in the nonextraction group.

Table 3 - Descriptive statistics of the parent sample of 150 cases.

Measures	Extraction group n = 89		Nonextraction group n = 61		t-value	p-value
	Mean	SD	Mean	SD		
SNA	82.09	2.45	81.72	3.02	0.82	0.4121
SNB	79.27	2.43	79.25	3.24	0.05	0.9592
ANB	2.81	1.09	2.48	1.21	1.77	0.0793
FMA	26.51	4.33	24.90	4.71	2.15*	0.0331
U1-SN	118.04	5.87	114.89	8.79	2.64**	0.0092
U1-NA (mm)	10.10	2.50	8.48	3.43	3.34**	0.0010
U1.NA (degrees)	35.36	5.36	32.59	7.76	2.59**	0.0107
L1-NB (mm)	9.52	2.50	7.21	2.42	5.63**	< 0.0001
L1.NB (degrees)	35.76	6.22	31.10	6.76	4.36**	< 0.0001
N-S-Ar	124.40	4.41	125.10	5.26	-0.87	0.3832
Z angle	72.37	5.65	72.36	5.43	0.01	0.9913
Llip-Eplane	4.23	3.28	2.13	2.85	4.06**	0.0001
L1-APog (mm)	7.41	2.68	5.79	3.03	3.45**	0.0007
Jarabak ratio	64.27	4.55	65.46	4.94	-1.52	0.1308
Overbite	2.83	1.65	2.80	1.85	0.10	0.9222
Overjet	3.88	2.00	3.50	2.52	1.03	0.3034
Max tooth-arch L	-5.89	3.98	-0.34	4.62	-7.86**	< 0.0001
Mand tooth-arch L	-6.50	3.67	-1.42	4.26	-7.80**	< 0.0001

* $p < 0.05$ (Significant at 5%).
** $p < 0.01$ (Significant at 1%).

Table 4 - Discriminant analysis: significance of the function differentiating extraction and nonextraction cases.

	Eigen-value	Canonical R	Wilks' Lambda	Chi-Sqr.	Df	p-value
0	0.8271	0.6728	0.5473	86.19	10	p < 0.0001
			Raw coefficient Root 1		Standardized coefficients Root 1	
FMA			0.0216		0.0970	
U1-SN			0.0139		0.0998	
U1-NA (mm)			0.0355		0.1035	
U1.NA (degrees)			0.0133		0.0855	
L1-NB (mm)			0.1422		**0.3504**	
L1.NB (degrees)			0.0405		0.2609	
Lower lip-E-plane			0.0066		0.0205	
L1-A Pog (mm)			-0.0440		-0.1244	
Max tooth-arch length			-0.1216		**-0.5168**	
Mand tooth-arch length			-0.1047		**-0.4104**	
Constant			-6.1884			

Table 5 - Borderline extraction sample: descriptive and inferential statistics of soft tissue analysis results.

Measures	Pre-treatment		Post-treatment		MD	Paired t-test	p-value
	Mean	SD	Mean	SD			
G'–Sn-Pg'	14.82	6.51	14.00	5.72	0.82	1.38	0.1806
Ls–E-plane	-0.39	3.22	-2.61	2.43	-2.23	5.02**	0.0001
Li–E-plane	2.89	3.36	0.30	2.93	-2.59	5.28**	< 0.0001
Ls–Sn-Pg' line	6.09	1.78	4.43	1.94	-1.66	5.28**	< 0.0001
Li–Sn-Pg' line	6.57	2.88	4.48	2.30	-2.09	4.06**	0.0006
Is-Stm	2.39	1.63	2.57	1.26	0.18	-0.74	0.4666
Is-Ls	12.20	2.34	15.61	2.08	3.41	-6.91**	< 0.0001
Ii-Li	13.84	2.06	15.34	1.55	1.50	-3.79**	0.0011
Max. sulcus - Sn'-Ls	2.27	0.74	2.23	0.77	-0.05	0.24	0.8120
Mand. sulcus - Li-Pg'	6.02	1.98	5.75	1.45	-0.27	0.98	0.3388
Nasolabial angle	93.36	8.64	102.77	9.46	9.41	-5.20**	< 0.0001
LLs–Me'	44.95	4.13	45.80	3.73	0.84	-1.30	0.2081
Sn'–ULi	21.18	2.39	21.64	2.22	-0.45	-1.46	0.1599
ULi–LLs	3.30	3.44	0.52	0.75	-2.77	4.07**	0.0006
G'Sn': Sn'Me'	0.99	0.12	1.00	0.09	0.01	-0.63	0.5333
ULi–Is	3.77	2.35	3.16	1.31	-0.61	1.61	0.1219
N'–Pn	23.45	4.18	23.93	4.26	0.48	-1.43	0.1685
N'–A'	8.27	3.88	7.68	3.99	-0.59	1.02	0.3205
N'–Ls	13.52	4.51	11.27	4.53	-2.25	2.92**	0.0081
N'–B'	1.09	4.60	0.45	3.98	-0.64	0.85	0.4028
N'–Li	11.30	4.98	8.80	4.29	-2.50	3.21**	0.0042
N'–Pg'	1.82	4.91	2.00	4.28	0.18	-0.29	0.7729

Table 6 - Borderline nonextraction sample: descriptive and inferential statistics of soft tissue analysis results.

Measures	Pre-treatment		Post-treatment		MD	Paired t-test	p-value
	Mean	SD	Mean	SD			
G'–Sn-Pg'	14.82	4.41	14.41	5.18	-0.41	0.58	0.5676
Ls–E-plane	-1.48	2.25	-2.02	2.46	-0.55	1.43	0.1666
Li–E-plane	1.91	2.93	1.95	2.75	0.05	-0.10	0.9240
Ls–Sn-Pg' line	5.64	1.90	5.27	2.02	0.36	1.21	0.2390
Li–Sn-Pg' line	6.11	2.45	6.20	2.60	0.09	-0.18	0.8626
Is-Stm	2.34	2.09	2.55	1.91	0.20	-0.71	0.4826
Is-Ls	12.09	2.85	14.02	2.55	1.93	-4.50**	0.0002
Ii-Li	14.11	2.93	14.91	2.60	0.80	-1.31	0.2056
Max. sulcus - Sn'-Ls	2.05	0.77	2.07	0.56	0.02	-0.19	0.8525
Mand. sulcus - Li-Pg'	5.80	1.62	5.86	1.54	0.07	-0.21	0.8364
Nasolabial angle	96.23	14.06	98.23	13.03	2.00	-0.98	0.3380
LLs–Me'	46.36	4.20	46.23	4.05	-0.14	0.40	0.6902
Sn'–ULi	21.86	1.78	22.34	2.46	0.48	-1.43	0.1665
ULi–LLs	1.93	1.54	1.55	1.66	-0.39	0.92	0.3694
G'Sn': Sn'Me'	1.05	0.16	1.02	0.14	-0.03	1.34	0.1943
ULi–Is	3.91	3.03	3.50	2.34	-0.41	0.99	0.3347
N'–Pn	23.30	4.24	23.55	4.42	0.25	-1.37	0.1850
N'–A'	8.64	4.54	8.52	4.65	-0.11	0.34	0.7344
N'–Ls	12.89	5.49	12.41	5.39	-0.48	1.02	0.3195
N'–B'	0.80	5.97	0.41	5.63	-0.39	0.69	0.4994
N'–Li	10.20	7.01	9.82	6.37	-0.39	0.68	0.5023
N'–Pg'	0.75	6.32	0.80	6.12	0.05	-0.16	0.8755

Table 7 - Descriptive and inferential statistics of mean value differences: extraction *versus* nonextraction.

Measures	Extraction mean difference	Nonextraction mean difference	MD	t-value	p-value
G'–Sn-Pg'	-0.82	-0.41	0.41	0.44	0.6587
Ls–E-plane	-2.23	-0.55	1.68	2.88**	0.0063
Li–E-plane	-2.59	0.05	2.64	3.88**	0.0004
Ls–Sn-Pg' line	-1.66	-0.36	1.30	2.98**	0.0048
Li–Sn-Pg' line	-2.09	0.09	2.18	2.99**	0.0047
Is-Stm	0.18	0.20	0.02	0.06	0.9522
Is-Ls	3.41	1.93	-1.48	-2.26*	0.0291
Ii-Li	1.50	0.80	-0.70	-0.97	0.3377
Max. sulcus - Sn'-Ls	-0.05	0.02	0.07	0.30	0.7624
Mand. sulcus - Li-Pg'	-0.27	0.07	0.34	0.79	0.4312
Nasolabial angle	9.41	2.00	-7.41	-2.72**	0.0095
LLs–Me'	0.84	-0.14	-0.98	-1.34	0.1879
Sn'–ULi	0.45	0.48	0.02	0.05	0.9605
ULi–LLs	-2.77	-0.39	2.39	2.98**	0.0048
G'Sn': Sn'Me'	0.01	-0.03	-0.04	-1.45	0.1541
ULi–Is	-0.61	-0.41	0.20	0.36	0.7180
N'–Pn	0.48	0.25	-0.23	-0.60	0.5542
N'–A'	-0.59	-0.11	0.48	0.71	0.4790
N'–Ls	-2.25	-0.48	1.77	1.97	0.0556
N'–B'	-0.64	-0.39	0.25	0.27	0.7901
N'–Li	-2.50	-0.39	2.11	2.20*	0.0337
N'–Pg'	0.18	0.05	-0.14	-0.20	0.8431

*$p < 0.05$ (Significant at 5%). **$p < 0.01$ (Significant at 1%).

Table 8 - Standard deviation of error for repeated measures.

Parameters	Standard deviation of error
G'–Sn-Pg'	0.7416
Ls–E-plane	0.1936
Li–E-plane	0.3162
Ls–Sn-Pg'	0.5916
Li–Sn-Pg'	0.2958
Is-Stm	0.3708
Is-Ls	1.0124
Ii-Li	0.5123
Max. sulcus (Sn'–Ls)	0.4031
Mand. sulcus (Li–Pg')	0.3873
Nasolabial angle	3.6125
Lower Lip length	0.5701
Upper lip length	0.6021
Interlabial gap	0.1936
G'Sn':Sn'Me'	0.0647
ULi-Is	0.3708
TVL N'–Pn	0.3708
TVL N'–A'	0.4472
TVL N'–Ls	0.9421
TVL N'–B'	0.6124
TVL N'–Li	0.3354
TVL N'–Pg'	0.3354

The values of standard deviation of error of the repeated measures for each of the soft tissue cephalometric measurement by means of Dahlberg's formula are listed in Table 8. These values were found to be comparable to those reported in the literature.[6,10,11]

DISCUSSION

There is probably no other aspect of orthodontic treatment that has caused as much controversy as the decision of whether to extract or not permanent teeth. Just like a pendulum, the popularity of premolar extractions has swung between the option of nonextraction at any cost and extraction treatment to achieve arbitrary cephalometric norms.

Borderline cases are those cases which are equally susceptible to both extraction and nonextraction treatment modalities. The aim of this study was to compare soft tissue changes in Class I borderline cases treated with extraction and nonextraction modalities and to identify those parameters which can act as guidelines to differentiate between these two treatment modalities in Class I borderline cases.

Considering the changes in the upper lip in relation to E-plane, the borderline extraction sample showed -2.23-mm retraction while the borderline nonextraction sample showed -0.55-mm retraction. Drobocky et al.[12] and Bravo[13], in their studies, reported -3.4 mm of upper lip retraction with extraction of maxillary first premolars. Kocadereli[14], in his study, showed that upper lip was retracted by -1.64 mm. Upper lip retraction in relation to the true vertical line was found to be -2.25 mm for the extraction group and -0.48 mm for the nonextraction group. In relation to the Sn-Pg' line, upper lip protrusion was reduced by -1.66 mm in the extraction group and was insignificant in the nonextraction group. Drobocky et al.[12] and Bravo[13] reported upper lip retraction in relation to Sn-Pg' line values to be of -2.12 mm and -2.4 mm, respectively. The insignificant reduction in lip protrusion in the nonextraction group is similar to the values seen in the studies by Kocadareli[14] and Konstantonis[15].

Upper lip thickness was increased by 3.41 mm in the extraction group and by 1.93 mm in the nonextraction group. These values are comparable to the study results of Talass et al[16] who reported an increase of upper lip thickness of 3.7 mm in the extraction group.

The nasolabial angle showed an increase of 9.41˚ in the extraction borderline group. Bravo reported an increase of 3.7˚ in nasolabial angle with the extraction of first premolars.[13] Ramos et al[17] reported an increase of 4˚ in their study which involved extraction of maxillary first premolars for treatment of Class II, Division 1 cases. The increase in the nasolabial angle was statistically insignificant in the nonextraction group. Contrary to the results obtained in our study, Waldman[18] reported that there was only a slight correlation (r = 0.42) between retraction of anterior teeth and change in the nasolabial angle.

The changes in lower lip showed significant difference between treatment groups. In relation to the E-plane, the lower lip was retracted by -2.59 mm in the extraction group. Drobocky et al.[12] reported a similar value of lower lip retraction with extraction of first premolars (-3.22 mm). In the nonextraction group, lower lip in relation to E-plane showed no change. Konstantonis[15], in his study, showed that the lower lip was brought forward by 0.67 mm. In contrast to these findings, Battagel, Finnoy et al and

Xu et al reported lower lip retraction with values of -1.44 mm, -2.2 mm and -0.4 mm, respectively.[10,19,20] With respect to the Sn-Pg' line, the lower lip showed -2.09-mm retraction in the extraction group and no change in the nonextraction group. The findings by Konstantonis[15] showed -2.55-mm retraction in the extraction group and 1.01-mm lower lip protraction. Young and Smith[11] found -0.58-mm lower lip retraction. The mean values of lower lip response to treatment vary between this study and the other studies discussed above. This can be due to factors such as variation in position of the maxillary incisor post-treatment, weak correlation between mandibular incisors retraction and lower lip position, as well as weaker correlation and ratio between lower lip change and underlying hard tissue change due to treatment. In relation to the true vertical line (TVL) the lower lip showed 3.21-mm retraction in the extraction group. The change in the nonextraction group was insignificant. These values were comparable to the values inferred from lower lip changes in relation to the Sn-Pg' line and E-plane. Hence, the relationship between soft tissue landmarks and the true vertical line (TVL) shows that it can be used as an adjunct parameter for assessing soft tissue changes with treatment.

The interlabial gap was found to reduce by 2.77 mm in the extraction group. This parameter did not show any significant change with nonextraction treatment. Jacobs[21], in his study, reported that the decrease in interlabial gap can be predicted by retraction and intrusion of maxillary incisors. The change in interlabial gap was found only in the extraction group, probably because of significant lower lip retraction (-2.59 mm in relation to E-plane). This inference can be confirmed with the results of a study by Yogosawa[22], which showed that to close interlabial gap, movement of lower lip must be four times the movement of upper lip. Contrary to these results, Janson et al[23] reported that nonextraction patients had greater interlabial gap reduction (2.7 mm) than observed in extraction patients (1.3 mm) in the long-term post-treatment period.

There exists a difference in treatment changes between this study and those carried out by other authors discussed herein. Soft tissue changes due to extraction or nonextraction treatment depend on the characteristics of the patients studied, sample size, the prescription used, anchorage considerations and treatment mechanics. Many of the studies discussed above have shown soft tissue changes associated with Class II malocclusions.[13,16-19] Moreover, treatment mechanics and anchorage considerations were not specified in many of those studies. This influences the amount of incisor retraction which, in turn, influences soft tissue changes.

In this study, all patients were treated by MBT prescription in 0.022-in slot with appropriate anchorage preparation. Few of the studies discussed have used Tweed's technique. It has been shown that patients treated with Tweed's technique have shown greater lip retraction.[12] These may be the reasons why the values of soft tissue changes of this study do not coincide with values observed in other studies.

CONCLUSION

From the results obtained in this study, it can be concluded that upper and lower lips were retracted more significantly, while upper lip thickness increased more significantly in the borderline extraction cases. The nasolabial angle became more obtuse and the interlabial gap was reduced in the borderline extraction cases. The other parameters, such as maxillary incisor exposure, upper and lower lip lengths, vertical height ratio and soft tissue changes at the chin, were found to be statistically insignificant in both extraction and nonextraction treatment groups.

The parameters which differentiate between extraction and nonextraction treatment modalities in Class I borderline cases are upper and lower lip protrusion in relation to E-plane and the Sn-Pg' line, lower lip protrusion in relation to the true vertical line (TVL), upper lip thickness, nasolabial angle and interlabial gap. These parameters can be used as guidelines in decision making to choose either extraction or nonextraction in Class I borderline cases.

REFERENCES

1. Riedel RA. Esthetics and its relation to orthodontic therapy. Angle Orthod. 1950 July;20(3):168-78.
2. Peck H, Peck S. A concept of facial esthetics. Angle Orthod. 1970 Oct;40(4):284-318.
3. Burstone CJ. The integumental profile. Am J Orthod. 1958;44(1):1-25.
4. Wuerpel EH. On facial balance and harmony. Angle Orthod. 1937;7(2):81-9.
5. Germec-Cakan D, Taner TU, Akan S. Arch-width and perimeter changes in patients with borderline Class I malocclusion treated with extractions or without extractions with air-rotor stripping. Am J Orthod Dentofacial Orthop. 2010 Juny;137(6):734.e1-7; discussion 734-5.
6. Luppanapornlarp S, Johnston LE Jr. The effects of premolar-extraction: a long-term comparison of outcomes in "clear-cut" extraction and nonextraction Class II patients. Angle Orthod. 1993 Winter;63(4):257-72.
7. Janson G, Fuziy A, Freitas MR, Castanha Henriques JF, Almeida RR. Soft-tissue treatment changes in Class II Division 1 malocclusion with and without extraction of maxillary premolars. Am J Orthod Dentofacial Orthop. 2007;132:729.e1-8.
8. Paquette DE, Beattie JR, Johnston LE Jr. A long-term comparison of nonextraction and premolar extraction edgewise therapy in "borderline" Class II patients. Am J Orthod Dentofacial Orthop. 1992 July;102(1):1-14.
9. Hair JF Jr, Anderson RE, Tatham RL, Black WC. Multivariate data analysis with readings. New York: MacMillan; 1992.
10. Battagel JM. The relationship between hard and soft tissue changes following treatment of Class II division 1 malocclusions using Edgewise and Fränkel appliance techniques. Eur J Orthod. 1990 May;12(2):154-65.
11. Young TM, Smith RJ. Effects of orthodontics on the facial profile: a comparison of changes during nonextraction and four premolar extraction treatment. Am J Orthod Dentofacial Orthop. 1993 May;103(5):452-8.
12. Drobocky OB, Smith RJ. Changes in facial profile during orthodontic treatment with extraction of four first premolars. Am J Orthod Dentofacial Orthop. 1989 Mar;95(3):220-30.
13. Bravo LA. Soft tissue facial profile changes after orthodontic treatment with four premolars extracted. Angle Orthod. 1994;64(1):31-42.
14. Kocadereli I. Changes in soft tissue profile after orthodontic treatment with and without extractions. Am J Orthod Dentofacial Orthop. 2002 July;122(1):67-72.
15. Konstantonis D. The impact of extraction vs nonextraction treatment on soft tissue changes in Class I borderline malocclusions. Angle Orthod. 2012 Mar;82(2):209-17.
16. Talass MF, Talass L, Baker RC. Soft-tissue profile changes resulting from retraction of maxillary incisors. Am J Orthod Dentofacial Orthop. 1987 May;91(5):385-94.
17. Ramos AL, Sakima MT, Pinto A dos S, Bowman SJ. Upper lip changes correlated to maxillary incisor retraction: a metallic implant study. Angle Orthod. 2005 July;75(4):499-505.
18. Waldman BH. Change in lip contour with maxillary incisor retraction. Angle Orthod. 1982 Apr;52(2):129-34.
19. Finnoy JP, Wisth PJ, Boe OE. Changes in soft tissue profile during and after orthodontic treatment. Eur J Orthod. 1987;9(1):68-78.
20. Xu TM, Liu Y, Yang MZ, Huang W. Comparison of extraction versus nonextraction orthodontic treatment outcomes for borderline Chinese patients. Am J Orthod Dentofacial Orthop. 2006 May;129(5):672-7.
21. Jacobs JD. Vertical lip changes from maxillary incisor retraction. Am J Orthod. 1978 Oct;74(4):396-404.
22. Yogosawa F. Predicting soft tissue profile changes concurrent with orthodontic treatment. Angle Orthod. 1990 Fall;60(3):199-206.
23. Janson G, Santos PBD, Garib DG, Francisconi MF, Baldo TO, Barros SE. Interlabial gap behaviour with time. J World Fed Orthod. 2013;2(4):e175-9.

15

Impact of two early treatment protocols for anterior dental crossbite on children's quality of life

Cristina Batista Miamoto[1], Leandro Silva Marques[2], Lucas Guimarães Abreu[1], Saul Martins Paiva[1]

Objective: To assess the impact of two early treatment protocols for anterior dental crossbite on children's quality of life. **Methods:** Thirty children, 8 to 10 years of age, with anterior dental crossbite, participated in this study. Individuals were divided into two groups: Group 1 – 15 children undergoing treatment with an upper removable appliance with digital springs; Group 2 – 15 children undergoing treatment with resin-reinforced glass ionomer cement bite pads on the lower first molars. Quality of life was evaluated using the Brazilian version of the *Child Perceptions Questionnaire* (CPQ_{8-10}), which contains four subscales: oral symptoms (OS), functional limitations (FL), emotional well-being (EW), and social well-being (SW). A higher score denotes a greater negative impact on children's quality of life. Children answered the questionnaire before treatment (T_1) and twelve months after orthodontic treatment onset (T_2). Descriptive statistics, the Wilcoxon test and analysis of covariance (ANCOVA) were performed. **Results:** Children's mean age was 9.07 ± 0.79 years in Group 1 and 9.00 ± 0.84 years in Group 2. For Group 1, the FL and EW subscale scores and the overall CPQ_{8-10} were significantly higher in T_1 as compared to T_2 ($p=0.004$, $p=0.012$ and $p=0.015$, respectively). For Group 2, there were no statistically significant differences. The ANCOVA showed no significant difference regarding quality of life at T_2 between groups, after controlling for quality of life measures at T_1. **Conclusions:** The difference regarding the impact on quality of life between groups is not related to the protocol used.

Keywords: Children. Malocclusion. Anterior crossbite. Interceptive orthodontics. Quality of life.

[1] Universidade Federal de Minas Gerais, Departamento de Odontopediatria e Ortodontia (Belo Horizonte/MG, Brazil).
[2] Universidade Federal dos Vales do Jequitinhonha e Mucuri, Departamento de Odontopediatria e Ortodontia (Diamantina/MG, Brazil).

» The authors report no commercial, proprietary or financial interest in the products or companies described in this article.

Lucas Guimarães Abreu
Rua Maranhão 1447 / 1101, Funcionários, Belo Horizonte/MG, Brasil
CEP: 30.150-338 – E-mail: lucasgabreu@bol.com.br

INTRODUCTION

The concept of oral health-related quality of life (OHRQoL) has been used to measure the impact of oral outcomes on the functions and quality of life of individuals.[1] Recently, one of the objectives of dental research has been to assess the OHRQoL of children and adolescents, since oral diseases, such as dental caries and malocclusion, have a negative effect on the physical and psychological well-being of young people.[2,3] Generally, the instruments used to assess OHRQoL are constructed in the form of surveys consisting of questions aimed at measuring how much oral outcomes affect people's lives and daily routines by means of responses organized in numerical scales.[4]

Anterior dental crossbite occurs when there is a change in the inclination of one or more anterior teeth with the upper incisor(s) positioned palatally in relation to the lingual surface of the lower teeth.[5] Studies evaluating these changes reported the possibility of periodontal problems in the lower incisors, the presence of discomfort, alteration in the anteroposterior position of the mandible, and problems with the temporomandibular joint (TMJ), when the problem is not treated early.[6,7] Interceptive orthodontic intervention in the mixed dentition allows the orthodontist to correct the anterior crossbite earlier in a way that promotes the harmonious growth of the bone bases,[8,9] mitigating the chances of severe disorders in the permanent dentition.

The impact of orthodontic treatment with fixed appliances on the quality of life of children and adolescents has been explored in depth in prior literature.[10,11] However, the association between interceptive orthodontic treatment and OHRQoL still needs to be properly investigated.[12,13] It is important to consider relevant aspects of the patient's quality of life during orthodontic treatment, such as potential psychosocial problems and functional disabilities caused by the wearing of orthodontic devices.[14] Therefore, the objective of this study was to assess the impact of two early treatment protocols for correction of the anterior dental crossbite (upper removable appliance with digital springs; and resin-reinforced glass ionomer cement bite pads on the lower first molars) on the quality of life of children. The null hypothesis was that there is no difference between both protocols regarding the impact on children's quality of life.

METHODS

Participants, study site, and eligibility criteria

The sample of this prospective study was selected from the registry of patients attending the Children's Clinic of the Federal University of the Valleys of Jequitinhonha and Mucuri (UFVJM), located in the city of Diamantina, Brazil. The study was conducted between March, 2014 and December, 2015. Individuals between 8 and 10 years of age and who presented anterior dental crossbite in the mixed dentition, with the presence of the four first permanent molars and at least one crossed permanent incisor, were included in this study. Exclusion criteria were: (I) impairment in general health based on medical history and physical examination, (II) anterior skeletal or functional crossbite, (III) posterior crossbite associated with anterior crossbite, (IV) presence of sucking habits or individuals who had stopped the habit less than a year before the study's onset, (V) previous history of orthodontic treatment, and (VI) individuals with any oral disease or those who had undergone any kind of dental treatment within the last month.

The sample consisted of 30 individuals, 8 to 10 years of age, with anterior dental crossbite in the mixed dentition. The participants were divided into two groups: Group 1 consisted of 15 patients undergoing treatment with an upper removable appliance with digital springs; Group 2 consisted of 15 patients undergoing treatment with resin-reinforced glass ionomer cement bite pads on the lower first molars. The distribution of 30 individuals between the two groups was performed randomly as follows: an envelope was prepared with 30 records with the names of the two treatment protocols, each mode containing 15 records. A card was selected from the envelope for each participant, indicating the group to which he/she belonged. This process was carried out by an assistant.

Ethical considerations

The research proposal was submitted to and approved by the Ethics Committee on Human Research from UFVJM (protocol #525.056). Children and their guardians were informed about the study and that their participation was entirely voluntary. The children who agreed to participate in the study signed an informed consent form, as did their parents or guardians. After the follow-up period, patients whose anterior dental crossbite had not been fully corrected continued the treatment or were subjected to a new type of therapy.

OHRQoL assessment tool

Participants' OHRQoL was assessed by means of the Brazilian version of the Child Perceptions Questionnaire (CPQ_{8-10}), which is a tool used to assess the impact of oral conditions on the quality of life of children from 8 to 10 years of age.[15] The CPQ_{8-10} consists of 25 questions divided into four subscales: oral symptoms (OS), with 5 questions; functional limitations (FL), with 5 questions; emotional well-being (EW), with 5 questions; and social well-being (SW), with 10 questions. An ordinal scale provides the following response options for each question: never (0), once/twice (1), sometimes (2), often (3), and every day/almost every day (4). The scores for each subscale are computed by adding up the scores for each question. The overall score is calculated by adding the scores of the four subscales. The overall score ranges from 0 to 100 points. Higher values indicate a more negative impact of the oral outcome on children's quality of life. The CPQ_{8-10} was translated and adapted cross-culturally for the Brazilian population with similar psychometric properties to the original version.[16]

Data were collected through surveys that were answered in an average time of 15 minutes in a separate room next door to the clinic. The subjects answered them on two occasions: the first occurred before placing the two types of protocols, for determining the baseline (T_1); the second assessment was carried out twelve months after the onset of the interceptive orthodontic treatment (T_2). Treatments were conducted by a specialist in orthodontics , who stressed the benefit of the early treatment of anterior dental crossbite for the children and their parents/caregivers. Shortly after the placement of the resin-reinforced glass ionomer cement bite pads or the upper removable appliance with digital springs, the participants and their parents/caregivers were given instruction on diet restrictions, hygiene, and the commitment required by orthodontic treatment. This information was emphasized again on subsequent monthly appointments. Parents/caregivers were asked to check their own commitments before scheduling consultations for their children, to avoid delays or missing the consultations. A telephone number was provided in case of need for emergency consultation due to breakage or loss of devices.

Early orthodontic protocols for anterior dental crossbite

Upper removable appliance with digital springs

The device presented two Adams clasps in the permanent upper first molars, two arrow clasps between the deciduous upper molars and a double spring adapted to the palatal surfaces of the teeth to be uncrossed, in addition to the vestibular arch (Fig 1). The posterior region presented an occlusal splint in an attempt to promote sufficient disocclusion, enabling the movement of the crossed teeth. The patients were advised to remove the appliance only to eat and during oral hygiene.

Resin-reinforced glass ionomer cement bite pads

Resin-reinforced glass ionomer cement bite pads (Riva Light Cure®, Bayswater, Australia) were placed on the occlusal surface of the permanent lower first molars (Fig 2). These devices contained dimensions that were sufficient to promote the disocclusion of all of the anterior teeth, which allowed enough space for the movement of the crossed teeth by tongue pressure.

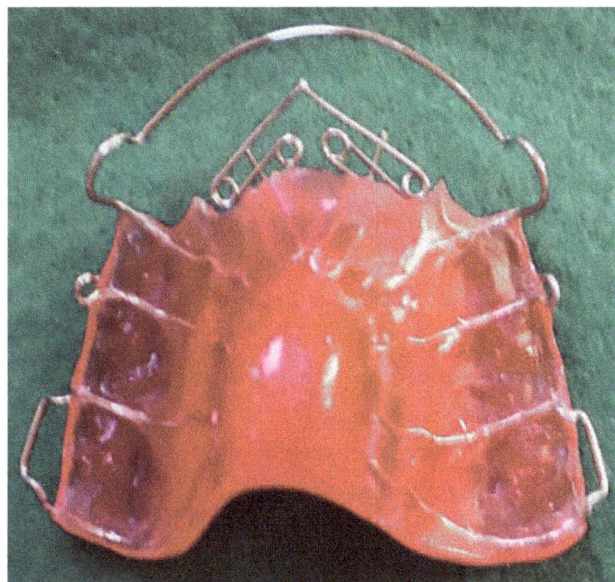

Figure 1 - The upper removable appliance with digital springs.

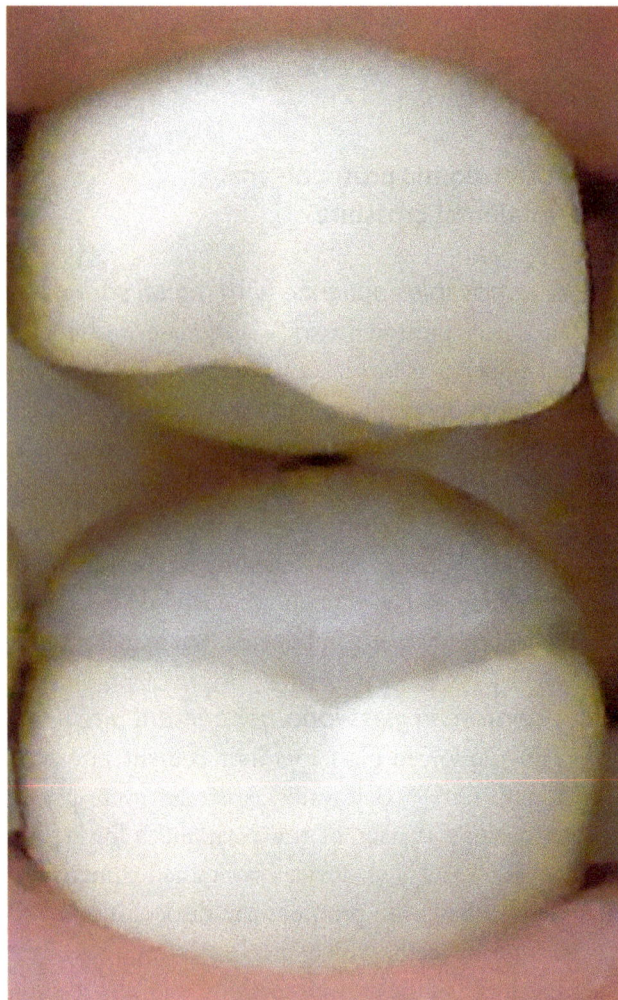

Figure 2 - Glass ionomer cement bite pads

Sample power calculation

The sample power calculation was carried out by means of the Power and Sample Size Calculation Program (PS, version 3.0, Nashville, Tenn, USA). The overall CPQ_{8-10} score was the outcome with which the sample power was calculated. For Group 1, the mean difference in the response of matched pairs was 15.53 and the standard deviation of this mean difference was 11.98. For Group 2, the mean difference in the response of matched pairs was 11.73 and the standard deviation of this mean difference was 10.68. The type I error was 0.05. Thus, the power of the study to identify significant differences between T_1 and T_2 was 99.4% for Group 1 and 97.3% for Group 2.

Orthodontic treatment need assessment

Children's orthodontic treatment need was as-

sessed using the Dental Aesthetic Index (DAI). The DAI consists of scores for 10 occlusal characteristics. The score of each occlusal characteristic is multiplied by a linear regression coefficient and added together to the constant value of 13, resulting in the DAI final score. Based on DAI cut-offs, the children were assigned to four groups: slight need of treatment (DAI ≤ 25); elective treatment (DAI = 26 to 30); highly desirable treatment (DAI = 31 to 35), and mandatory treatment (DAI ≥ 36).[17] Before study's commencement, a training and calibration exercise guaranteed accuracy for the use of DAI.

Monthly family income

The monthly family income was categorized in terms of the Brazilian minimum wage (BZMW), which was R$788.00 at the time of the study and was established as the sum of monthly income of all economically active members of that family. The children were then categorized as follows: those whose families had a monthly income of ≤ 1 BZMW; > 1 BZMW and ≤ 2 BZMWs; > 2 BZMWs and ≤ 5 BZMWs and those whose families had a monthly income of > 5 BZMWs and ≤ 10 BZMWs.

Data analysis

Data from both groups were analyzed using the *Statistical Package for Social Sciences* (SPSS for Windows, version 20.0; SPSS Inc., Chicago, IL, USA). Descriptive statistics were calculated with the aim of providing the sample characteristics. The Shapiro-Wilk test was used to determine the distribution of data and the result showed that the data had non-normal distribution. Inter-group comparisons regarding children's sociodemographic characteristics, orthodontic treatment need and CPQ_{8-10} scores at T_1 were carried out using the Chi-square test and the Mann-Whitney test.

The Wilcoxon signed-rank test was used to assess statistical differences between T_1 and T_2 for the subscales and overall CPQ_{8-10} score. For the overall score, the level of statistical significance was $p < 0.05$. The Bonferroni correction was used with the subscales for which the level of statistical significance was $p < 0.013$.

Evaluation of the relationship between the type of treatment protocol and the OHRQoL scores at T_2, controlling for confounding variables was carried out by means of the analysis of covariance (ANCOVA). Confounding variables with a $p < 0.20$ in the inter-group comparisons were incorporated in the model. Again, the level of significance for the overall score was $p < 0.05$ and for the subscales, a $p < 0.013$ was considered statistically significant.

RESULTS

Of the 15 children in Group 1, 11 were male (73.3%) and 4 were female (26.7%); the mean age of these children was 9.07 ± 0.79 years. Of the 15 children in Group 2, 7 were male (46.7%) and 8 were female (53.3%); the mean age was 9.00 ± 0.84 years. The socio-demographic characteristics of the participants are presented in Table 1.

Group 1 scores for the FL and EW subscales and the overall CPQ_{8-10} score were significantly higher in T_1 as compared to T_2 ($p = 0.004$, $p = 0.012$, and $p = 0.015$, respectively). There were no significant statistical differences in Group 2 (Table 2).

The results of the ANCOVA showed no significant difference in the subscale and CPQ_{8-10} overall scores at T_2 between the two types of treatment protocol (Group 1 and Group 2), after controlling the model for children's measures of quality of life at T_1 (Table 3).

Table 1 - Children's sociodemographic characteristics, orthodontic treatment needs and quality of life before treatment.

	Group 1	Group 2	Intergroup comparison (p value)
Gender of the children			
Boys	11 (73.3)	07 (46.7)	0.264*
Girls	04 (26.7)	08 (53.3)	
Age of the children (years)			
8	04 (26.6)	05 (33.3)	
9	06 (40.0)	05 (33.3)	0.999**
10	05 (33.4)	05 (33.4)	
Orthodontic treatment needs			
Slight	01 (06.7)	02 (13.3)	
Elective	05 (33.3)	02 (13.3)	
Highly desirable	04 (26.7)	08 (53.4)	0.999**
Mandatory	05 (33.3)	03 (20.0)	
Family income (BZMW)			
Up to 1 BZMW	01 (06.7)	01 (06.7)	
From 1 to 2 BZMWs	07 (46.7)	10 (66.7)	
From 2 to 5 BZMWs	06 (40.0)	04 (26.7)	0.412**
From 5 to 10 BZMWs	01 (06.7)	00 (00.0)	
CPQ_{8-10} (T_1)			
OS[1]	7.47 (7.00)[2]	4.40 (3.00)[2]	0.067***
FL[1]	6.13 (7.00)[2]	2.40 (1.00)[2]	0.011***
EW[1]	6.33 (6.00)[2]	2.40 (0.00)[2]	0.019***
SW[1]	7.80 (6.00)[2]	2.33 (1.00)[2]	0.032***
OL[1]	27.87 (35.0)[2]	11.13 (7.00)[2]	0.008***

BZMW = Brazilian monthly wage.
CPQ_{8-10} = Child Perceptions Questionnaire. T_1 = before beginning treatment.
OS = oral symptoms; FL = functional limitations; EW = emotional well-being; SW = social well-being; OL = overall score.
[1] Analyzed as a continuous variable. [2] Mean (Median). *Pearson chi-square. **Linear by linear chi-square. ***Mann-Whitney test.

Table 2 - Comparison of the medians and modes of CPQ$_{8-10}$ subscale and overall scores for the two early treatment protocols of anterior dental crossbite.

	CPQ$_{8-10}$ Variation	Median T$_1$	Mode T$_1$	Median T$_2$	Mode T$_2$	p value T$_1$ – T$_2$
Group 1						
OS	0 – 20	7.00	12	4.00	6	0.032*
FL	0 – 20	7.00	8	1.00	0	0.004*
EW	0 – 20	6.00	0	1.00	0	0.012*
SW	0 – 40	6.00	0	4.00	0	0.269*
OL	0 – 100	35.00	36	12.00	3	0.015**
Group 2						
OS	0 – 20	3.00	2	5.00	8	0.441*
FL	0 – 20	1.00	0	2.00	0	0.590*
EW	0 – 20	0.00	0	3.00	0	0.683*
SW	0 – 40	1.00	0	1.00	0	0.570*
OL	0 – 100	7.00	2	8.00	0	0.589**

CPQ$_{8-10}$ = Child Perceptions Questionnaire.
T$_1$ = before beginning treatment. T$_2$ = 12 months after beginning treatment.
OS = oral symptoms; FL = functional limitations; EW = emotional well-being; SW = social well-being; OL = overall score.
* Wilcoxon signed-rank test and Bonferroni correction. Significance level < 0.013.
** Wilcoxon signed-rank test. Significance level < 0.05.

Table 3 - ANCOVA models demonstrating contribution of covariates to overall and subscale CPQ$_{8-10}$ scores at T$_2$.

	OS F statistics	OS p value*	FL F statistics	FL p value*	EW F statistics	EW p value*	SW F statistics	SW p value*	OL F statistics	OL p value**
CPQ$_{8-10}$ (T$_1$)	1.5	0.231	7.3	0.012	7.24	0.012	17.98	0.001	7.49	0.011
Treatment protocol	0.96	0.335	0.02	0.9	0.65	0.424	0.36	0.553	0.76	0.39

CPQ$_{8-10}$ = Child Perceptions Questionnaire.
T$_1$ = before beginning treatment; T$_2$ = 12 months after beginning treatment.
OS = oral symptoms; FL = functional limitations; EW = emotional well-being; SW = social well-being; OL = overall score.
*Significance level < 0.013. **Significance level < 0.05.

DISCUSSION

The results of this study confirmed that no statistical difference was found in the OS, FL, EW and SW subscales as well as in the overall CPQ$_{8-10}$ score between children wearing an upper removable appliance with digital springs and children who were treated with resin-reinforced glass ionomer cement bite pads on the lower first molars. The covariate that contributed most for individuals' OHRQoL at T$_2$ was the measures of quality of life at T$_1$ in the FL, EW and SW subscales as well as in the overall CPQ$_{8-10}$ score.

Within interceptive orthodontics, recent studies have shown the positive effect of orthodontic therapy on the OHRQoL of treated patients.[12,18] It is important to understand that an improved function is not the only reason why many individuals seek treatment.[19,20] The effects of malocclusion on emotional and social well-being are also important justifications for seeking orthodontic treatment,[21] and these are the motivations that subjective indices, such as the CPQ$_{8-10}$, also assess. OHRQoL has been considered a multidimensional construct, in regards to the frequency of the impact that oral conditions may have on physical aspects, such as oral symptoms and functional limitations. This construct also concerns the effects of oral outcomes on individuals' psychosocial aspects.[22] It has been recognized that malocclusion has a negative impact on children's and adolescents' quality of life, mostly on emotional and social well-beings[23] and orthodontic treatment, on the other hand, improves OHRQoL with positive repercussions on functioning[18] and self-esteem.[12]

OHRQoL assessment becomes relevant in the participants' age group, especially with regard to anterior dental crossbite, given that correction in mixed dentition are recommended to avoid compromising the dentofacial condition, which could result in the development of periodontal issues due to traumatic occlusion[24] or a skeletal Class III malocclusion.[8,9] These findings may indicate the need for the orthodontist to prioritize the early correction of this irregularity[25] and any other irregularities, such as the presence of crowding in the anterior region,[26] to improve the patients' perception in regard to their dental appearance. This work highlights the importance of diagnosis and early intervention for anterior dental crossbite using orthodontic devices that seem to correct this malocclusion quickly and effectively, with minimal discomfort to the child.[27]

This study has limitations that need to be acknowledged. The first regards the income of the families. Most participants belonged to families with monthly income of less than 5 BZMWs. The present evaluation would have benefited of a more equalized sample in terms of socioeconomic characteristics. Although some factors that could influence the results were controlled, such as having treatments performed by only one practitioner, other factors were not controlled, such as differences (intragroups) regarding the severity of malocclusion.[28] Moreover, children in the second assessment did not demonstrate the same stage of correction in their anterior dental crossbite.

A systematic review[29] on the treatment of anterior dental crossbite showed that most of the articles published about therapy protocols for this malocclusion are case reports. Moreover, none of the included studies evaluated patients' perceptions and the impact of treatment on their OHRQoL. There are several fixed or removable devices used to correct anterior dental crossbite. The choice of a particular type of treatment depends on a close examination of various factors, such as the severity of malocclusion, the patient's tolerance of discomfort caused by the treatment, and the professional skill of the orthodontist performing the treatment. Therefore, future research should be conducted addressing the impact of different early treatment protocols for anterior dental crossbite. Evidence-based dentistry, in the last 20 years, has been understood as the standard for oral health care worldwide.[30] Clinicians should consider in their clinical routine both clinical experience and the best available evidence. However, awareness of patients' needs and preferences is also an important component of orthodontic practice. The psychosocial characteristics of individuals along with their perceptions, expectations and values need to be taken into account when practitioners are providing orthodontic treatment.[31]

CONCLUSION

While the quality of life of children undergoing treatment with upper removable appliance with digital springs improved, no change was observed in the quality of life of children submitted to treatment with resin-reinforced glass ionomer cement bite pads. This difference regarding the impact on OHRQoL, however, is unrelated to the protocol used.

REFERENCES

1. Sischo L, Broder HL. Oral health-related quality of life: what, why, how and future implications. J Dent Res. 2011 Nov;90(11):1264-70.

2. Martins-Júnior PA, Oliveira M, Marques LS, Ramos-Jorge ML. Untreated dental caries: impact on quality of life of children of low socioeconomic status. Pediatr Dent. 2012 May-June;34(3):49-52.

3. Ukra A, Foster Page LA, Thomson WM, Farella M, Tawse Smith A, Beck V. Impact of malocclusion on quality of life among New Zealand adolescents. N Z Dent J. 2013 Mar;109(1):18-23.

4. Wallander JL, Schmitt M, Koot HM. Quality of life measurement in children and adolescents: issues, instruments, and applications. J Clin Psychol. 2001 Apr;57(4):571-85.

5. Jirgensone I, Liepa A, Abeltins A. Anterior crossbite correction in primary and mixed dentition with removable inclined plane (Bruckl appliance). Stomatologija. 2008;10(4):140-4.

6. Valentine F, Howitt JW. Implication of early anterior crossbite correction. ASDC J Dent Child. 1970 Sept-Out;37(5):420-7.

7. Vadiakas G, Viazis AD. Anterior crossbite correction in the early deciduous dentition. Am J Orthod Dentofacial Orthop. 1992 Aug;102(2):160-2.

8. Karaiskos N, Wiltshire WA, Odlum O, Brothwell D, Hassard TH. Preventive and interceptive orthodontic treatment needs of an inner-city group of 6- and 9-year-old Canadian children. J Can Dent Assoc. 2005 Oct;71(9):649.

9. Schopf P. Indication for and frequency of early orthodontic therapy or interceptive measures. J Orofac Orthop. 2003 May;64(3):186-200.

10. Zhang M, McGrath C, Hagg U. Changes in oral health-related quality of life during fixed orthodontic appliance therapy. Am J Orthod Dentofacial Orthop. 2008 Jan;133(1):25-9.

11. Abreu LG, Melgaço CA, Lages EM, Abreu MH, Paiva SM. Effect of year one orthodontic treatment on the quality of life of adolescents, assessed by the short form of the Child Perceptions Questionnaire. Eur Arch Paediatric Dent. 2014 Dec;15(6):435-41.

12. Souki BQ, Figueiredo DS, Lima IL, Oliveira DD, Miguel JA. Two-phase orthodontic treatment of a complex malocclusion: giving up efficiency in favor of effectiveness, quality of life, and functional rehabilitation? Am J Orthod Dentofacial Orthop. 2013 Apr;143(4):547-58.

13. Abraham KK, James AR, Thenumkal E, Emmatty T. Correction of anterior crossbite using modified transparente aligners: An esthetic approach. Contemp Clin Dent 2016 Jul-Sept;7(3):394-7.

14. Piassi E, Antunes LS, Andrade MR, Antunes LA. Quality of life following orthodontic therapy for anterior crossbite: report of cases in twin boys. Case Rep Dent. 2016;2016:3685693.

15. Jokovic A, Locker D, Tompson B, Guyatt G. Questionnaire for measuring oral health-related quality of life in eight- to ten-year-old children. Pediatr Dent. 2004 Nov-Dec;26(6):512-8.

16. Martins MT, Ferreira FM, Oliveira AC, Paiva SM, Vale MP, Allison PJ, et al. Preliminary validation of the Brazilian version of the Child Perceptions Questionnaire 8-10. Eur J Paediatr Dent. 2009 Sept;10(3):135-40.

17. Jenny J, Cons NC. Establishing malocclusion severity levels on the Dental Aesthetic Index (DAI) scale. Aust Dent J. 1996 Feb;41(1):43-6.

18. Seehra J, Newton JT, Dibiase AT. Interceptive orthodontic treatment in bullied adolescents and its impact on self-esteem and oral-health-related quality of life. Eur J Orthod. 2013 Oct;35(5):615-21.

19. Bernabé E, Sheiham A, Tsakos G, Messias de Oliveira C. The impact of orthodontic treatment on the quality of life in adolescents: a case-control study. Eur J Orthod. 2008 Oct;30(5):515-20.

20. Liu Z, McGrath C, Hägg U. The impact of malocclusion/orthodontic treatment need on the quality of life: a systematic review. Angle Orthod. 2009 May;79(3):585-91.

21. Wedrychowska-Szulc B, Syrynska M. Patient and parent motivation for orthodontic treatment--a questionnaire study. Eur J Orthod. 2010 Aug;32(4):447-52.

22. Cella DF. Quality of life: concepts and definition. J Pain Symptom Manage. 1994 Apr;9(3):186-92.

23. Dimberg L, Arnrup K, Bondemark L. The impact of malocclusion on the quality of life among children and adolescents: a systematic review of quantitative studies. Eur J Orthod. 2015 June;37(3):238-47.

24. Eismann D, Prusas R. Periodontal findings before and after orthodontic therapy in cases of incisor cross-bite. Eur J Orthod. 1990 Aug;12(3):281-3.

25. Nagarajan S, Pushpanjali K. The relationship of malocclusion as assessed by the Dental Aesthetic Index (DAI) with perceptions of aesthetics, function, speech and treatment needs among 14- to 15-year-old schoolchildren of Bangalore, India. Oral Health Prev Dent. 2010;8(3):221-8.

26. Marques LS, Ramos-Jorge ML, Paiva SM, Pordeus IA. Malocclusion: esthetic impact and quality of life among Brazilian schoolchildren. Am J Orthod Dentofacial Orthop. 2006 Mar;129(3):424-7.

27. Proffitt WR. The timing of early treatment: an overview. Am J Orthod Dentofacial Orthop. 2006 Apr;129(4 Suppl):S47-9.

28. Joury E, Marcenes W, Johal A. The role of psychosocial factors in predicting orthodontic treatment outcome at the end of 1 year of active treatment. Eur J Orthod. 2013 Apr;35(2):205-15.

29. Borrie F, Bearn D. Early correction of anterior crossbites: a systematic review. J Orthod. 2011 Sept;38(3):175-84.

30. Richards D, Lawrence A. Evidence-based practice. Br Dent J. 1996 Sept;181(5):165.

31. Yao J, Li DD, Yang YQ, McGrath CP, Mattheos N. What are the patients' expectations of orthodontic treatment: a systematic review. BMC Oral Health. 2016 Feb;16:19.

16

Influence of the socioeconomic status on the prevalence of malocclusion in the primary dentition

Thiene Silva Normando[1], Regina Fátima Feio Barroso[2,] David Normando[3]

Objective: To assess the influence of socioeconomic background on malocclusion prevalence in primary dentition in a population from the Brazilian Amazon. **Methods:** This cross-sectional study comprised 652 children (males and females) aged between 3 to 6 years old. Subjects were enrolled in private preschools (higher socioeconomic status - HSS, n = 312) or public preschools (lower socioeconomic status - LSS, n = 340) in Belém, Pará, Brazil. Chi-square and binomial statistics were used to assess differences between both socioeconomic groups, with significance level set at $P < 0.05$. **Results:** A high prevalence of malocclusion (81.44%) was found in the sample. LSS females exhibited significantly lower prevalence (72.1%) in comparison to HSS females (84.7%), particularly with regard to Class II ($P < 0.0001$), posterior crossbite ($P = 0.006$), increased overbite ($P = 0.005$) and overjet ($P < 0.0001$). Overall, malocclusion prevalence was similar between HSS and LSS male children ($P = 0.36$). Early loss of primary teeth was significantly more prevalent in the LSS group (20.9%) in comparison to children in the HSS group (0.9%), for both males and females ($P < 0.0001$). **Conclusion:** Socioeconomic background influences the occurrence of malocclusion in the primary dentition. In the largest metropolitan area of the Amazon, one in every five LSS children has lost at least one primary tooth before the age of seven.

Keywords: Malocclusion. Primary dentition. Socioeconomic factors.

» The authors report no commercial, proprietary or financial interest in the products or companies described in this article.

[1] Master's student in Dentistry, Federal University of Pará (UFPA).
[2] Associate professor, UFPA.
[3] Adjunct professor, UFPA.

Thiene Silva Normando
E-mail: thienenormando@gmail.com

INTRODUCTION

Literature reveals the prevalence of malocclusion in approximately 80-90% of Brazilian children in mixed and permanent dentition,[1-5] while these data are conflicting for the primary dentition, ranging from 50% to 80%.[6-12] This discrepancy may be explained by the various diagnostic criteria employed,[9] the examiner's background, as well as research subjects' age and ethnicity. Additionally, the socioeconomic background of the studied population seems to be another relevant etiologic factor.[3] Despite the large number of epidemiologic investigations regarding malocclusion prevalence, only a few have examined the etiologic factors that could be controlled by health measures.[13]

Brazil has one of the steepest socioeconomic disparities around the world.[14] Only a few studies have investigated the influence of this variable on malocclusion prevalence. The main difficulty appears to be the access to the most economically privileged groups, particularly because they usually refuse to participate in this kind of investigation.[7,9] Data on primary dentition in children are contradictory and restricted to cities in São Paulo state, the wealthiest Brazilian state, in which socioeconomic imbalance is not as evident as in other regions. Studies conducted in São Paulo have not identified any influence of patients' socioeconomic background on malocclusion,[7] except for a study conducted in Bauru city (São Paulo state),[9] which reported a higher risk of malocclusion prevalence in children studying in public schools (lower socioeconomic status).

A limited number of studies have investigated the socioeconomic influence on malocclusion prevalence in populations in primary dentition around the world. In developed countries,no significant influence of patients' socioeconomic background has been identified.[15,16] However, in underdeveloped areas, a significantly higher prevalence of posterior crossbite is observed among children belonging to higher socioeconomic classes.[17] Moreover, children with lower socioeconomic status (LSS) had significantly greater early primary tooth loss.

Cities located in the Brazilian Amazon are characterized by trihybrid ethnic miscegenation involving Latin/European Caucasians, Brazilian African-descendants, and Amerindians.[18] Furthermore, there is a clear socioeconomic imbalance among people living in this region. Determining the actual prevalence of malocclusion in such a population should elucidate the influence of socioeconomic status on malocclusion.

MATERIAL AND METHODS

A random selection of children were examined, males and females, with complete primary dentition. Subjects ranged in age from 3 to 6 years old, and were enrolled in preschools in Belém (Pará, Brazil), city with mean population of 1.5 million.

In general, the richer population in Brazil attends private schools, while the poor one attends public schools.[19] This criterion was used to assess the groups of the present study. The sample was divided into two groups: The first one comprising children attending public preschools (representing children from a lower socioeconomic status), and the second group comprising children attending private preschools (representing children from a higher socioeconomic status). Comparative analysis between groups was carried out to assess potential differences in malocclusion prevalence.

Sample size calculation was carried out on the basis of the school population data obtained from the Municipal Secretary of Education. In total, 14,356 children were enrolled in Belém kindergarten schools: 6,898 of which were enrolled in private schools whereas 7,458 were enrolled in public schools. A value of P = 0.5 was used for sample size calculation (estimated malocclusion prevalence),[6] confidence level at 95% and sample error of 4%. These calculations indicated that it would be necessary a sample comprising 576 children, 276 from private schools and 300 from public schools.

This study was submitted to the Federal University of Pará Ethics Committee on Human Research, and approved under protocol #143/06 CEP-ICS/UFPA. The study was also approved by the kindergarten coordination staff and children's parents. Students were selected to represent the entire metropolitan area encompassed by the city of Belém, Pará, located in the Brazilian Amazon region.

The schools selected were the ones which presented the highest number of children enrolled in the age range established for this study and which also allowed this research to be conducted. Four public schools (n = 4) were selected. All of them were located at the city suburb (the poorest area).

The private schools (n = 5) were located in the central area of Belém (the wealthiest area). The sample was collected at the schools approving the collection of data, since the access with scientific research purposes is frequently denied by Brazilian private schools.

Children's clinical examinations were performed by one single specialist in Orthodontics. Overjet, overbite, transverse dental arch relationship, early tooth loss, and occlusal relationship (Class I, II and III) were all examined. The normal characteristics of dentition were assessed as described in the literature.[6,9]

Inter-group comparative analysis was performed by means of chi-square test. Binomial test was used to compare the populations of public and private schools with regard to different morphological types of malocclusion. The level of confidence in all statistical analyses was 95% (P < 0.05). Reproducibility of clinical examination was verified by means of Kappa's statistics.

RESULTS

To assess reproducibility of clinical examination, Kappa test was applied in 8.6% (n = 56) of the sample. Results revealed satisfactory reproducibility (Kappa = 0.72, P < 0.01).

The prevalence of malocclusion found in this study was 81.44% (Table 1). Class II malocclusion was the most prevalent, occurring in 67.5% of cases. Class I malocclusion was observed in 9.4% of children, whereas Class III prevalence was observed among 4.5% of cases (Table 1).

Regarding the influence of socioeconomic factors on malocclusion prevalence, the overall findings revealed that high socioeconomic status (HSS) children showed higher prevalence of malocclusion (OR=0.59, 95% CI= 0.39-0.88, Table 1). Class II malocclusion, overbite and increased overjet were less prevalent among female children in public preschools, as compared to their counterparts in private preschools (P < 0.0001, Table 1). With regard to male children, we did not observe any significant differences in the prevalence of malocclusion, when represented by the sagittal canine relationship (P = 0.12, Table 1). Nevertheless, increased overbite was significantly more frequent in the lower level socioeconomic group (P = 0.048).

When the various types of morphological malocclusion were analyzed, overbite was observed in 23.15% of the total sample. On the other hand, anterior open bite was observed in only 7.5% of children, with no significant influence of socioeconomic status (Table 1).

Anterior crossbite appeared in a very similar manner in both socioeconomic status, for both males (P = 0.085) and females (P = 0.805) (Table 1), with relatively low occurrence (4.60%). However, posterior crossbite presented higher prevalence among children attending private schools (HSS), for both males

Table 1 - Frequency distribution of children enrolled in public preschools (lower socioeconomic status; LSS) or private preschools (higher socioeconomic status; HSS), according to the sex and malocclusion characteristics.

	Male (n = 341)		P-value (Male)	Female (n = 311)		P-value (Female)	LSS (n = 340)	HSS (n = 312)	Odds ratio Male + Female	Total (n = 652)
	LSS (n = 186)	HSS (n = 155)	LSS x HSS	LSS (n = 154)	HSS (n = 157)	LSS X HSS	Male + Fem	Male + Fem	LSS X HSS	Male+ Fem
Normal x Malocclusion										
Normal	33 (17.7%)	21 (13.5%)	0.36 (ns)	43 (27.9%)	24 (15.3%)	0.01**	76 (22.4%)	45 (14.4%)	0.59* (0.4-0.9)	121 (18.6%)
Malocclusion	153 (82.3%)	134 (86.5%)		111 (72.1%)	133 (84.7%)		264 (77.6%)	267 (85.6%)		531 (81.4%)
Malocclusion classification										
Class I	18 (9.7%)	16 (10.3%)		20 (13.1%)	7 (4.5%)	0.013*	38 (11.2%)	23 (7.4%)		61 (9.4%)
Class II	121 (65.1%)	114 (73.6%)	0.12 (ns)	80 (51.9%)	125 (79.6%)	< 0.0001***	201 (59.1%)	239 (76.6%)		440 (67.5%)
Class III	14 (7.5%)	4 (2.6%)		11 (7.1%)	1 (0.6%)	0.007**	25 (7.3%)	5 (1.6%)		30 (4.5%)
Malocclusion type										
Overbite >	38 (20.4%)	46 (29.7%)	0.048*	23 (14.9%)	44 (28%)	0.005**	61 (17.9%)	90 (28.8%)	0.54* (0.4-0.8)	151 (23.2%)
Open bite	12 (6.5%)	8 (11.6%)	0.09 (ns)	11 (7.1%)	18 (11.5%)	0.19 (ns)	23 (6.8%)	26 (8.3%)	0.80 (0.5-1.4)	49 (7.5%)
Overjet >	27 (14.5%)	25 (16.1%)	0.68 (ns)	8 (5.2%)	27 (17.2%)	< 0.0001***	35 (10.2%)	52 (16.7%)	0.57* (0.4-0.9)	87 (13.3%)
Anterior crossbite	12 (6.5%)	9 (5.8%)	0.80 (ns)	7 (4.5%)	2 (1.3%)	0.09 (ns)	19 (5.6%)	11 (3.52%)	1.62 (0.8-3.5)	30 (4.6%)
Posterior crossbite	7 (3.8%)	15 (9.7%)	0.026 *	3 (1.9%)	14 (8.9%)	0.006**	10 (2.9%)	29 (9.3%)	0.30* (0.1-0.6)	39 (6.0%)
Early tooth loss	40 (21.5%)	3 (1.9%)	< 0.0001***	31 (20.1%)	0 (0%)	< 0.0001***	71 (20.9%)	3 (1.0%)	27.2** (8.5-87.3)	74 (11.3%)

(ns)= not significant; *P < 0.05; **P < 0.01; ***P < 0.001.

and females (P = 0.006; and P = 0.026, Table 1). Posterior crossbite was observed in 6% of the sample.

Early primary tooth loss was present in less than 1% of high socioeconomic status children and in 21% of low socioeconomic status children (OR = 27.19, 95% CI = 8.46-87.31).

DISCUSSION

Malocclusion prevalence in primary dentition observed in the present investigation (81.44%) is one of the highest reported in the literature.[6-12,21] This high prevalence of malocclusion may be related to the high level of genetic miscegenation in Brazilian Amazon cities.[8] This matter should be addressed in future investigations.

Results revealed that high socioeconomic status (HSS) children showed a higher prevalence of malocclusion. These data conflict with most previous studies on the same topic,[7,15,16] which did not report any significant influence of socioeconomic background. Further investigations should explore environmental factors associated with socioeconomic background, such as sucking habits and breast-feeding,[13,22,23] and their impact on the development of malocclusion.

One single study performed in a Venezuelan school[17] found that children from public schools had a considerably higher prevalence of primary tooth loss, while posterior crossbite was significantly more prevalent among children from private preschools (high socioeconomic status). On the other hand, another study performed on a population of Brazilian children[9] found a higher prevalence of anterior open bite and deleterious oral habits in children belonging to lower socioeconomic status. The present findings corroborate the findings obtained in Venezuela,[17] since a significantly lower frequency of posterior crossbite (OR = 0.3, 95% CI = 0.14-0.62) and a significantly higher frequency of early tooth loss were observed in the lower socioeconomic group of children (OR = 27.19, 95% CI = 8.47-87.1). However, open bite does not seem to be related to socioeconomic background.

The reduced frequency of Class II and related malocclusions (overbite and increased overjet) among LSS female children is an interesting finding that cannot be explained by the data obtained herein. This tendency was also observed for male children, but was only significant in the case of overbite. Factors related to deleterious oral health must be investigated. A previous report[2]

stated that, while female children whose mothers had formal jobs had a significantly higher frequency of sucking habits, while no significant effect was observed for the male group.

Overbite was observed in one of every four children. This prevalence is higher than what was reported by previously published reports.[11,24] On the other hand, anterior open bite was observed in only 7.5% of children, with no significant influence of socioeconomic status (Table 1). This open bite frequency seems to be lower than it is in previously published data[13,22]. The lower frequency of open bite and the higher level of overbite may be linked to the facial skeletal characteristics of the Amazon population, mainly the striking indigenous influence over the formation of urban populations.[18]

Anterior crossbite prevalence was similar in previous data.[6,9,11] However, posterior crossbite was more prevalent among children attending private preschools (HSS), for both males and females (P = 0.006; and P = 0.026, Table 1). Posterior crossbite was observed in 6% of the examined sample, lower than typically reported.[6,9-12] The fact that posterior crossbite is directly related to the presence of deleterious oral habits[9,22,25] suggests that private preschool children are more likely to present these habits while breathing or sucking. Once again, this matter should be investigated in further studies, since there was no difference regarding anterior open bite between LSS and HSS groups. Non-breast-fed children presented significantly greater chances of having anterior open bite[26] and posterior crossbite[27] when compared with those who were breast-fed for periods longer than 12 months.

Literature describes lower prevalence of early primary tooth loss in other Brazilian regions.[9,24] The present findings showed that one in every five LSS children in the largest Brazilian Amazon city had early loss of at least one primary tooth before the age of seven. The reasons for the trends outlined herein include lack of access by this part of the population to basic dental services, as well as deficient oral hygiene and a deficient public health system. The National Brazilian Social Project 2003[28] showed that children in the northern region of the country present the highest frequency of untreated tooth decay. The DMF was approximately 27% higher in this region than in the southeast of Brazil, the wealthiest area. A longitudinal study[29] revealed that children with loss of primary molars before 7 1/2 years old developed more crowding than children without losses or with losses after 7 1/2 years of age. Thus, the high incidence of primary tooth loss among children belonging to lower socioeconomic groups set a worrying picture for the future. It is expected that the current high prevalence of malocclusion undergoes even greater increase.

CONCLUSION

Malocclusion is highly prevalent in the primary dentition of urban Brazilian Amazon children. The influence of socioeconomic background on the prevalence of malocclusion varies according to the morphological classification of malocclusion. Class II, increased overbite and overjet, as well as posterior crossbite were significantly more frequent among children at a higher socioeconomic status. Furthermore, in Belém, the largest city in Brazilian Amazon, one in every five LSS children has lost at least one primary tooth before the age of seven. These results indicate the need for oral health policies that include preventive care so as to improve the dental health of this segment of the population.

REFERENCES

1. Silva CHT, Araújo TM. A prevalência de más oclusões na ilha do governador, Rio de Janeiro. Parte I. Classe I, II e III (Angle) e mordida cruzada. Ortodontia. 1983;16:10-6.

2. Silva Filho OG, Freitas SF, Cavassan AO. Oclusão: escolares de Bauru-Prevalência de oclusão normal e má oclusão na mista em escolares da cidade de Bauru (São Paulo). Rev Assoc Paul Cir Dent. 1989;43:287-90.

3. Silva Filho OG, Freitas SF, Cavassan AO. Prevalência de oclusão normal e má oclusão em escolares da cidade de Bauru (São Paulo). Parte II: Influência da estratificação sócio-Econômica. Rev Odontol Univ São Paulo. 1990;4:189-96.

4. Brandão AMM, Normando ADC, Galon GM, Botelho PCE, Almeida HG, Freitas EM. Oclusão normal e Má oclusão na Dentição Mista: um estudo epidemiológico em escolares do município de Belém-PA. Rev Paraense Odontol. 1997;2:13-9.

5. Normando ADC, Brandão AMM, Matos JNR, Cunha AVR, Mohry O, Jorge STM, et al. Má oclusão e oclusão normal na dentição permanente: um estudo epidemiológico em escolares do Município de Belém-PA. Rev Paraense Odontol. 1999;4:21 6.

6. Brandão AMM, Normando ADC, Sinimbu CMB, Milhomem SC, Esteves RA. Oclusão normal e má oclusão na dentição decídua: um estudo epidemiológico em pré-escolares do município de Belém-PA. Rev Paraense Odontol. 1996;1:13-7.

7. Martins JCR, Sinimbu CMB, Dinelli TCS, Martins LPM. Prevalência de má-oclusão em pré-escolares de Araraquara: relação da dentição decídua com hábitos e nível sócio econômico. Rev Dental Press Ortod Ortop Facial. 1998;3(6):35-43.

8. Tomita NE, Bijella MFTB, Silva SMB, Bijella VT, Lopes ES, Novo NF, et al. Prevalência de má oclusão em pré-escolares de Bauru – SP – Brasil. Rev Fac Odontol Bauru. 1998;6:35-44.

9. Silva Filho OG, Silva PRB, Rego MVNN, Silva FPL, Cavassan AO. Epidemiologia da má oclusão da dentadura decídua. Ortodontia. 2002;25:22-33.

10. Lenci PRJ. Trabalho sobre a incidência de má oclusão entre crianças de 3 a 6 anos. Rev Dental Press Ortod Ortop Facial. 2002;7(1):81-3.

11. Chevitarese ABA, Valle DD, Moreira TC. Prevalence of malocclusion in 4-6 year old Brazilian children. J Clin Pediatr Dent. 2002;27:81-6.

12. Thomaz EBAF, Valença AMG. Prevalência de má oclusão e fatores relacionados à sua ocorrência em pré-escolares da cidade de São Luís- MA- Brasil. Rev Pós-Grad. 2005;12(2):212-21.

13. Peres KG, Latorre MRO, Sheiham A, Peres MA, Victora CG, Barros FC. Social and biological early life influences on the prevalence of open bite in Brazilian 6-year-olds. Int J Paediatr Dent. 2007;17:41-9.

14. Diaz MDM. Desigualdades socioeconômicas na saúde. Rev Bras Econ. 2003;57:7-25.

15. Calisti LJP, Cohen MM, Fales MH. Correlation between malocclusion, oral habits, and socio-economic level of preschool children. J Dent Res. 1960;39:450-4.

16. Popovich F. The prevalence of sucking habit and its relationship to malocclusion. Oral Health. 1967;57:498-9.

17. Morón AB, Baez A, Rivera L, Hernandez N, Rivera N, Luchese E. Perfil de la oclusion Del ninõ en edad preescolar. Factores de benefício y riesgo. Acta Odontol Venez. 1997;35:12-5.

18. Galvão CAAN, Pereira CB, Bello DRM. Prevalência de maloclusões na América Latina e considerações antropológicas. Ortodontia. 1994; 27(1):51-8.

19. Farias ES, Lanza MB, Ferreira CRT, Carvalho WRG, Guerra-Júnior G. Maturação sexual em Escolares de baixo nível socioeconômico da cidade de Rio Branco-AC. Rev Bras Cineantropom Desempenho Hum. 2006;8(3):45-50.

20. Piovesan C, Pádua MC, Ardenghi TM, Mendes FM, Bonini GC. Can type of school be used as an alternative indicator of socioeconomic status in dental caries studies? A cross-sectional study. BMC Med Res Methodol. 2011 Apr 2;11:37.

21. Stecksén-Blicks C, Holm AK. Dental caries, tooth trauma, malocclusion, fluoride usage, toothbrushing and dietary habits in 4-year-old Swedish children: changes between 1967 and 1992. Int J Paediatr Dent. 1995;5:143-8.

22. Tomita NE, Sheiham A, Bijella VT, Franco LJ. Relação entre determinantes socioeconômicos e hábitos bucais de risco para más-oclusões em pré-escolares. Pesq Odont Bras. 2000;14:169-75.

23. Thomaz EBAF, Ely MR, Lira CC, Moraes ES, Valença AMG. Prevalência de protrusão dos incisivos superiores, sobremordida profunda, perda prematura de elementos dentários e apinhamento na dentição decídua. J Bras Odontopediatr Odontol Bebê. 2002;5(26):276-82.

24. Bueno SB, Bittar TO, Vazquez FL, Meneghim MC, Pereira AC. Association of breastfeeding, pacifier use, breathing pattern and malocclusions in preschoolers. Dental Press J Orthod. 2013;18(1):30.e1-6.

25. Romero CC, Scavone-Junior H, Garib DG, Cotrim-Ferreira FA, Ferreira RI. Breastfeeding and non-nutritive sucking patterns related to the prevalence of anterior open bite in primarydentition. J Appl Oral Sci. 2011;19(2):161-8.

26. Brasil. Ministério da Saúde. Projeto SB Brasil 2003: condições de saúde bucal da população brasileira 2002-2003- Resultados Principais. Brasília, DF: Secretaria de Atenção à Saúde; Departamento de Atenção Básica; Coordenação Nacional de Saúde Bucal; 2004.

27. Kobayashi HM, Scavone H Jr, Ferreira RI, Garib DG. Relationship between breastfeeding duration and prevalence of posterior crossbite in the primary dentition. Am J Orthod Dentofacial Orthop. 2010;137(1):54-8.

17

Dentoskeletal effects of Class II malocclusion treatment with the Twin Block appliance in a Brazilian sample

Luciano Zilio Saikoski[1], Rodrigo Hermont Cançado[2], Fabrício Pinelli Valarelli[3], Karina Maria Salvatore de Freitas[2]

Objective: The aim of this study was to assess the dentoskeletal effects of Class II malocclusion treatment performed with the Twin Block appliance. **Methods:** The experimental group comprised 20 individuals with initial mean age of 11.76 years and was treated for a period of 1.13 years. The control group comprised 25 individuals with initial mean age of 11.39 years and a follow-up period of 1.07 years. Lateral cephalograms were taken at treatment onset and completion to assess treatment outcomes. Intergroup comparison was performed by means of the chi-square and independent t tests. **Results:** The Twin Block appliance did not show significant effects on the maxillary component. The mandibular component showed a statistically significant increase in the effective mandibular length (Co-Gn) and significant improvement in the maxillomandibular relationship. The maxillary and mandibular dentoalveolar components presented a significant inclination of anterior teeth in both arches. The maxillary incisors were lingually tipped and retruded, while the mandibular incisors were labially tipped and protruded. **Conclusions:** The Twin Block appliance has great effectiveness for correction of skeletal Class II malocclusion in individuals with growth potential. Most changes are of dentoalveolar nature with a large component of tooth inclination associated with a significant skeletal effect on the mandible.

Keywords: Angle Class II malocclusion. Skull circumference. Functional orthodontic appliances. Prospective studies. Treatment outcome.

[1] MSc in Orthodontics, Ingá College (UNINGÁ).
[2] Adjunct professor, Department of Orthodontics, postgraduate program, (UNINGÁ).
[3] Adjunct professor, Department of Orthodontics, Ingá College (UNINGÁ).

Rodrigo Hermont Cançado
Rua do Amparo, nº 100 - Centro - Diamantina-MG — Brazil
CEP: 39100-000 - E-mail: rohercan@uol.com.br

INTRODUCTION

Functional appliances have been widely used for treatment of skeletal Class II malocclusion. Even though a few clinicians do not recognize the great effectiveness of these appliances, scientific evidence about the fact that these appliances promote changes in jaw growth remains undefined.[1,2]

Some authors believe that there is little evidence to support the fact that functional appliances significantly alter mandibular growth.[3,4] Conversely, other authors suggest that these appliances may have a significant influence over mandibular growth, when used in proper timing.[5,6,7]

The main changes caused by functional appliances are of dentoalveolar nature, including distalization of the maxillary posterior segment, lingual inclination of maxillary incisors, mesialization of the mandibular posterior segment and buccal inclination of mandibular incisors.[8] The main vertical changes comprise restriction of vertical development of maxillary molars and stimulation of vertical development of mandibular molars.[8]

However, most of the aforementioned results have been obtained from retrospective studies, and a relatively small number of studies which aimed at assessing dentoskeletal changes were considered as prospective.[9-12] Thus, this study prospectively assessed the dentoskeletal effects of the Twin Block appliance for treatment of the Class II malocclusion .

MATERIAL AND METHODS
Sample

This study was approved by the Institutional Review Board of Ingá College and all subjects in the sample signed an informed consent form before treatment onset. Sample size calculation was performed to determine the minimum number of individuals in each group. It was calculated considering α = 5% (type I error), β = 20% (type II error), estimated variability (s) of 1.5[13] and a minimum difference of 2 mm to be detected (d) between the control and experimental groups. The results revealed a sample of 17 individuals in each group (accounting for occasional losses), with a test power of 80%. A sample of 19 individuals in each group allows a test power of 85%.

The prospective sample comprised 20 dental casts obtained at treatment onset (T_1) and 40 lateral cephalograms obtained at onset (T_1) and completion (T_2) of orthopedic treatment of 20 individuals with Class II division 1 malocclusion. Twenty-five dental casts and 50 lateral cephalograms obtained from 25 individuals with Class II division 1 malocclusion, who did not receive treatment, comprised the control group. The cephalograms and dental casts in the control group were obtained from the files of the Department of Orthodontics of School of Dentistry — University of São Paulo/Bauru.

The experimental group comprised 20 individuals, 11 males and 9 females, with initial mean age of 11.76 ± 1.64 years presenting Class II division 1 malocclusion at treatment onset and who were treated with the modified Twin Block functional orthopedic appliance. The mean treatment time was 1.13 ± 0.40 years and the final mean age was 12.89 ± 1.56 years. With regard to the initial severity of anteroposterior relationship between the permanent first molars assessed on the dental casts, 9 individuals presented full Class II, 3 presented ¾ of Class II, 7 presented ½ Class II and 1 presented ¼ of Class II.

The control group comprised 25 untreated individuals, 14 males and 11 females, with Class II division 1 malocclusion, with initial mean age of 11.39 ± 1.35 years. The mean follow-up time was 1.07 ± 0.17 years and the final mean age was 12.46 ± 1.38 years. As for the initial severity of anteroposterior relationship between the permanent first molars assessed on the dental casts, 4 individuals presented full Class II, 6 presented ¾ of Class II, 9 presented ½ Class II and 6 presented ¼ of Class II.

The inclusion criteria for the experimental group were: 1) presence of Class II division 1 malocclusion assessed on the dental casts and clinically confirmed (no cephalometric criterion was used to determine that individuals presented skeletal Class II with ANB values greater than 4 degrees); 2) crowding in the mandibular arch not greater than 4 mm; 3) no previous orthodontic treatment; 4) presence of clinically observable facial convexity.

Description of the modified Twin-Block appliance

Maxillary portion — composed of an acrylic base covering the hard palate, open at the midpalatal suture line with a Dentaurum® 6.5 mm expanding screw, allowing transverse expansion of the maxillary arch. It contains an anterior Hawley bow used to enhance retention, retract the lip musculature and control the inclinations of maxillary incisors. The appliance has simple coils on the palatal region of maxillary central and lateral incisors for tongue pressure control and teeth uprighting. The appliance retention is achieved in posterior teeth with Benac clasps, which allow activation and present good flexibility due to the great amount of wire employed for fabrication. The acrylic blocks are placed on the occlusal surface of posterior teeth with enough height to allow disocclusion of anterior teeth. The anterior portion of planes present an angle of 70 degrees, which, in combination with the mandibular planes, keeps the mandible protruded (Figs 1 and 2).

The mandibular portion is composed of an acrylic base on the lingual alveolar ridge, with anterior Hawley bow to control the inclination of incisors. The presence of a Dentaurum® 5.5-mm expanding screw on the midline allows correction of small lingual inclinations of posterior teeth. Benac clasps are used for appliance retention on the posterior portion, and, if the bow is not sufficient in the anterior portion, an acrylic coverage should be applied on the edges of mandibular incisors. The planes are located ahead, at the region of the first premolars, and are extended up to the canines in order to achieve greater strength. They are fabricated at 70 degrees to fit with the maxillary portion of the appliance, keeping the mandible in a more anterior position. Plane height is compatible with the upper plane, without contact with teeth

in the maxillary arch (Figs 1 and 2). The individuals were instructed to use the modified Twin Block for an approximate period of 20h/day.

Lateral cephalograms

Aiming to verify the dentoskeletal changes of the modified Twin Block appliance, lateral cephalograms obtained at treatment onset and completion were assessed and compared to the control group. All radiographic images were obtained with the lips at rest and in maximum intercuspation, with the aid of the Broadbent cephalostat to standardize head positioning. All cephalograms in the sample were performed in three difference machines and the magnification of each appliance was determined in order to allow greater accuracy of results. The different machines presented distinct magnification percentages which ranged from 6% to 10.94%.

Cephalometric tracing and achievement of measurements

The cephalograms were digitized at a resolution of 9600 x 4800 dpi in a Microtek ScanMaker i800 scanner (Microtek International, Inc., Carson, CA, USA) connected to a Pentium microcomputer. The images were transferred to the Dolphin Imaging Premium 10.5 software (Dolphin Imaging & Management Solutions, Chatsworth, CA, USA) through which the cephalometric points of interest were marked and measurements involving the planes and lines were obtained.

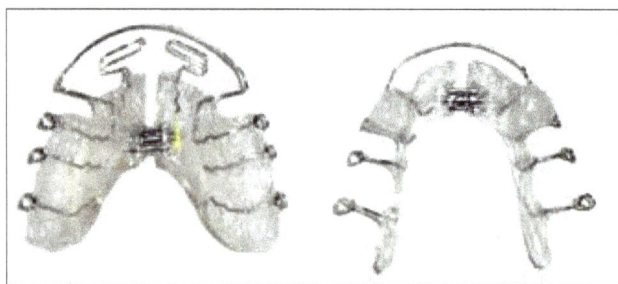

Figure 1 - Modified Twin Block appliance.

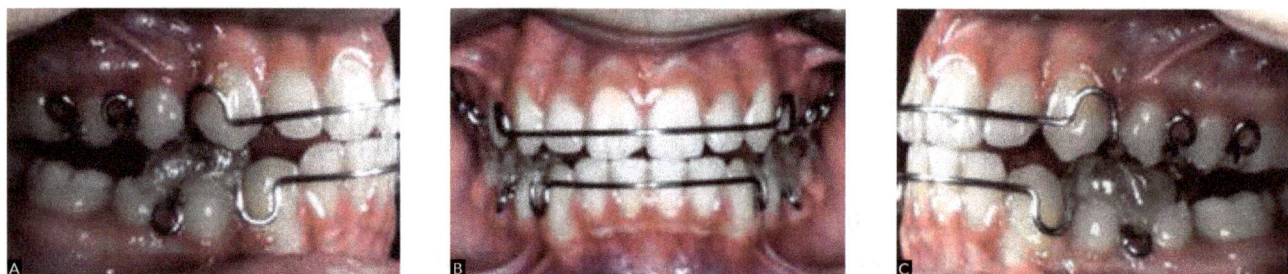

Figure 2 - Twin Block appliance in use - **A)** Right lateral view. **B)** Frontal view. **C)** Left lateral view.

Cephalometric measurements employed (Figs 3, 4, 5 and 6)

The following cephalometric measurements were used in this study:

1. Maxillary component: SNA, A-Nperp and Co-A.
2. Mandibular component: SNB, P-Nperp and Co-Gn.
3. Maxillomandibular relationship: ANB and Wits.
4. Growth pattern: SN.GoGn, SN.GoMe, SN.Ocl, FMA and LAFH.
5. Maxillary dentoalveolar component: 1.NA, 1-NA, 1-Aperp, 1.PP and 1-PP.
6. Mandibular dentoalveolar component: 1.NB, 1-NB, 1-AP and IMPA.
7. Dental relationships: overjet, overbite and molar relationship.

STATISTICAL ANALYSIS
Method error

To evaluate the intra-examiner error, all measurements were repeated by the same investigator on 30 lateral cephalograms randomly selected after a three-week interval. Application of the mathematical formula proposed by Dahlberg ($Se^2 = \Sigma d^2/2n$) allowed estimation of casual errors.[14] Systematic errors were assessed by the dependent t test.[15,16]

Intergroup comparison

The Kolmogorov-Smirnov test was applied to analyze if cephalometric data in the experimental and control groups presented normal distribution. The results revealed that the cephalometric variables presented normal distribution in both groups and in all periods analyzed ($P > 0.05$). Thus, parametric tests were used for intergroup comparison. The compatibility between experimental and control groups in relation to the initial (T_1) and final mean ages (T_2) and the treatment/follow-up time was assessed by the independent t test. The chi-square test was used to verify the compatibility between groups with regard to gender distribution and anteroposterior severity existing between molars.

The independent t test was used for intergroup comparison at the initial (T_1) and final periods (T_2) and to assess changes between the initial and final periods (T_2-T_1) in both groups. Bonferroni correction was used for false-positive control (type I error), and differences were considered statistically significant at $P < (0.05/24) = 0.002$.

All statistical tests were performed by means of the Statistica for Windows 7.0 software (Stat Soft Inc., Tulsa, Oklahoma, USA).

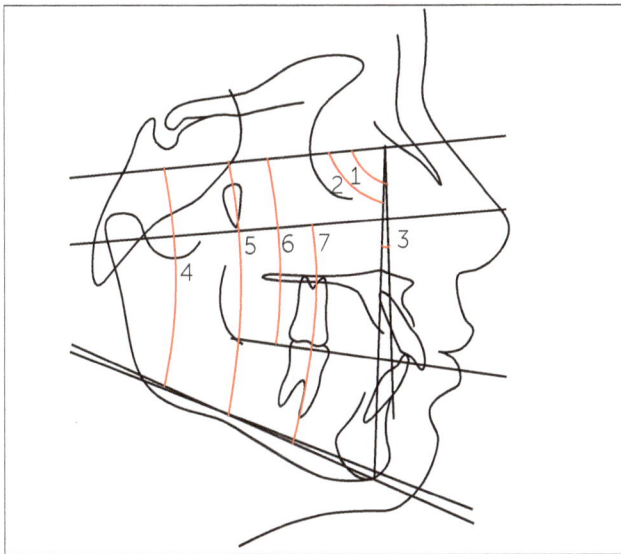

Figure 3 - Skeletal angular cephalometric measurements: 1) SNA; 2) SNB; 3) ANB; 4) SN.GoMe; 5) SN.GoGn; 6) SN.Ocl; 7) FMA.

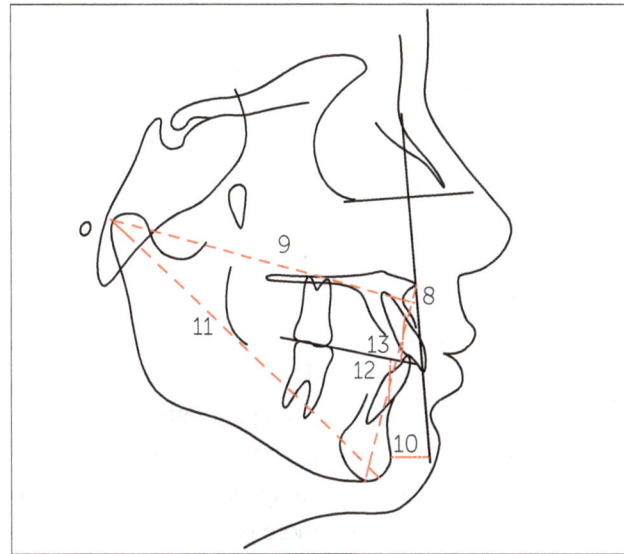

Figure 4 - Linear skeletal cephalometric measurements: 8) A-Nperp; 9) Co-A; 10) P-Nperp; 11) Co-Gn ;12) Wits; 13) LAFH.

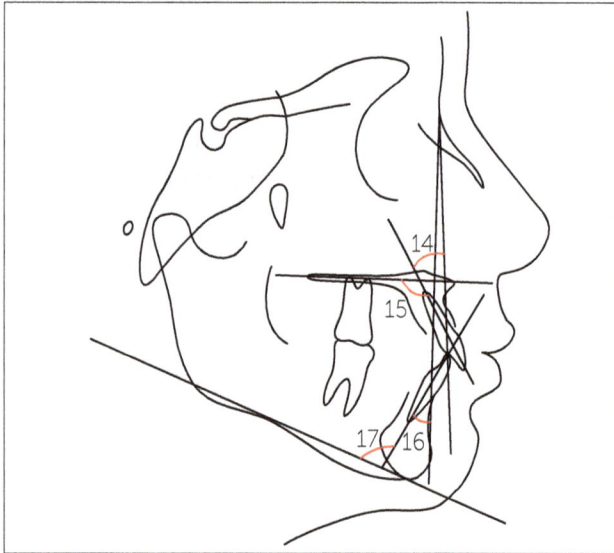

Figure 5 - Angular dental cephalometric measurements: 14) 1.NA; 15) 1.PP; 16) 1.NB; 17) IMPA.

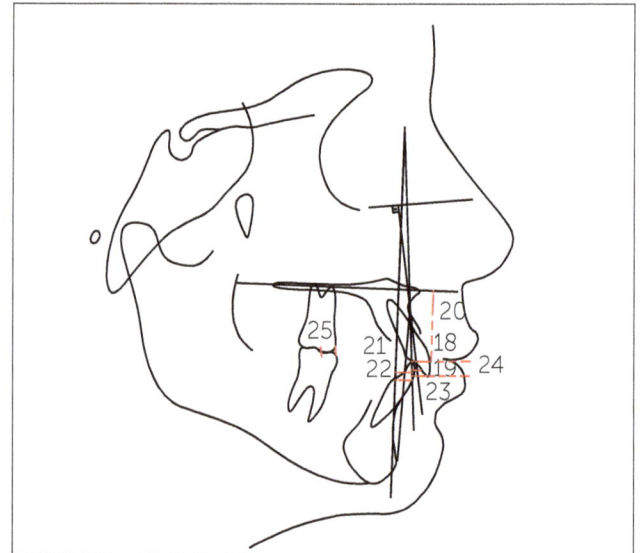

Figure 6 - Linear dental cephalometric measurements: 18) 1-NA; 19) 1-Aperp; 20) 1-PP; 21) 1-NB; 22) 1-AP; 23) overjet; 24) overbite; 25) molar relationship.

RESULTS

Three variables (SNA, SN.GoGn and LAFH) presented systematic error ($P < 0.05$) and the amplitude of casual errors ranged from 0.32 (ANB) to 2.39 (LAFH).

The experimental and control groups were compatible in initial and final age, treatment/follow-up time, gender distribution and severity of anteroposterior relationship existing between molars (Tables 1, 2 and 3).

At treatment onset (T_1), the experimental and control groups presented moderate cephalometric compatibility, with the variables ANB and Wits in the maxillomandibular relationship component presenting the worst relationship between jaws in the experimental group ($P < 0.002$). In the maxillary dentoalveolar component, the 1-Aperp variable revealed that maxillary incisors in the experimental group were significantly more buccally inclined and protruded in the maxilla ($P < 0.002$). As for the dental relationship component, the overjet variable significantly increased in relation to the control group ($P < 0.002$) (Table 4).

At treatment completion (T_2), the growth pattern, evaluated by the LAFH variable, was significantly greater in the experimental group in comparison to the control group. In the mandibular dentoalveolar component, the experimental group presented significantly more protruded and buccally inclined mandibular incisors in comparison to the control group. In the evaluation of dental relationships, the experimental group presented significantly smaller molar relationship in comparison to the control group (Table 5).

Comparison of dentoskeletal changes (T_2-T_1) between the experimental and control groups revealed that, in relation to the mandibular component, the experimental group exhibited a significantly greater increase in mandibular length (Co-Gn). As for the growth pattern component, the Sn.Ocl variable exhibited significantly greater increase in the experimental group in comparison to the control group. With regard to the maxillary dentoalveolar component, the experimental group presented greater and significant lingual inclination and retrusion of maxillary incisors in comparison to the control group. In the mandibular dentoalveolar component, the experimental group exhibited greater and significant buccal inclination and protrusion of mandibular incisors in comparison to the control group. In the analysis of dental relationships, the experimental group exhibited significantly greater reduction in overjet and molar relationship when compared to the control group (Table 6).

DISCUSSION

The use of removable functional orthopedic appliances in growing individuals with skeletal Class II has demonstrated to have some advantages promoted by treatment of Class II malocclusion in two stages (functional orthopedics and fixed appliance).[11,17] Reduction in overjet at early ages, better relationship between the jaws, reduction in facial convexity and shorter treatment time with fixed appliances are factors that encourage treatment of Class II malocclusion in two stages.[9]

Table 1 - Evaluation of compatibility between groups considering initial age, final age and treatment/follow-up time (independent t test).

Variables (years)	Experimental group (n = 20) Mean ± S.D.	Control group (n = 25) Mean ± S.D.	P
Initial age	11.76 ± 1.64	11.39 ± 1.35	0.4063
Final age	12.89 ± 1.56	12.45 ± 1.38	0.3239
Treatment/follow-up time	1.13 ± 0.40	1.07 ± 0.17	0.4773

Table 2 - Comparison of sex distribution in the two groups (chi-square test).

Group	Sex Female	Sex Male	Total
Experimental	9	11	20
Control	11	14	25
Total	20	25	45

$\chi^2 = 0.005$; df = 1; P = 0.9465

Table 3 - Result of the chi-square test for comparison between experimental and control groups with regard to the severity of existing anteroposterior molar relationship.

Severity	Experimental group (n = 20)	Control group (n = 25)
¼ Class II	1	6
½ Class II	7	9
¾ Class II	3	6
Full Class II	9	4

$\chi^2 = 6.2663$; df = 3; P = 0.0993

Table 4 - Results of the independent t test for comparison between experimental and control groups at the initial period (T_1).

Variables	Experimental Group (T_1) (n = 20) Mean ± S.D.	Control Group (T_1) (n = 25) Mean ± S.D.	P
Maxillary component			
SNA (degrees)	84.51 ± 3.51	83.30 ± 3.16	0.2270
A-Nperp (mm)	0.78 ± 2.98	-0.18 ± 2.70	0.2618
Co-A (mm)	85.45 ± 3.38	83.67 ± 4.80	0.1686
Mandibular component			
SNB (degrees)	77.33 ± 4.10	78.59 ± 3.49	0.2723
P-Nperp (mm)	-8.95 ± 6.64	-6.30 ± 4.83	0.1287
Co-Gn (mm)	108.49 ± 6.60	108.14 ± 6.27	0.8570
Maxillomandibular relationship			
ANB (degrees)	7.19 ± 2.27	4.69 ± 1.66	**0.0001**
Wits (mm)	3.84 ± 2.65	0.50 ± 2.34	0.0001
Growth pattern			
SN.GoGn (degrees)	30.46 ± 5.24	29.88 ± 4.95	0.7049
SN.Ocl (degrees)	13.00 ± 5.20	14.57 ± 2.99	0.2095
FMA (degrees)	26.58 ± 4.85	25.83 ± 4.06	0.5743
LAFH (mm)	61.16 ± 4.03	58.49 ± 4.55	0.0461
Maxillary dentoalveolar component			
1.NA (degrees)	29.48 ± 6.75	24.73 ± 6.29	0.0190
1-NA (mm)	5.03 ± 2.10	3.44 ± 1.87	0.0107
1-Aperp (mm)	6.23 ± 1.74	4.40 ± 1.05	**0.0001**
1.PP (degrees)	120.68 ± 5.63	115.20 ± 5.80	0.0027
1-PP (mm)	26.35 ± 1.86	25.37 ± 2.76	0.1837
Mandibular dentoalveolar component			
1-NB (mm)	5.14 ± 2.44	3.92 ± 1.97	0.0713
1.NB (degrees)	26.18 ± 6.98	24.40 ± 6.34	0.3760
1-AP (mm)	-0.15 ± 2.12	0.37 ± 2.16	0.4213
IMPA (degrees)	95.92 ± 8.16	93.47 ± 6.59	0.2715
Dental relationships			
Overjet (mm)	9.16 ± 2.10	5.61 ± 2.61	**0.0000**
Overbite (mm)	4.59 ± 2.50	3.29 ± 1.73	0.0464
Molar relationship (mm)	1.90 ± 1.54	0.40 ± 1.55	0.0024

Table 5 - Results of the independent t test for comparison between experimental and control groups at the final period (T$_2$).

Variables	Experimental Group (T$_2$) (n = 20) Mean ± S.D.	Control Group (T$_2$) (n = 25) Mean ± S.D.	p
Maxillary component			
SNA (degrees)	84.18 ± 4.55	82.99 ± 3.26	0.3117
A-Nperp (mm)	0.50 ± 3.36	-0.48 ± 2.51	0.2728
Co-A (mm)	87.26 ± 3.68	84.84 ± 4.39	0.0562
Mandibular component			
SNB (degrees)	78.61 ± 4.66	78.84 ± 3.90	0.8523
P-Nperp (mm)	-7.08 ± 7.14	-5.93 ± 4.81	0.5256
Co-Gn (mm)	115.00 ± 6.72	110.48 ± 6.21	0.0242
Maxillomandibular relationship			
ANB (degrees)	5.59 ± 1.83	4.14 ± 1.69	0.0087
Wits (mm)	1.67 ± 3.15	0.16 ± 3.02	0.1083
Growth pattern			
SN.GoGn (degrees)	29.94 ± 5.39	28.96 ± 4.79	0.5223
SN.Ocl (degrees)	14.37 ± 5.13	13.70 ± 3.02	0.5823
FMA (degrees)	25.91 ± 4.58	25.26 ± 3.40	0.5885
LAFH (mm)	64.34 ± 4.00	59.02 ± 4.43	**0.0014**
Maxillary dentoalveolar component			
1.NA (degrees)	22.42 ± 5.11	25.13 ± 3.92	0.0502
1-NA (mm)	3.25 ± 1.78	4.04 ± 1.61	0.1265
1-Aperp (mm)	4.78 ± 1.52	4.88 ± 1.22	0.8001
1.PP (degrees)	113.68 ± 4.38	114.96 ± 4.19	0.3221
1-PP (mm)	27.84 ± 2.09	26.02 ± 2.67	0.0167
Mandibular dentoalveolar component			
1-NB (mm)	7.10 ± 2.27	4.10 ± 1.74	**0.0000**
1.NB (degrees)	32.35 ± 6.28	25.25 ± 5.10	**0.0001**
1-AP (mm)	2.85 ± 2.10	0.74 ± 2.00	**0.0013**
IMPA (degrees)	101.43 ± 6.95	94.68 ± 5.02	**0.0005**
Dental relationships			
Overjet (mm)	3.88 ± 1.46	5.43 ± 2.09	0.0071
Overbite (mm)	3.04 ± 1.44	3.30 ± 1.53	0.5633
Molar relationship (mm)	-1.87 ± 2.24	0.42 ± 1.22	**0.0001**

Conversely, some authors have demonstrated that treatment of Class II malocclusion performed in one stage in the permanent dentition (fixed appliance) is more efficient in comparison to treatment performed in two stages, given that similar occlusal results are obtained in significantly shorter treatment time.[18,19,20]

Investigations into the actual dentoskeletal changes obtained with the Twin Block appliance in the first treatment stage did not reveal any restriction of anterior maxillary displacement (Table 6). This result suggests that treatment of Class II malocclusion with the Twin Block did not present any significant extraoral effect, as reported in previous studies.[17,21]

Evaluation of the mandibular component revealed a statistically significant increase of 4.17 mm in the mandibular length (Co-Gn) with anterior displacement of the Gonion, two changes that are desirable in the treatment of individuals with skeletal Class II malocclusion (Table 6). It was not possible to determine if the increase in the Co-Gn variable was caused by an increase in mandibular length or mandibular repositioning. Some authors have also evidenced similar changes in relation to mandibular length.[9,11,17,22] However, the functional orthopedic appliances promote a greater increase in mandibular length within shorter treatment time, yet the final mandibular length at completion of the growth period is not significantly greater in

Table 6 - Results of the independent t test for comparison of changes (T_2-T_1) between experimental and control groups.

Variables	Experimental Group (T_2) (n = 20) Mean ± S.D.	Control Group (T_2) (n = 25) Mean ± S.D.	P
Maxillary component			
SNA (degrees)	-0.33 ± 1.69	-0.30 ± 1.47	0.9564
A-Nperp (mm)	-0.29 ± 2.46	-0.29 ± 1.90	0.9915
Co-A (mm)	1.80 ± 2.60	1.17 ± 1.23	0.2870
Mandibular component			
SNB (degrees)	1.27 ± 1.41	0.26 ± 1.29	0.0152
P-Nperp (mm)	1.88 ± 4.35	0.37 ± 2.82	0.1674
Co-Gn (mm)	6.51 ± 3.13	2.34 ± 1.56	**0.0000**
Maxillomandibular relationship			
ANB (degrees)	-1.60 ± 1.55	-0.54 ± 1.10	0.0108
Wits (mm)	-2.16 ± 2.78	-0.34 ± 2.30	0.0210
Growth pattern			
SN.GoGn (degrees)	-0.53 ± 1.67	-0.92 ± 2.09	0.4911
SN.Ocl (degrees)	1.37 ± 2.38	-0.87 ± 1.87	**0.0010**
FMA (degrees)	-0.68 ± 2.21	-0.57 ± 2.57	0.8877
LAFH (mm)	3.18 ± 3.12	1.49 ± 1.44	0.0201
Maxillary dentoalveolar component			
1.NA (degrees)	-7.06 ± 6.11	0.40 ± 4.38	**0.0000**
1-NA (mm)	-1.77 ± 1.62	0.60 ± 1.45	**0.0000**
1-Aperp (mm)	-1.44 ± 1.33	0.49 ± 1.16	**0.0000**
1.PP (degrees)	-7.00 ± 6.41	-0.24 ± 3.93	**0.0001**
1-PP (mm)	1.50 ± 1.64	0.65 ± 1.27	0.0583
Mandibular dentoalveolar component			
1-NB (mm)	1.96 ± 1.83	0.18 ± 0.95	**0.0001**
1.NB (degrees)	6.17 ± 5.96	0.85 ± 3.29	**0.0004**
1-AP (mm)	3.00 ± 1.97	0.36 ± 1.10	**0.0000**
IMPA (degrees)	5.51 ± 6.33	1.20 ± 3.53	0.0060
Dental relationships			
Overjet (mm)	-5.29 ± 2.20	-0.18 ± 1.28	**0.0000**
Overbite (mm)	-1.55 ± 2.73	0.01 ± 1.39	0.0169
Molar relationship (mm)	-3.76 ± 2.32	0.02 ± 1.39	**0.0000**

comparison to untreated individuals. This characteristic of functional appliances is known in the literature as the mortgage of mandibular growth.[2,23] Improvement in mandibular retrognathism was also observed in individuals in the experimental group, who presented a greater increase in the SNB variable (1.01 degrees) when compared to the control group (Table 6). This change probably contributed to reduce facial convexity in individuals in the experimental group.

A probable lingual movement of the roots of mandibular incisors may promote alveolar remodeling, changing the position of point B to a more posterior position and, as a consequence, reducing the SNB variable. The mandibular incisors presented significant buccal inclination and protrusion, yet evidenced an increase in the SNB angle (Table 6). Previous studies also found similar changes in the evaluation of cephalometric effects promoted by the use of functional appliances.[11,21]

Evaluation of the maxillomandibular relationship component revealed that mandibular growth and/or repositioning did not promote significant changes in ANB and Wits variables with consequent reduction in skeletal discrepancy between jaws in individuals in the experimental group (Table 6). This result does not agree with previous studies, since several studies in the literature demonstrate the great effectiveness of functional appliances in achieving a better relationship between maxilla and mandible.[17,24,25]

With regard to growth pattern, there was a non-significant increase in LAFH (1.69 mm) in individuals in the experimental group compared to the control group, with consequent clockwise rotation of the occlusal plane, as observed by the significant increase in the SN.Ocl variable (Table 6). These effects were probably caused by selective wear of the acrylic in contact with the mandibular posterior teeth, allowing greater vertical development of these teeth, which contributes for correction of Class II relationship, curve of Spee and deep bite in the individuals.[26,27,28]

The maxillary and mandibular dentoalveolar components presented a significant component of inclination of anterior teeth in both arches. The maxillary incisors were lingually inclined and retruded, while the mandibular incisors were buccally inclined and protruded (Table 6). These dentoalveolar changes significantly contributed for correction of the overjet.[9,17,22] However, excessive inclination of incisors should be carefully controlled, since they substantially reduce the potential of changes of orthopedic nature.[9]

In the evaluation of dental relationships, there was a significant reduction of 5.11 mm in the overjet and of 3.78 mm in molar relationship in comparison to the control group. These changes contribute to correct the anteroposterior discrepancy in individuals with Class II malocclusion (Table 6). These results represent a desirable consequence of treatment of skeletal Class II malocclusion, and are established by the combination of dentoalveolar and skeletal changes that occurred in the experimental group.[29,30]

CONCLUSION

Based on the methods applied and the results achieved, it is reasonable to conclude that the Twin Block appliance presented great effectiveness for correction of Class II malocclusion in growing individuals. Most changes were of dentoalveolar nature with a marked component of dental inclination associated with a significant skeletal effect on the mandible.

REFERENCES

1. Woodside DG. Do functional appliances have an orthopedic effect? Am J Orthod Dentofacial Orthop. 1998;113(1):11-4.
2. Chen JY, Will LA, Niederman R. Analysis of efficacy of functional appliances on mandibular growth. Am J Orthod Dentofacial Orthop. 2002;122(5):470-6.
3. Björk A. The principles of the Andresen method of orthodontic treatment: a discussion based on cephalometric x-ray analysis of treated cases. Am J Orthod. 1951;37(6):437-58.
4. Pancherz H. A cephalometric analysis of skeletal and dental changes contributing to Class II correction in activator treatment. Am J Orthod. 1984;85(2):125-34.
5. DeVincenzo JP. Changes in mandibular length before, during and after successful orthopaedic correction of Class II malocclusions using a functional appliance. Am J Orthod Dentofacial Orthop. 1991;99(3):241-57.
6. Windmiller EC. The acrylic-splint Herbst appliance: a cephalometric evaluation. Am J Orthod Dentofacial Orthop. 1993;104(1):73-84.
7. Olibone VLL, Guimarães AS, Atta JY. Influência do aparelho propulsor Twin Block no crescimento mandibular: revisão sistemática da literatura. Rev Dental Press Ortod Ortop Facial. 2006;11(1):19-27.
8. Hirzel HC, Grewe JM. Activators: a practical approach. Am J Orthod. 1974;66(5):557-70.
9. Lund DI, Sandler PJ. The effects of Twin Blocks: a prospective controlled study. Am J Orthod Dentofacial Orthop. 1998;113(1):104-10.
10. Gill DS, Lee RT. Prospective clinical trial comparing the effects of conventional Twin-block and mini-block appliances: Part 1. Hard tissue changes. Am J Orthod Dentofacial Orthop. 2005;127(4):465-72; quiz 517.
11. Illing HM, Morris DO, Lee RT. A prospective evaluation of Bass, Bionator and Twin Block appliances. Part I--The hard tissues. Eur J Orthod. 1998;20(5):501-16.
12. Brunharo IHVP, Quintão CA, Almeida MAO, Motta A, Barreto SYN. Alterações dentoesqueléticas decorrentes do tratamento com aparelho ortopédico funcional Twin Block em pacientes portadores de má oclusão de Classe II esquelética. Dental Press J Orthod. 2011;16(5):40.e1-8.

13. Antonarakis GS, Kiliaridis S. Short-term anteroposterior treatment effects of functional appliances and extraoral traction on class II malocclusion. A meta-analysis. Angle Orthod. 2007;77(5):907-14.
14. Dahlberg G. Statistical methods for medical and biological students. New York: Interscience; 1940.
15. Baumrind S, Frantz RC. The reliability of head film measurements. 1. Landmark identification. Am J Orthod. 1971;60(2):111-27.
16. Houston WJ. The analysis of errors in orthodontic measurements. Am J Orthod. 1983;83(5):382-90.
17. Jena AK, Duggal R, Parkash H. Skeletal and dentoalveolar effects of Twin-block and bionator appliances in the treatment of Class II malocclusion: a comparative study. Am J Orthod Dentofacial Orthop. 2006;130(5):594-602.
18. Dolce C, McGorray SP, Brazeau L, King GJ, Wheeler TT. Timing of Class II treatment: skeletal changes comparing 1-phase and 2-phase treatment. Am J Orthod Dentofacial Orthop. 2007;132(4):481-9.
19. Ghafari J, Shofer FS, Jacobsson-Hunt U, Markowitz DL, Laster LL. Headgear versus function regulator in the early treatment of Class II, division 1 malocclusion: a randomized clinical trial. Am J Orthod Dentofacial Orthop. 1998;113(1):51-61.
20. Tulloch JF, Phillips C, Proffit WR. Benefit of early Class II treatment: progress report of a two-phase randomized clinical trial. Am J Orthod Dentofacial Orthop. 1998;113(1):62-72.
21. DeVincenzo JP, Huffer RA, Winn MW. A study in human subjects using a new device designed to mimic the protrusive functional appliances used previously in monkeys. Am J Orthod Dentofacial Orthop. 1987;91(3):213-24.
22. Mills CM, McCulloch KJ. Treatment effects of the twin block appliance: a cephalometric study. Am J Orthod Dentofacial Orthop. 1998;114(1):15-24.
23. Johnston LE Jr. Functional appliances: a mortgage on mandibular position. Aust Orthod J. 1996;14(3):154-7.
24. Kalha A. Early treatment with the twin-block appliance is effective in reducing overjet and severity of malocclusion. Evid Based Dent. 2004;5(4):102-3.

25. O'Brien K, Wright J, Conboy F, Sanjie Y, Mandall N, Chadwick S, et al. Effectiveness of early orthodontic treatment with the Twin-block appliance: a multicenter, randomized, controlled trial. Part 1: Dental and skeletal effects. Am J Orthod Dentofacial Orthop. 2003;124(3):234-43.

26. Clark WJ. The Twin Block technique. A functional orthopedic appliance system. Am J Orthod Dentofacial Orthop. 1988;93(1):1-18.

27. Clark WJ. The Twin Block technique. Part 2. Funct Orthod. 1992;9(6):45-9.

28. Clark WJ. The Twin Block technique. Part 1. Funct Orthod. 1992;9(5):32-4, 36-7.

29. Lee RT. How orthodontic functional appliances work. Prim Dent Care. 2000;7(2):67-73.

30. Bishara SE, Ziaja RR. Functional appliances: a review. Am J Orthod Dentofacial Orthop. 1989;95(3):250-8.

18

Interproximal wear *versus* incisors extraction to solve anterior lower crowding

Natália Valli de Almeida[1], Giordani Santos Silveira[1], Daniele Masterson Tavares Pereira[2], Claudia Trindade Mattos[3], José Nelson Mucha[4]

Objective: To determine by means of a systematic review the best treatment, whether interproximal wear or incisor extraction, to correct anterior lower crowding in Class I patients in permanent dentition. **Methods:** A literature review was conducted using MEDLINE, Scopus and Web of Science to retrieve studies published between January 1950 and October 2013. In selecting the sample, the following inclusion criteria were applied: studies involving interproximal wear and/or extraction of mandibular incisors, as well as Class I cases with anterior lower crowding in permanent dentition. **Results:** Out of a total of 943 articles found after excluding duplicates, 925 were excluded after abstract analysis. After full articles were read, 13 were excluded by the eligibility criteria and one due to methodological quality; therefore, only fours articles remained: two retrospective and two randomized prospective studies. Data were collected, analyzed and organized in tables. **Conclusion:** Both interproximal wear and mandibular incisor extraction are effective in treating Class I malocclusion in permanent dentition with moderate anterior lower crowding and pleasant facial profile. There is scant evidence to determine the best treatment option for each case. Clinical decision should be made on an individual basis by taking into account dental characteristics, crowding, dental and oral health, patient's expectations and the use of set-up models.

Keywords: Incisor. Angle Class I malocclusion. Tooth extraction.

» The authors report no commercial, proprietary or financial interest in the products or companies described in this article.

[1] Masters student of Orthodontics, Fluminense Federal University (UFF).
[2] Specialist in Library science, Integrated Colleges of Jacarepaguá (FIJ)
[3] Adjunct professor, Department of Orthodontics, UFF.
[4] Full professor, Department of Orthodontics, UFF.

Claudia Trindade Mattos
E-mail: claudiatrindademattos@gmail.com

INTRODUCTION

A pleasant smile and proper alignment of anterior teeth are the main motivation for patients seeking orthodontic treatment.[1] In permanent dentition, the mandibular anterior region is most susceptible[2] to patient's dissatisfaction. It is the most common complaint, particularly among older adult patients due to greater exposure of mandibular teeth at smiling.[3]

Orthodontic planning for this type of deficiency may involve permanent teeth extraction[1,4-26] or other approaches that do not involve extractions, such as interproximal wear,[6-11,14,19,23,24,27-31] dental expansion,[7-11,14] distraction osteogenesis of the mandibular symphysis,[32,33] as well as a combination of different techniques.[14]

The treatment of choice should be based on a number of features, such as type of malocclusion, negative discrepancy,[17,34] facial profile,[8,10,11,17] Bolton's ratio,[5] dental and periodontal conditions,[1,5,14] and patient's chief complaint. For a better prognosis, diagnostic,[1,5,13,14,19] or virtual set-ups[18] are indicated.

The aim of this study was to determine — in cases in which there is doubt as to the most appropriate procedure — the best treatment option between interproximal wear and incisor extraction to correct anterior lower crowding in Class I patients in permanent dentition and to achieve good facial esthetics.

MATERIAL AND METHODS

The guidelines and directives set by the Preferred Reporting Items for Systematic Reviews and Meta-Analysis, the PRISMA Statement, were adopted for this review.[35]

The search, as well as the inclusion/exclusion criteria, were based on PICO format (Table 1).

For sample selection, the following inclusion criteria were applied: studies involving interproximal wear and/or extraction of mandibular incisors in cases of anterior lower crowding and Class I malocclusion in permanent dentition. The exclusion criteria were: case reports; case series; laboratory studies; epidemiological studies; narrative reviews; opinion articles; studies involving orthognathic surgery, distraction osteogenesis, extraction of premolars, syndromic and/or cleft patients, supernumerary teeth and/or abnormal shape of teeth, transverse deficiencies, anterior crossbite, use of auxiliary devices; primary or mixed dentition and/or Class II or III malocclusion.

The literature review was conducted using MEDLINE (via PubMed), Scopus and Web of Science to retrieve studies that met the eligibility criteria and had been published from January 1950 to October 2013, without language restrictions. The combinations of words or terms used are described in Table 2.

Duplicate articles were eliminated from the final search results. Titles and abstracts were read independently by two reviewers who analyzed the articles in light of the inclusion and exclusion criteria. All articles found to be compatible and somehow related to the question (Table 1) were reviewed. Disagreements between reviewers were settled in a consensus meeting held with a third investigator. The articles selected were fully read. The references of the articles included in the research were also analyzed in search of potential relevant articles that might not have been found in the selected databases.

The articles selected were assessed for methodological quality according to a list based on CONSORT,[36] whenever applicable, and modified by the reviewers (Table 3). Disagreements were solved in consensus meetings, and articles were classified into high (≥ 13), moderate (<13 and ≥ 9) and low (<9) methodological quality.

Data were extracted from the articles by two reviewers.

Table 1 - PICO format.

P = Population	Angle Class I patients in permanent dentition presenting with lower anterior crowding.
I = Intervention	Subjected to orthodontic treatment involving interproximal wear or extraction of a lower incisor.
C = Comparison	Between the two types of treatment and the original characteristics of each malocclusion.
O = Outcome	The best solution for each malocclusion.
Question	What is the best treatment for lower anterior crowding in patients with Class I malocclusion in permanent dentition, interproximal wear or incisor extraction?
Null hypothesis	One treatment is no better than the other.

Table 2 - List of search parameters used in each database..

Databases	Search parameters
MEDLINE	(wear[tw] OR enamel reduction[tw] OR bolton[tw] OR reproximation[tw] OR reaproximation[tw] OR slenderizing OR tooth wear*[tw] OR tooth wear[MeSH Terms] OR dental wear*[tw] OR dental wear[MeSH Terms] OR tooth attrition[MeSH Terms] OR dental abrasion[MeSH Terms] OR dental abrasion*[tw] OR dental enamel[MeSH Terms] OR dental enamel*[tw] OR non-extraction[tw] OR nonextraction[tw] OR non extraction[tw]) OR (incisor[MeSH Terms] OR incisor*[tw] OR tooth[MeSH Terms] OR tooth[tw] OR teeth[tw] OR tooth extraction*[tw] OR teeth extraction*[tw] OR incisor extraction*[tw] OR extraction*[tw]) AND (tooth crowding[tw] OR tooth crowding[MeSH Terms] OR arch length discrepancy[tw] OR deficiency arch length[tw] OR lower jaw[tw] OR dental irregularity[tw] OR space deficiency[tw] OR lower crowding[tw] OR mandibular crowding[tw] OR incisor crowding[tw] OR crowded[tw]) AND (malocclusion, angle class I[MeSH Terms] OR angle class I[tw]) Filters: ppublication date from 1950/01/01
Scopus	(((ALL(wear) OR ALL("enamel reduction") OR ALL(bolton) OR ALL(reproximation) OR ALL(reaproximation) OR ALL(slenderizing) OR ALL("tooth wear") OR ALL("tooth wears") OR ALL("dental wear") OR ALL("dental wears") OR ALL("tooth attrition") OR ALL("dental abrasion") OR ALL("dental abrasions") OR ALL("dental enamel") OR ALL("dental enamels") OR ALL("non-extraction") OR ALL(nonextraction) OR ALL("non extraction"))) OR ((ALL(incisor) OR ALL(incisors) OR ALL(tooth) OR ALL(teeth) OR ALL("tooth extraction") OR ALL("tooth extractions") OR ALL("teeth extractions") OR ALL("teeth extraction") OR ALL("incisor extraction") OR ALL("incisor extractions") OR ALL(extraction) OR ALL(extractions)))) AND ((ALL("tooth crowding") OR ALL("arch length discrepancy") ORA LL("deficiency arch length") OR ALL("lower jaw") OR ALL("dental irregularity") OR ALL("space deficiency") OR ALL("lower crowding") OR ALL("mandibular crowding") OR ALL("incisor crowding") OR ALL("crowded"))) AND((ALL("malocclusion angle class I") OR ALL("angle class I") OR ALL("class I")))
Web of Science	#1 = TS=(wear) OR TS=(enamel reduction) OR TS=(bolton) OR TS=(reproximation) OR TS=(reaproximation) OR TS=(slenderizing) OR TS=(tooth wear*) OR TS=(dental wear*) OR TS=(tooth attrition) OR TS=(dental abrasion) OR TS=(dental enamel*) OR TS=(non-extraction) OR TS=(non extraction) OR TS=(nonextraction) #2 = TI=(wear) OR TI=(enamel reduction) OR TI=(bolton) OR TI=(reproximation) OR TI=(reaproximation) OR TI=(slenderizing) OR TI=(tooth wear*) OR TI=(dental wear*) OR TI=(tooth attrition) OR TI=(dental abrasion) OR TI=(dental enamel*) OR TI=(non-extraction) OR TI=(non extraction) OR TI=(nonextraction) #3 = TS=(incisor) OR TS=(tooth) OR TS=(teeth) OR TS=(tooth extraction*) OR TS=(teeth extraction*) #4 = TI=(incisor) OR TI=(tooth) OR TI=(teeth) OR TI=(tooth extraction*) OR TI=(teeth extraction*) #5 = TS=(tooth crowding) OR TS=(tooth crowding) OR TS=(arch length discrepancy) OR TS=(deficiency arch length) OR TS=(lower jaw) OR TS=(dental irregularity) OR TS=(space deficiency) OR TS=(lower crowding) OR TS=(mandibular crowding) OR TS=(incisor crowding) OR TS=(crowded) #6 = TI=(tooth crowding) OR TI=(tooth crowding) OR TI=(arch length discrepancy) OR TI=(deficiency arch length) OR TI=(lower jaw) OR TI=(dental irregularity) OR TI=(space deficiency) OR TI=(lower crowding) OR TI=(mandibular crowding) OR TI=(incisor crowding) OR TI=(crowded) #7 TS=(malocclusion angle class I) OR TS=(angle class I) OR TS=(class I) #8 TI=(malocclusion angle class I) OR TI=(angle class I) OR TI=(class I) #1 OR #2 = #9 / #3 OR #4 = #10 / #5 OR #6 = # 11 / #7 OR #8 = #12 / #9 OR #10 = #13 / #13 AND #11 AND #12 Time period covered by searches = 1950-2013

RESULTS

The search in the literature identified 1,094 studies, 706 from MEDLINE, 240 from Scopus and 148 from Web of Science, which are all presented in a "Prism Flow Diagram"[35] (Fig 1). After excluding 151 repeated articles, all titles and abstracts were read and those found to be unrelated to the review were eliminated. Eighteen preselected articles were read in full and the inclusion and exclusion criteria were applied. Five articles remained and were classified according to the methodological quality assessment.

One article was assigned as presenting low methodological quality[22] and was, therefore, not included in this study. Four articles showed moderate quality,[23-26] and none presented high quality (Table 4). Most articles offered insufficient sample description, both demographically and in terms of sample size calculation.

Of the four studies included, two were randomized prospective[23,24] and two were retrospective studies.[25,26] Only one article presented sample size calculation.[25] In the study by Ileri et al,[25] only the sample data for incisor extraction (IE) were considered, given that no wear was mentioned in the non extraction (NE) group, and although the authors were contacted by e-mail, no response was given. Only the data from groups of interest were extracted from the articles.[23-26]

All information regarding the author, year, study type, sample, type of treatment, statistical analysis, data evaluated and total treatment time, was gleaned from the included articles and described in Table 5.

Table 3 - Methodological quality assessment - based on CONSORT.[35]

	Methodological quality features assessed in the included studies	Score
A	Description of study objectives	1
B	Study design (retrospective = 0 point; prospective = 1 point; randomized prospective = 2 points)	2
C	Description of sample inclusion/exclusion criteria	1
D	Intervention clearly described (reason for choosing the extracted tooth/performing the wear)	1
E	Measures for evaluating the results described	1
F	Determining the sample size (sample size calculation)	1
G	Description of statistical analysis methods	1
H	Sample description (demographic - age, sex and ethnicity)	1
I	Sample description (overjet, overbite, perimeter discrepancy, Bolton, tooth form, oral health, profile) (0.5 point/item. More than 6 items = 3 points)	3
J	Description of treatment duration and follow-up (1 point each)	2
K	Description of limitations, biases and inaccuracies of the study	1
L	Operator calibration	1

Table 4 - Methodological quality scores for the selected articles. Items A to L are described in Table 3.

Studies	A	B	C	D	E	F	G	H	I	J	K	L	Points	Quality
Dacre[26]	1	0	0.5	0	1	0	1	0.5	2	2	0	1	9	Moderate
Biondi[22]	0	0	0	1	1	0	0	0.5	1	0	0	0	3.5	Low
Germeç et al[23]	1	2	1	1	1	0	1	0.5	2	1	0	1	11.5	Moderate
Germec-Cakan et al[24]	1	2	1	1	1	0	1	0.5	1	1	1	1	11.5	Moderate
Ileri et al[25]	1	0	1	0	1	1	1	0.5	2	1	1	1	10.5	Moderate

Data analyzed in each study varied widely. Ileri et al[25] assessed changes in the PAR index and Bolton ratio, and treatment included mandibular incisor extraction. Dacre[26] correlated cephalometric measurements, overjet, overbite and initial intercanine width also involving mandibular incisor extraction. Germeç et al[23] analyzed the effect of interproximal wear on cephalometric measurements, overbite and overjet. Germec-Cakan et al[24] compared intercanine and intermolar widths, as well as pre and posttreatment arch perimeter after interproximal wear. Only one study[26] described sample follow-up. Three studies[24,25,26] mentioned treatment time.

Given that studies included different data, it was impossible to compare them directly and/or perform meta-analysis.

DISCUSSION

By the end of this research, only one systematic review[37] with indications, contraindications and

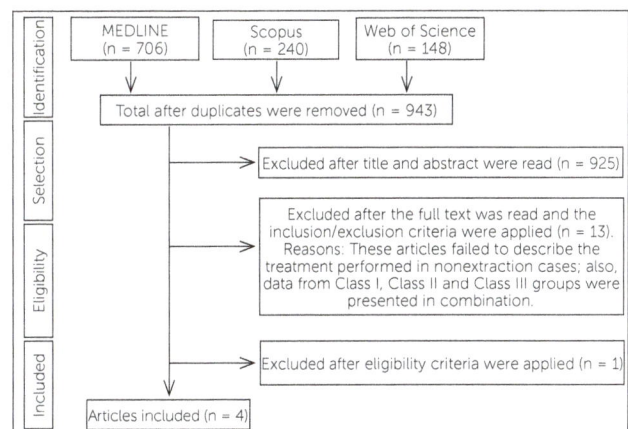

Figure 1 - PRISMA flow diagram of database research results.

effects of extracting a mandibular incisor in patients with different malocclusions, was found. Our review, however, had a different goal: to determine the advantages and disadvantages as well as the indications and contraindications of interproximal wear *versus* incisor extraction for correction of anterior

Table 5 - Data obtained from articles included.

	Dacre,[26] 1985	Germeç et al,[23] 2008	Germec-Cakan et al,[24] 2010	Ileri et al,[25] 2012
Study type	Retrospective	Randomized prospective	Randomized prospective	Retrospective
n / sex	8F/8M	11F/2M	11F/2M	13F/7M
Mean age (years)	15.0 ± 2.7	17.8 ±2.4	17.8 ± 2.4	14.3 ± 2.9
Treatment type	IE	NE = Air rotor wear (AIR) from mesial of 1st molar to mesial of 1st molar	NE = Air rotor wear (AIR) from mesial of 1st molar to mesial of 1st molar	IE
Statistical analysis	Dahlberg's formula Snedecor's F ratio T-test	Wilcoxon test Mann-Whitney U test Dahlberg's formula T-test	Wilcoxon test Mann-Whitney U test Dahlberg's formula	ANOVA Tukey HSD Mann-Whitney U test
Treatment duration (years)	1.8 ± 1.4	ND	17.0 ± 4.6	1.6 ± 0.9
Author's conclusion	Overjet and overbite increased mildly after incisor extraction with clinical significance varying from patient to patient. Posterior occlusion was not affected.	In determining treatment for borderline Class I patients the following should be considered: Treatment duration with premolar extraction, AIR limitations (enamel thickness, tooth morphology, convexity of the proximal surface), and in facial changes resulting from growth.	In Class I borderline patients with moderate crowding the extraction of premolars with minimum anchorage does not result in a narrower arch. Furthermore, in treatments without extraction both the intercanine width and the arch perimeter are preserved.	Treatments without extraction yield better results than those involving extraction of 4 first premolars, or extraction of incisors in Class I patients with moderate to severe crowding. Tooth size discrepancy should be considered to ensure satisfactory interdigitation of upper and lower teeth.

F = females; M = males; IE = incisor extraction; NE = nonextraction (interproximal wear); ND = not declared.

lower crowding in patients in permanent dentition and Class I malocclusion.

Several clinical cases[1,2,5,9,12-15,17-21,30,31,38] reported interproximal wear or mandibular incisor extraction as potential therapies for mild or moderate anterior lower crowding in patients in permanent dentition, with Class I malocclusion and a pleasant facial profile. Nevertheless, there are yet few clinical trials or randomized controlled trials addressing this issue.

Of the 943 articles found after duplicates removal, only eighteen were selected for full reading. The articles excluded after title and abstract reading included case reports or epidemiological research. Either that or the sample had undergone treatment for crossbite, distal movement of molars, surgical treatment and extraction of other permanent teeth. Some articles addressed mixed and primary dentition, or only Class II or Class III malocclusion.

Of the eighteen[16,22-26,37,39-49] articles included for full reading, only five[22-26] were selected for methodological quality assessment. The reasons for exclusion were: no description of treatment used when referring to nonextraction; lack of clear information on

whether or not interproximal wear had been performed; treatment including dental arch expansion or incisor protrusion;[39,40,42-49] use of auxiliary appliances;[40] systematic review performed using some other approach;[37] description of clinical cases;[16] and whenever data from Class I, II and III groups were presented together, which precluded the use of data from Class I patients, only.[41]

Only one[22] out of the five articles selected for methodological assessment was excluded due to low methodological quality and also because it failed to report the final results. Two out of the four articles included after qualifying addressed treatment with incisor extraction[25,26] while two reported using interproximal wear.[23,24]

Mandibular wear performed in the study by Germeç et al[23] measured 5.1 ± 0.9 mm, with 2.0 ± 0.5 mm in anterior lower teeth, only. To solve crowding of 4 mm to 8 mm, Sheridan[50] advocates interproximal reduction carried out mostly, but not exclusively, in the anterior segment. Wear should be limited to about 0.5 mm on each side of anterior teeth, and 0.8 mm on posterior teeth.[9,28] It should not exceed

Table 6 - Data obtained from articles included.

Author / year	Data assessed			
		T₁	T₂	
Dacre,²⁶ 1985	SNA	81.7±4.27	82.5±4.41	
	SNB	78.2±3.72	79.1±3.78	
	SNI	82.4±4.36	82.5±4.60	
	Overjet	3.30±1.27	4.40±1.69	
	Overbite	3.10±1.59	3.90±1.85	
	CD	24.7±1.42	22.5±1.42	

Crowding

	Severe	Moderate	Mild	Aligned	Space
Initial	9	6	1	-	-
Final	-	1	7	5	3

Crowding (mm)

NE = -5.9 ± 1.3
ARS performed

Upper: 5.4±1.7 (2.6±0.9 mm ant / 2.8±1.0 mm post)

Lower: 5.1±0.9 (2.0±0.5 mm ant / 3.1±0.9 mm post)

	T₁	T₂	P
Overjet	3.1±0.8	2.9±0.8	0.578
Overbite	2.4±1.6	3.0±0.9	0.280
Cephalometric measurements			
FMA (°)	24.5±3.9	24.3±4.1	0.186
AFI (°)	46.4±2.3	46.3±2.4	0.765
SNA (°)	79.5±3.6	79.5±2.9	0.821
SNB (°)	77.2±2.2	76.9±2.5	0.490
Pog-NB (mm)	2.0±1.6	2.5±2.0	0.027*
IMPA (°)	94.9±6.9	88.7±6.3	0.002**
Nasolabial ang (°)	108.5±8.9	109.9±10.4	0.366
UL-E-plane (mm)	-5.4±1.7	-6.4±1.8	0.046*
LL-E-plane (mm)	-2.4±1.6	-3.6±2.1	0.013*
L1-NB (°)	26.8±4.2	20.9±4.7	0.002**
UL-PTV (mm)	71.1±3.3	71.0±3.5	0.721
LL-PTV (mm)	69.0±4.0	68.9±4.0	0.479

Germeç et al,²³ 2008

*P < 0.05 **P < 0.01

Crowding

NE = -5.9 ± 1.3

	T₁	T₂	P
CD upper	34.02±2.98	33.78±2.04	0.78
MD upper	50.49±2.79	49.42±2.13	0.011*
P upper	75.46±4.91	75.15±3.36	0.469
CD lower	24.60±2.25	25.52±1.45	0.173
MD lower	43.07±3.29	41.81±2.34	0.046*
P lower	63.46±3.91	64.15±3.05	0.214

Germec-Cakan et al,²⁴ 2010

*P < 0.05

	Mean ± SD	ANOVA
PAR %	80.3±18	*(P < 0.05)
Anterior ratio	81.7±4.5	***(P < 0.01)
Overall ratio	94.2±2.9	**(P < 0.001)
PAR score	T₁	T₂
	21.5±11.5	3.8±3.52

Ileri et al,²⁵ 2012

T₁ = pretreatment; T₂ = post-treatment; PAR% = PAR index = T₂-T₁ x 100/PAR T₁; MD = intermolar distance; CD = intercanine distance; P = arch perimeter.

50% of total enamel thickness.[7] The areas of mandibular teeth where enamel thickness is greater are the distal surfaces of lateral incisors[2,7] and the mesial and distal surfaces of canines.[2]

Germec-Cakan et al[24] observed that cases in which interproximal wear was carried out had a decrease in intermolar width whereas intercanine width and arch perimeter remained unchanged. This treatment allows the creation of a contact area between teeth, which favors stability.[6] When performed carefully, interproximal wear yields a healthy dentition, which is not susceptible to periodontal disease and tooth decay.[29,51] There is a certain degree of concern, however, that a thin interdental alveolar septum might accelerate gingival attachment loss and the spread of periodontal disease.[52]

According to Ileri et al,[25] a PAR index comparison showed that malocclusions were corrected by extracting mandibular incisors, which was indicated in cases with mandibular anterior Bolton[53] discrepancy whereby the anterior ratio equals to 81.7 ± 4.5,25, thereby corroborating other articles.[5,13,16,17,18,25,37,38,54] This seems to suggest that in cases in which mandibular dental volume excess is smaller, the best alternative may be interproximal wear.[15,16] The other groups compared by Ileri et al[25] (premolar extraction and treatment without extraction) were assigned better scores after treatment, perhaps due to difficult intercuspation and/or overjet remaining in cases involving mandibular incisor extraction.[25] Thus, in these cases, interproximal wear is indicated on maxillary anterior teeth to correct remaining overjet.[1,5] Priority should be given to extracting incisors in patients with decreased overjet and overbite.[13,16,18,20,37,38]

Dacre[26] showed in a follow-up of 16 patients, after mandibular incisor extraction and retainer removal, that only five cases preserved good alignment, while seven had mild crowding relapse, one had moderate relapse, and three showed space opening. Intercanine width was slightly reduced, since extraction caused canines to move closer to the region where the dental arch is narrower.[26]

Selection of the incisor to be extracted is usually based on malposition, periodontal involvement, color change, decay and/or fracture,[1,18] factors which are less likely to induce changes in profile,[5,12] and arch length.[13] Loss of interdental papilla or formation of triangular space are examples of common undesirable effects.[13,16,37] From an esthetic point of view, teeth with a triangular shape[2,31] may benefit from interproximal wear while those with a rectangular shape respond better to extraction.

Total treatment time was similar between the studies by Ileri et al[25] and Germec-Cakan et al;[24] and both were shorter when compared to the group in which premolars were extracted. Other authors also reported decreased treatment time due to incisor extraction.[5,14,17,54]

Patients with the following characteristics may benefit from mandibular incisor extraction: Bolton's tooth-size discrepancies ≥ 4 mm,[5,12,13,16,17,18,25,37,38,54] mild to moderate mandibular crowding,[5,13,14,17-21,23,28,29,4] a tendency towards or moderate Class III,[1,16,37] Class I,[1,12,13,16,17,18,20,25,26] or Class II malocclusion,[55] a pleasant facial profile,[5,12,18,20] decreased overjet and overbite,[13,16,18,20,37,38] structurally and periodontally compromised teeth, teeth with a rectangular shape,[1,18,19,37] supernumerary incisors,[37] ectopic eruption,[37] TMD involving a retropositioned mandible,[37] mild or nonexistent maxillary crowding,[1,16,17,18,20] absence of or abnormality in the shape of maxillary central or lateral incisors,[17-20] patients with complete growth,[18,20] and treatment confirmed by set-up model tests.[1,5,13,14,18,19]

Interproximal wear should be given priority when aiming at conservative treatment[2,30] with minor changes in a pleasant profile,[2,23,30] in Class I cases,[2,9,23,24,30] cases without mandibular dental excess (Bolton ≤ 3 mm),[15,16] mild to moderate mandibular crowding,[2,16,23,24,30,31] normal overjet and overbite, low incidence of caries,[2] proper oral hygiene,[31] teeth with a triangular shape,[2,31] potential for maxillary wear, and treatment confirmed by set-up model tests.[1,5,13,14,18,19]

Several case reports[1,2,5,9,12-15,17-21,30,31,38] addressing the issue were not included, given their low evidence and inference that these cases were successful. Lack of high-methodological-quality articles is a limitation of the present study. Nevertheless, no studies have been found with good methodological quality comparing the two treatments in patients with Class I malocclusion, moderate crowding and pleasant facial profile. However, there is credible evidence[23,24,25] showing that treatment involving interproximal wear and incisor extraction do help to improve malocclusion.

CONCLUSIONS

» Both mandibular incisor extraction and interproximal wear are effective to treat patients with Class I malocclusion with moderate anterior lower crowding, in permanent dentition and with a pleasant facial profile. There is, however, scant evidence to determine the best treatment approach.

» Decreased overjet, overbite and Bolton's tooth-size discrepancy were the most decisive parameters used to indicate mandibular incisor extraction.

» Clinical decision should be made on an individual basis by taking into account patient's dental anatomical characteristics, crowding, dental and oral health conditions, expectations and the use of set-up models.

REFERENCES

1. Kokich VO Jr. Treatment of a Class I malocclusion with a carious mandibular incisor and no Bolton discrepancy. Am J Orthod Dentofacial Orthop. 2000;118(1):107-13.

2. Harfin J. Interproximal wear for the treatment of adult crowding. J Clin Orthod. 2000;34(7):424-33.

3. Motta AFJ, Souza MMG, Bolognese AM, Guerra CJ, Mucha JN. Display of the incisors as functions of age and gender. Aust Orthod J. 2010;26(1):27-32.

4. Pithon MM, Santos AM, Couto FS, Coqueiro RDS, Freitas LMA, Souza RA, et al. Perception of the esthetic impact of mandibular incisor extraction treatment on laypersons, dental professional, and dental students. Angle Orthod. 2012;82(4):732-8.

5. Kokich VG, Shapiro PA. Lower incisor extraction in orthodontic treatment. Angle Orthod. 1984;54(2):139-53.

6. Tuverson DL. Anterior interocclusal relations. Part I. Am J Orthod Dentofacial Orthop. 1980;78(4):361-70.

7. Araújo SGA, Motta AFJ, Mucha JN. A espessura do esmalte interproximal dos incisivos inferiores. Rev SOB. 2005;5(2):93-106.

8. Germec-Cakan D, Taner TU, Akan S. Arch-width and perimeter changes in patients with borderline Class I malocclusion treated with extractions or without extractions with air-rotor wear. Am J Orthod Dentofacial Orthop. 2010;137(6):734.e1-7.

9. Mondelli AL, Siqueira DF, Freitas MRd, Almeida RR. Desgaste interproximal: opção de tratamento para o apinhamento. Rev Clin Ortod Dental Press. 2002;1(3):5-17.

10. Guerrero CA, Bell WH, Contasti GI, Rodriguez AM. Mandibular widening by intraoral distraction osteogenesis. Br J Oral Maxillofac Surg. 1997;35(6):383-92.

11. Del Santo Júnior M, English JD, Wolford LM, Gandini LG. Midsymphyseal distraction osteogenesis for correcting transverse mandibular discrepancies. Am J Orthod Dentofacial Orthop. 2002;121(6):629-38.

12. Grob DJ. Extraction of a mandibular incisor in a Class I malocclusion. Am J Orthod Dentofacial Orthop. 1995;108(5):533-41.

13. Bayram M, Özer M. Mandibular incisor extraction treatment of a Class I malocclusion with Bolton Discrepancy: a case report. Eur J Dent. 2007;1(1):54-9.

14. Valinot JR. Mandibular incisor extraction therapy. Am J Orthod Dentofacial Orthop. 1994;105(2):107-16.

15. Raju DS, Veereshi A, Naidu DL, Raju BR, Goel M, Maheshwari A. Therapeutic extraction of lower incisor for orthodontic treatment. J Contemp Dent Pract. 2012;13(4):574-7.

16. Uribe F, Nanda R. Considerations in mandibular incisor extraction cases. J Clin Orthod. 2009;43(1):45-51.

17. Bahreman A-A. Lower incisor extraction in orthodontic treatment. Am J Orthod Dentofacial Orthop. 197;72(5):560-7.

18. Miller RJ, Duong TT, Derakhshan M. Lower incisor extraction treatment with the Invisalign System. J Clin Orthod. 2002;36(2):95:102.

19. Tuverson DL. Anterior interocclusal relations. Part II. Am J Orthod. 1980;78(4):371-93.

20. Owen AH. Single lower incisor extractions. J Clin Orthod. 1993;27(3):153-60.

21. Sheridan JJ, Hastings J. Air-rotor wear and lower incisor extraction treatment. J Clin Orthod. 1992;26(1):18-22.

22. Biondi G. Extraction of a lower incisor in adult orthodontic treatment: An acceptable compromise? L'extraction d'une incisive inférieure dans le traitement orthodontique de l'adulte: Un compromis acceptable? Int Orthod. 2006;4:63-72.

23. Germeç D, Taner TU. Effects of extraction and nonextraction therapy with air-rotor wear on facial esthetics in postadolescent borderline patients. Am J Orthod Dentofacial Orthop. 2008;133(4):539-49.

24. Germec-Cakan D, Taner TU, Akan S. Arch-width and perimeter changes in patients with borderline Class I malocclusion treated with extractions or without extractions with air-rotor wear. Am J Orthod Dentofacial Orthop. 2010;137(6):734.e1-7.

25. Ileri Z, Basciftci FA, Malkoc S, Ramoglu SI. Comparison of the outcomes of the lower incisor extraction, premolar extraction and non-extraction treatments. Eur J Orthod. 2012;34(6):681-85.

26. Dacre JT. The long term effects of one lower incisor extraction. Eur J Orthod. 1985;7(2):136-44.

27. Peck H, Peck S. An index for assessing tooth shape deviations as applied to the mandibular incisors. Am J Orthod Dentofacial Orthop. 1972;61(4):384-401.

28. Sheridan JJ, Ledoux PM. Air-rotor wear and proximal sealants. J Clin Orthod. 1989;23(12):790-4.

29. Zachrisson BU, Nyoygaard L, Mobarak K. Dental health assessed more than 10 years after interproximal enamel reduction of mandibular anterior teeth. Am J Orthod Dentofacial Orthop. 2007;131(2):162-9.

30. Capelli Júnior J, Cardoso M, Rosembach G. Tratamento do apinhamento ântero-inferior por meio de desgaste interproximal. Rev Bras Odontol. 1999;56(4):107-3.

31. Nojima LI. Tratamento conservador de uma má oclusão Classe I de Angle, com atresia maxilar e apinhamento anterior. Dental Press J Orthod. 2011;16(5):163-71.

32. Del Santo M Jr, Guerrero CA, Buschang PH, English JD, Samchukov ML, Bell WH. Long-term skeletal and dental effects of mandibular symphyseal distraction osteogenesis. Am J Orthod Dentofacial Orthop. 2000;118(5):485-93.

33. Maia LGM, Gandini Jr LG, Gandini MREAS, Moraes ML, Monini AC. Distração osteogênica da sínfese mandibular como opção de tratamento ortodôntico: relato de caso. Rev Dental Press Ortod Ortop Facial. 2007;12(5):34-45.

34. Uysal T, Yagci A, Ozer T, Veli I, Ozturk A. Mandibular anterior bony support and incisor crowding: Is there a relationship? Am J Orthod Dentofacial Orthop. 2012;142(5):645-53.

35. Moher D, Liberati A, Tetzlaff J, Altman DG, Group Prisma. Preferred Reporting Items for Systematic Reviews and Meta-Analyses: The PRISMA Statement. Ann Int Med. 2009;151(4):264-70.

36. Moher D, Hopewel S, Schul KF, Montori V, Gøtzsche PC, Devereaux PJ, et al. CONSORT 2010 Explanation and Elaboration: updated guidelines for reporting parallel group randomised trials. J Clin Epidemiol. 2010;63(8):e1-37.

37. Zhylich D, Suri S. Mandibular incisor extraction: a systematic review of an uncommon extraction choice in orthodontic treatment. J Orthod. 2011;38(3):185-95.

38. Matsumoto MAN, Romano FL, Ferreira JTL, Tanaka S, Morizono EN. Lower incisor extraction: an orthodontic treatment option. Dental Press J Orthod. 2010;15(6):143-61.

39. Konstantonis D. The impact of extraction vs nonextraction treatment on soft tissue changes in Class I borderline malocclusions. Angle Orthod. 2012;82(2):209-17.

40. Weinberg M, Sadowsky C. Resolution of mandibular arch crowding in growing patients with Class I malocclusions treated nonextraction. Am J Orthod Dentofacial Orthop. 1996;110(4):359-64.

41. Uribe F, Holliday B, Nanda R. Incidence of open gingival embrasures after mandibular incisor extractions: a clinical photographic evaluation. Am J Orthod Dentofacial Orthop. 2011;139(1):49-54.

42. Aksu M, Kocadereli I. Arch width changes in extraction and nonextraction treatment in class I patients. Angle Orthod. 2005;75(6):948-52.

43. Basciftci FA, Usumez S. Effects of extraction and nonextraction treatment on class I and class II subjects. Angle Orthod. 2003;73(1):36-42.

44. Ismail SF, Moss JP, Hennessy R. Three-dimensional assessment of the effects of extraction and nonextraction orthodontic treatment on the face. Am J Orthod Dentofacial Orthop. 2002;121(3):244-56.

45. Hayasaki SM, Castanha Henriques JF, Janson G, Freitas MR. Influence of extraction and nonextraction orthodontic treatment in Japanese-Brazilians with class I and class II division 1 malocclusions. Am J Orthod Dentofacial Orthop. 2005;127(1):30-6.

46. Akyalcin S, Hazar S, Guneri P, Gogus S, Erdinc AM. Extraction versus non-extraction: evaluation by digital subtraction radiography. Eur J Orthod. 2007;29(6):639-47.

47. Wes Fleming J, Buschang PH, Kim KB, Oliver DR. Posttreatment occlusal variability among angle Class I nonextraction patients. Angle Orthod. 2008;78(4):625-30.

48. Erdinc AE, Nanda RS, Işiksal E. Relapse of anterior crowding in patients treated with extraction and nonextraction of premolars. Am J Orthod Dentofacial Orthop. 2006;129(6):775-84.

49. Bowman SJ, Johnston LE. The esthetic impact of extraction and nonextraction treatments on Caucasian patients. Angle Orthod. 2000;70(1):3-10.

50. Sheridan JJ. Air-rotor Wear Update. J Clin Orthod. 1987;21(11):781-8.

51. Artun J, Kokich VG, Osterberg SK. Long-term effect of root proximity on periodontal health after orthodontic treatment. Am J Orthod Dentofacial Orthop. 1987;91(2):125-30.

52. Vermylen K, Quincey GNTd, Wolffe GN, Hof MAVt, Renggli HH. Root proximity as a risk marker for periodontal disease: a case-control study. J Clin Periodol. 2005;32(3):260-5.

53. Bolton WA. Disharmony in tooth size and its relation to the analysis and treatment of malocclusion. Angle Orthod. 1958;28(3):113-30.

54. Safavi SM, Namazi AH. Evaluation of mandibular incisor extraction treatment outcome in patients with Bolton discrepancy using peer assessment rating index. J Dent. 2012;9(1):27-34.

55. Borzabadi-Farahani A. A review of the oral health-related evidence that supports the orthodontic treatment need indices. Prog Orthod. 2012;13(3):314-25.

19

Dental and skeletal changes in patients with mandibular retrognathism following treatment with Herbst and pre-adjusted fixed appliance

Fabio de Abreu Vigorito[1], Gladys Cristina Dominguez[2], Luís Antônio de Arruda Aidar[3]

Objective: To assess the dentoskeletal changes observed in treatment of Class II, division 1 malocclusion patients with mandibular retrognathism. Treatment was performed with the Herbst orthopedic appliance during 13 months (phase I) and pre-adjusted orthodontic fixed appliance (phase II). **Methods:** Lateral cephalograms of 17 adolescents were taken in phase I onset (T_1) and completion (T_2); in the first thirteen months of phase II (T_3) and in phase II completion (T_4). Differences among the cephalometric variables were statistically analyzed (Bonferroni variance and multiple comparisons). **Results:** From T_1 to T_4, 42% of overall maxillary growth was observed between T_1 and T_2 (P < 0.01), 40.3% between T_2 and T_3 (P < 0.05) and 17.7% between T_3 and T_4 (n.s.). As for overall mandibular movement, 48.2% was observed between T_1 and T_2 (P < 0.001) and 51.8% between T_2 and T_4 (P < 0.01) of which 15.1% was observed between T_2 and T_3 (n.s.) and 36.7% between T_3 and T_4 (P < 0.01). Class II molar relationship and overjet were properly corrected. The occlusal plane which rotated clockwise between T_1 and T_2, returned to its initial position between T_2 and T_3 remaining stable until T_4. The mandibular plane inclination did not change at any time during treatment. **Conclusion:** Mandibular growth was significantly greater in comparison to maxillary, allowing sagittal maxillomandibular adjustment. The dentoalveolar changes (upper molar) that overcorrected the malocclusion in phase I, partially recurred in phase II, but did not hinder correction of the malocclusion. Facial type was preserved.

Keywords: Angle Class II malocclusion. Orthopedics. Orthodontics.

[1] PhD in Orthodontics, School of Dentistry, University of São Paulo (USP).
[2] Full professor, Department of Orthodontics, University of São Paulo (USP).
[3] Full professor, Department of Orthodontics, University of Santa Cecília (UNISANTA).

» The authors report no commercial, proprietary or financial interest in the products or companies described in this article.

Gladys Cristina Dominguez
Rua Dr. Alceu de Campos Rodrigues, 247 – Vila Nova Conceição
São Paulo/SP — Brazil
CEP: 04.544-000 – E-mail: gcdrodri@usp.br

INTRODUCTION

Growing patients with Class II malocclusion and mandibular retrognathism may be treated with a variety of techniques, as described in the literature. Some of the techniques include treatment performed with an orthopedic phase employing appliances such as the Herbst. This treatment has been widely studied by Pancherz[1-4] and other researchers[5-22] who took several aspects into consideration and revealed that this type of treatment not only represents an alternative to the correction of Class II malocclusion, but also preserves the stomatognathic system. However, with regard to Brazilian individuals, these results are questioned: Are treatment effects skeletal or dentoalveolar? Is the mandibular growth curve modified when stimulated by the Herbst appliance? Are the obtained results lost after the appliance is removed? The complexity of clarifying the referred doubts lays in the difficulty of performing longitudinal studies in homogeneous casuistries. With a view to eliminating the tendency towards including only successful cases and, thus, confuse the results, the ideal would be that prospective studies were conducted with groups of consecutive patients. From this point of view, in 2007, a study[23] was carried out to assess and compare, in patients treated during growth spurt, the dentoskeletal changes observed in the Herbst active phase and during a period of same duration after the appliance had been removed. The obtained results were the motivation to perform the present study which aims at assessing full treatment performed in adolescents in two phases: phase I – orthopedic with Herbst appliance and phase II – orthodontic with pre-adjusted fixed appliance.

MATERIAL AND METHODS

The sample comprised 17 Brazilian adolescent patients (12 men and 5 women), with mean age of 12 years and 4 months ± 1 year and 2 months, and bone age corresponding to the growth spurt, as revealed by a hand-wrist radiograph. The patients were selected according to the following inclusion criteria: individuals with mandibular retrognathism and Angle Class II, division 1 malocclusion greater than half-cusp (> 3 mm); individuals with overjet > 5 mm (permanent dentition); with model discrepancy under 4 mm; with clinical recommendation for mandibular advancement to be performed with functional orthopedic appliance. Individuals with absence of teeth, dental fractures and dental caries were excluded. Treatment was carried out in two phases. Initially, the orthopedic phase (phase I) was

performed with Herbst functional orthopedic appliance placed onto acrylic splints associated with maxillary expansion screw.[24] The objective was to correct the transversal discrepancy,[25] activating the expansion screw during the first month of treatment. The appliance was made according to a wax bite registration obtained with 6 mm of initial advancement, and progressive advancements of 2 mm every 2 months, according to individual needs. This phase lasted for an average of 13.9 ± 2.1 months. Thereafter, the orthodontic phase (phase II) was performed with pre-adjusted fixed appliance and aimed at leveling and aligning the upper and lower teeth as well as at obtaining functional occlusion with adequate overjet and overbite. This phase lasted for 46 months.

Complete orthodontic documentation (panoramic and hand-wrist radiographs, lateral and frontal cephalograms; intra and extraoral photographs; study casts) was prepared for all patients at four stages: T_1, immediately before treatment onset; T_2, after 13 months using the Herbst appliance, which represented the end of phase I; T_3, 13 months after phase II or orthodontic phase had begun; and T_4, phase II completion, totalizing a period of 33 months. All 68 lateral cephalograms were manually traced by the same operator at monthly intervals. They were analyzed with regard to the cephalometric variables of sagittal changes analysis (SO-analysis) suggested by Pancherz[4] (Figs 1 and 2).

Patients' guardians signed an informed consent form, agreeing with all stages of the study and the posterior disclosure of results. The project was approved by the Institutional Review Board of the School of Dentistry/ USP and registered under protocol 109/06.

STATISTICAL ANALYSIS

Method error assessment (Dahlberg[26]) was performed in 11.8% of the sample.

The values of each measure and the relation of each moment assessed by means and standard deviations were expressed and compared to the measurements taken between the moments of assessment using the analysis of variance carried out with repeated measures. For measurements that presented statistically significant differences between the moments of assessment, Bonferroni multiple comparisons were performed. They revealed in which moments these differences occurred. The tests were performed with a significance level set at 5%.

RESULTS

For a better understanding of the characteristics of each moment of growth (Fig 2) and the differences between them, the results are presented in three tables. Table 1 presents the measures, the relation between measurements at each moment of assessment and the result of the analysis of variance.

The results of Bonferroni multiple comparisons are presented in Table 2, whereas the results presenting differences in the relation between measures are shown in Table 3.

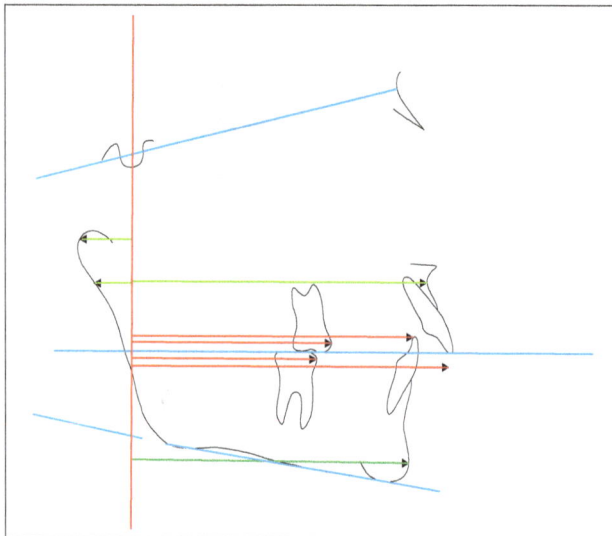

Figure 1 - Analysis of sagittal changes (SO-analysis) of Pancherz.

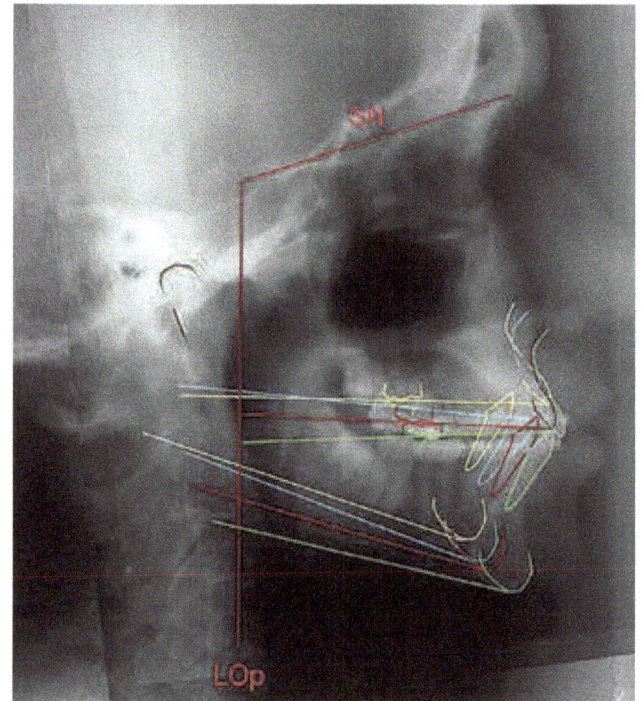

Figure 2 - Superimposition of tracings (according to analysis of Pancherz[4]), of one of the patients from the sample, in all four observation stages: T_1 = yellow, T_2 = blue, T_3 = red and T_4 = green.

Table 1 - Measures and relations between values obtained at each moment of assessment and result of the analysis of variance.

Variable	Orthopedic phase		Orthodontic phase		N	p
	T_1 Mean ± S.D.	T_2 Mean ± S.D.	T_3 Mean ± S.D.	T_4 Mean ± S.D.		
SN.PM	32.59 ± 5.42	32.56 ± 5.59	31.88 ± 5.36	32.03 ± 6.26	17	0.439
ui/Lop	90.77 ± 5.18	90.47 ± 6.55	92.15 ± 6.78	93.79 ± 6.28	17	<0.001
li/Lop	81.62 ± 5.95	87.82 ± 6.50	87.97 ± 6.60	90.06 ± 6.20	17	<0.001
um/Lop	57.12 ± 4.31	57.21 ± 5.02	59.56 ± 4.91	62.35 ± 5.45	17	<0.001
lm/Lop	55.53 ± 4.70	61.32 ± 5.24	62.59 ± 5.14	65.59 ± 5.61	17	<0.001
ss/Lop	81.24 ± 3.47	82.50 ± 3.94	83.71 ± 4.06	84.24 ± 4.40	17	<0.001
pg/Lop	83.15 ± 5.30	87.59 ± 5.85	88.59 ± 6.04	91.68 ± 6.19	17	<0.001
ar/Lop	10.59 ± 3.73	10.24 ± 3.70	10.44 ± 4.12	9.88 ± 4.14	17	0.241
co/Lop	12.94 ± 3.62	12.91 ± 3.58	13.29 ± 3.63	13.56 ± 4.08	17	0.319
SN.LO	20.29 ± 3.72	23.15 ± 4.63	20.79 ± 4.47	19.06 ± 4.72	17	<0.001
ui/Lop-li/Lop	9.15 ± 2.74	2.65 ± 1.23	4.18 ± 1.20	3.74 ± 0.90	17	<0.001
um/Lop-lm/Lop	1.59 ± 1.61	-4.12 ± 2.10	-3.03 ± 1.58	-3.24 ± 1.15	17	<0.001
pg/Lop+ar/Lop	93.74 ± 5.18	97.82 ± 5.76	99.03 ± 6.74	101.56 ± 7.66	17	<0.001
pg/Lop+co/Lop	96.09 ± 5.12	100.50 ± 5.69	101.88 ± 6.62	105.24 ± 7.95	17	<0.001
ui/Lop-ss/Lop	9.53 ± 2.70	7.97 ± 3.12	8.44 ± 3.28	9.56 ± 2.93	17	0.022
li/Lop-pg/Lop	-1.53 ± 5.83	0.24 ± 5.86	-0.62 ± 5.61	-1.62 ± 5.63	17	0.031
um/Lop-ss/Lop	-24.12 ± 2.24	-25.29 ± 2.30	-24.15 ± 2.18	-21.88 ± 2.71	17	<0.001
lm/Lop-pg/Lop	-27.62 ± 3.74	-26.26 ± 4.20	-26.00 ± 4.46	-26.09 ± 4.92	17	0.008

Table 2 - Result of Bonferroni multiple comparisons for measurements that presented differences during treatment.

Variable	Comparison	Mean difference	Standard error	p	CI (95%) Lower	Upper
ui/Lop	$T_1 - T_2$	0.29	0.56	> 0.999	-1.40	1.99
	$T_1 - T_3$	-1.38	0.76	0.516	-3.66	0.89
	$T_1 - T_4$	-3.03	0.70	0.003	-5.14	-0.92
	$T_2 - T_3$	-1.68	0.49	0.020	-3.14	-0.21
	$T_2 - T_4$	-3.32	0.73	0.002	-5.51	-1.14
	$T_3 - T_4$	-1.65	0.52	0.034	-3.20	-0.10
li/Lop	$T_1 - T_2$	-6.21	0.48	< 0.001	-7.66	-4.75
	$T_1 - T_3$	-6.35	0.65	< 0.001	-8.30	-4.41
	$T_1 - T_4$	-8.44	0.86	< 0.001	-11.01	-5.87
	$T_2 - T_3$	-0.15	0.56	> 0.999	-1.83	1.54
	$T_2 - T_4$	-2.24	0.79	0.072	-4.61	0.14
	$T_3 - T_4$	-2.09	0.59	0.016	-3.86	-0.31
um/Lop	$T_1 - T_2$	-0.09	0.40	> 0.999	-1.29	1.11
	$T_1 - T_3$	-2.44	0.44	< 0.001	-3.75	-1.13
	$T_1 - T_4$	-5.24	0.74	< 0.001	-7.45	-3.02
	$T_2 - T_3$	-2.35	0.37	< 0.001	-3.46	-1.25
	$T_2 - T_4$	-5.15	0.85	< 0.001	-7.70	-2.59
	$T_3 - T_4$	-2.79	0.65	0.003	-4.74	-0.85
lm/Lop	$T_1 - T_2$	-5.79	0.50	< 0.001	-7.29	-4.30
	$T_1 - T_3$	-7.06	0.57	< 0.001	-8.76	-5.36
	$T_1 - T_4$	-10.06	1.02	< 0.001	-13.13	-6.99
	$T_2 - T_3$	-1.27	0.45	0.073	-2.61	0.08
	$T_2 - T_4$	-4.27	0.98	0.003	-7.22	-1.31
	$T_3 - T_4$	-3.00	0.69	0.003	-5.07	-0.93
ss/Lop	$T_1 - T_2$	-1.27	0.30	0.004	2.17	-0.36
	$T_1 - T_3$	-2.47	0.45	< 0.001	-3.82	-1.12
	$T_1 - T_4$	-3.00	0.66	0.002	-4.99	-1.01
	$T_2 - T_3$	-1.21	0.37	0.032	-2.33	-0.08
	$T_2 - T_4$	-1.74	0.64	0.094	-3.67	0.20
	$T_3 - T_4$	-0.53	0.43	> 0.999	-1.81	0.75
pg/Lop	$T_1 - T_2$	-4.44	0.53	< 0.001	-6.02	-2.86
	$T_1 - T_3$	-5.44	0.71	< 0.001	-7.57	-3.31
	$T_1 - T_4$	-8.53	1.11	< 0.001	-11.86	-5.20
	$T_2 - T_3$	-1.00	0.46	0.280	-2.40	0.40
	$T_2 - T_4$	-4.09	1.00	0.005	-7.10	-1.08
	$T_3 - T_4$	-3.09	0.70	0.003	-5.19	-0.99
SN.LO	$T_1 - T_2$	-2.85	0.85	0.023	-5.40	-0.31
	$T_1 - T_3$	-0.50	0.75	> 0.999	-2.76	1.76
	$T_1 - T_4$	1.24	0.78	0.801	-1.12	3.59
	$T_2 - T_3$	2.35	0.32	< 0.001	1.39	3.32
	$T_2 - T_4$	4.09	0.86	0.001	1.51	6.67
	$T_3 - T_4$	1.74	0.61	0.068	-0.09	3.56

Table 3 - Result of Bonferroni multiple comparisons for relations between measures that presented differences during treatment.

Variable	Comparison	Mean difference	Standard error	p	CI (95%)	
					Lower	Upper
ui/Lop-li/Lop	$T_1 - T_2$	6.50	0.71	< 0.001	4.37	8.64
	$T_1 - T_3$	4.97	0.78	< 0.001	2.64	7.31
	$T_1 - T_4$	5.41	0.75	< 0.001	3.16	7.66
	$T_2 - T_3$	-1.53	0.49	0.041	-3.01	-0.05
	$T_2 - T_4$	-1.09	0.43	0.129	-2.37	0.20
	$T_3 - T_4$	0.44	0.30	0.963	-0.46	1.34
um/Lop-lm/Lop	$T_1 - T_2$	5.71	0.47	< 0.001	4.30	7.11
	$T_1 - T_3$	4.62	0.43	< 0.001	3.33	5.90
	$T_1 - T_4$	4.82	0.40	< 0.001	3.61	6.03
	$T_2 - T_3$	-1.09	0.24	0.002	-1.81	-0.37
	$T_2 - T_4$	-0.88	0.47	0.482	-2.30	0.54
	$T_3 - T_4$	0.21	0.33	> 0.999	-0.78	1.19
pg/Lop+ar/Lop	$T_1 - T_2$	-4.09	0.44	< 0.001	-5.42	-2.75
	$T_1 - T_3$	-5.29	0.69	< 0.001	-7.36	-3.23
	$T_1 - T_4$	-7.82	1.05	< 0.001	-10.98	-4.67
	$T_2 - T_3$	-1.21	0.56	0.286	-2.90	0.49
	$T_2 - T_4$	-3.74	0.96	0.008	-6.61	-0.86
	$T_3 - T_4$	-2.53	0.56	0.002	-4.22	-0.84
pg/Lop+co/Lop	$T_1 - T_2$	-4.41	0.37	< 0.001	-5.52	-3.30
	$T_1 - T_3$	-5.79	0.61	< 0.001	-7.63	-3.96
	$T_1 - T_4$	-9.15	1.12	< 0.001	-12.52	-5.77
	$T_2 - T_3$	-1.38	0.51	0.096	-2.93	0.16
	$T_2 - T_4$	-4.74	1.06	0.002	-7.91	-1.56
	$T_3 - T_4$	-3.35	0.71	0.001	-5.50	-1.21
ui/Lop-ss/Lop	$T_1 - T_2$	1.56	0.49	0.035	0.08	3.03
	$T_1 - T_3$	1.09	0.71	0.857	-1.04	3.21
	$T_1 - T_4$	-0.03	0.70	> 0.999	-2.12	2.06
	$T_2 - T_3$	-0.47	0.44	> 0.999	-1.80	0.86
	$T_2 - T_4$	-1.59	0.59	0.095	-3.36	0.18
	$T_3 - T_4$	-1.12	0.46	0.155	-2.49	0.25
li/Lop-pg/Lop	$T_1 - T_2$	-1.77	0.44	0.006	-3.08	-0.45
	$T_1 - T_3$	-0.91	0.76	> 0.999	-3.20	1.37
	$T_1 - T_4$	0.09	0.77	> 0.999	-2.24	2.41
	$T_2 - T_3$	0.85	0.59	> 0.999	-0.92	2.63
	$T_2 - T_4$	1.85	0.66	0.076	-0.13	3.84
	$T_3 - T_4$	1.00	0.37	0.092	-0.11	2.11
um/Lop-ss/Lop	$T_1 - T_2$	1.18	0.30	0.008	0.27	2.09
	$T_1 - T_3$	0.03	0.39	> 0.999	-1.13	1.19
	$T_1 - T_4$	-2.24	0.45	0.001	-3.60	-0.88
	$T_2 - T_3$	-1.15	0.33	0.019	-2.14	-0.15
	$T_2 - T_4$	-3.41	0.58	< 0.001	-5.16	-1.67
	$T_3 - T_4$	-2.27	0.58	0.008	-4.02	-0.51
lm/Lop-pg/Lop	$T_1 - T_2$	-1.35	0.41	0.026	-2.58	-0.12
	$T_1 - T_3$	-1.62	0.53	0.045	-3.21	-0.03
	$T_1 - T_4$	-1.53	0.62	0.156	-3.41	0.35
	$T_2 - T_3$	-0.27	0.26	> 0.999	-1.05	0.52
	$T_2 - T_4$	-0.18	0.47	> 0.999	-1.59	1.24
	$T_3 - T_4$	0.09	0.35	> 0.999	-0.97	1.15

DISCUSSION

All patients that comprised this study presented, in T_1, typical characteristics of Class II division 1 malocclusion, as confirmed by the initial cephalometric variables that describe the molar relationship (um/Lop - lm/Lop: 1.59 ± 1.61 mm) and the overjet (ui/Lop - li/Lop: 9.15 ± 2.74 mm). According to the inclusion criteria, all patients clinically presented mandibular retrognathism and accepted treatment that included mandibular advancement.

The results yielded by the present study are in agreement with previous studies that used similar methods.[9,12,23,27] Both the maxilla (SS/Lop) and mandible (PPg/Lop) were anteriorly projected, but since mandibular growth increment was 3.5 times greater, there was a favorable sagittal maxillomandibular adjustment. In order to identify the contribution of mandibular growth, measurements of the absolute mandibular length (pg/Lop+co/Lop and pg/Lop+ar/Lop) were assessed and significant growth increment was observed, although the condylar (co/Lop) and articular (ar/Lop) points did not present any alterations.

The registered amount of skeletal growth allowed better a understanding of how the teeth varied in their sagittal spatial position. Overcorrection of the observed molar relationship (um/Lop-lm/Lop: 5.71 mm) was due to the association between maintenance of upper molars position (um/Lop: -0.09) while the maxilla was anteriorly projected (SS/Lop: -1.27 mm), and mesialization of lower molars (lm/Lop: -5.79 mm) along with mandibular anterior projection (pg/Lop: -4.44 mm). Overjet was significantly reduced from 9.5 mm to 2.65 mm, as a result of mandibular anterior projection (pg/Lop: -4.44 mm) and buccal inclination of lower incisors in their bone base (li/Lop: -6.21 mm). The mechanical effect observed in the inclination of lower incisors restricts the recommendation of this type of therapy to individuals who do not present increased inclination at treatment onset.

The occlusal plane (SN.LO), which in the beginning presented a mean value that is typical of a mesofacial pattern (32.59 ± 5.42°), was rotated clockwise (2.85°) by the presence of interocclusal acrylic splints. This might have caused the effect of molar intrusion, since, when the appliance was removed, an important posterior disocclusion was observed in all patients. This speculation can be done because, differently from the occlusal plane,

the inclination of the mandibular plane (SN.PM) did not undergo any alterations, thus confirming that it was just a dentoalveolar effect and not a skeletal one, therefore, the facial type did not change.

In the following 13 months after the Herbst appliance had been removed, which corresponded to orthodontic treatment onset (T_2-T_3), the maxilla continued to be anteriorly projected (ss/Lop: -1.21 mm), whereas mandibular projection was little significant (pg/Lop: -1 mm). It was observed that partial recurrence of molar relationship (um/Lop-lm/Lop: -1.09 mm) occurred as a result of mesialization of upper molars (um/Lop-ss/Lop: -1.15 mm) along with non-significant mesialization of lower molars (lm/Lop-pg/Lop: -027). However, considering that a relation of overcorrection of molar relationship was observed in T_2 (um/Lop-lm/Lop: -4.12 mm), this recurrence was favorable to adjust the molars in Class I relation (um/Lop-lm/Lop: -3.03 mm). Additionally, there was a partial recurrence of 1.53 mm in overjet (ui/Lop-li/Lop) as a result of differential growth of the maxilla, which led the upper incisors to occupy a more anterior spatial position (is/Lop: -1.68 mm). This could not have been due to the insignificant uprighting of lower incisors (li/Lop: -0.15 mm) because, in this case, they did not change their position (li/Lop-pg/Lop: 0.85 mm).

The occlusal plane (SL.LO) rotated counterclockwise, since, from T_2 to T_3, with the removal of the Herbst appliance, the molars were free from the interocclusal splints and, additionally, were actively leveled to the orthodontic appliance, restoring the vertical spatial position that they presented at treatment onset. These data corroborate data found in the literature,[9,10] thus confirming that this movement happened without affecting the inclination of the mandibular plane (SN-PM), therefore, with preservation of facial type.

The complementary assessment carried out in this study, between the thirteen-month interval after removal of the Herbst appliance and the end of the active orthodontic treatment (T_3-T_4), showed that, while the maxilla was not significantly anteriorly projected (SS/Lop: -0.53 mm), the mandible resumed its growth (pg/Lop: -3.09 mm), significantly anteriorly projecting itself. Molar relationship (um/Lop-lm/Lop: 0.21 mm) remained stable in Class I. Moreover, no expressive changes were observed for the overjet (ui/Lop-li/Lop: 0.44mm).

Nevertheless, when analyzing the maintenance of dental stability, during a period in which there was significant expression of mandibular growth and absence of significant maxillary growth, it could be observed that tooth movement was compensatory, maintaining both molar and overjet relations. While the upper incisors (ui/Lop: -1.65 mm) and the upper molars (um/Lop: -2.79 mm) were anteriorly projected in the absence of significant maxillary growth (ss/Lop: -053 mm), the lower incisors (li/Lop: -2.09 mm) and lower molars (lm/Lop:-3 mm) were also spatially anteriorly projected, however, in association with significant mandibular growth (pg/Lop: -3.09 mm). Thus, it can be concluded by means of the differential calculus (dental movement minus skeletal movement) that only the upper molars had a significant movement of mesialization, regardless of the growth of its bone base (um/Lop-ss/Lop: -2.27 mm). This movement was necessary to maintain Class I molar relationship. The occlusal plane remained stable (SN.LO: 1.74°). This fact can be explained because in T_3, the molars already presented interocclusal contact and there were no additional vertical movements until T_4. The mandibular plane remained unchanged, revealing a uniform behavior during the entire treatment, thus, preserving facial type.

When considering the series of changes observed from the beginning to the end of treatment (T_1-T_4), it is verified that out of the total of maxillary anterior projection (3 mm), 42% happened during the orthopedic phase (T_1-T_2) and 58% during the orthodontic phase (T_2-T_4), of which the most part (40.3%) happened during the first 13 months (T_2-T_3) and the rest (17.7%), an insignificant increase, between T_3 and T_4. As shown in Tables 1 to 3, the mandibular anterior displacements (Pg/Lop) were compatible to the corresponding increment of the mandibular absolute growth (Pg/Lop+ar/Lop and Pg/Lop+co/Lop). When analyzing the variable Pg/Lop+co/Lop, it is verified that 48.2% of mandibular growth happened during the 13 months of the orthopedic phase (T_1-T_2) as a response to the stimulus provided by the Herbst appliance, in a period when the potential growth was intense; whereas 51.8% happened during the orthodontic phase (T_2-T_4). However, it must be emphasized that during the 13 months after the Herbst appliance was removed (T_2-T_3), there was growth deceleration, with slight, non-significant growth increment (15.1%) and, therefore, without anterior projec-

tion. Significant growth was soon resumed, expressing the remaining 36.7% in the following months until T_4. This type of response agrees with previous studies.[4,9] It was very important to assess the amount of growth during the orthodontic phase (T_2-T_4) as proposed in this study. Moreover, dividing observation into two periods, T_2-T_3 (13 months) and T_3-T_4 (33 months), was important to understand whether or not the curve of mandibular growth could modify its usual course before the stimulus given by the use of the Herbst appliance. Franchi et al[28] claim that mandibular growth follows the physical growth spurt and it is characterized by a gradual increase in the amount of increments until it reaches its maximum, when the greatest amount of growth is expressed. Afterwards, it gradually decelerates again, however, linearly, until growth is complete. In the present study, it was observed that during the 13 months of stimulus (T_1-T_2) provided by the Herbst appliance, the increments were intense. Nevertheless, a deceleration in the following 13 months (T_2-T_3), and then, a resumption of growth (T_3-T_4), explain that the growth verified between T_1 and T_2 represents the favorable expression of the present growth potential, for being in its maximum (as revealed by the hand-wrist radiograph in T_1), which is summed up to the anticipation of growth in the subsequent 13 months, which, without the use of the appliance, would not have manifested at that moment, thus, modifying the behavior of the descendant curve of growth spurt in adolescence.

As for growth complexity and mandibular spatial projection in the face, our results can be explained by those observed by Pancherz et al[29] who assessed the "effective condylar growth" and its influence over the spatial position of the symphysis in the face. Their findings reveal that condylar growth triplicated during the active phase of six months in which the Herbst appliance was used, decelerated in a similar period after the removal of the appliance, and soon resumed its normal growth in the subsequent 30 months. Comparison between total mandibular and maxillary projection, from T_1 to T_4, revealed that the mandible (pg/Lop: 8.47 mm) was projected 2.8 times more than the maxilla (ss/Lop: 3 mm), a fact that favored sagittal maxillomandibular adjustment.

With regard to dentoalveolar correction of Class II malocclusion, a favorable response was observed between T_1 and T_4, i.e., Class II molar relationship and the increase in overjet that patients presented at treatment onset were ideally corrected. In T_4, all of them showed characteristics of normal occlusion, with good molar relationship and adequate overjet, thus, achieving the purpose of the treatment. In order to produce such results, treatment evolved from sagittal overcorrection of molar relationship, which was associated with great reduction in overjet during the 13-month orthopedic phase; partially relapsed at the beginning of the orthodontic phase and became stable in the following 33 months until the end of the treatment.

Based on the aforementioned observations, it is important to emphasize that: First, the recurrence of the overcorrected molar relationship between T_2 and T_3 was necessary for molars to obtain cusp-to-fossa relationship instead of cusp-to-cusp, which probably contributed to offer the stability observed in the subsequent period. Additionally, despite being significant, the degree of overjet relapse registered between T_2 and T_3, did not prevent the values from being within the clinical parameters of normality by the end of the treatment. The second aspect is with regard to the stability observed in T_3 and T_4, a period of 33 months. The advantage of lasting nearly two times longer than each previous period allowed the stability of results to be assessed.

Clockwise rotation of the occlusal plane was significant during the orthopedic phase (T_1-T_2) and it happened as a result of the presence of interocclusal splints. In the subsequent phase (T_2-T_3), it rotated counterclockwise, therefore, relapsing by the removal of the splints and active orthodontic leveling, thus, restoring intermaxillary occlusal contacts. This pattern of counterclockwise rotation continued in the following 33 months, however, insignificantly. As for the changes that occurred in opposite directions, the comparison between orthopedic and orthodontic phases reveal that they did not present any adverse clinical effect, since the changes occurred without influencing the inclination of the mandibular plane. On the other hand, the occlusal plane restored its initial inclination in T_3 and remained stable until T_4. The mandibular plane (SN.PM), which defines the facial type, was maintained in all periods of assessment, a fact that is favorable to the stability achieved in the long term, all of which agreed with other authors in the literature.[9,30]

The size of the sample is a limitation of this study. However, it is of great value considering that it is a prospective study carried out with consecutive patients and that had never been performed with Brazilian patients. The results obtained from assessing these patients by means of the treatment protocol allowed us to visualize not only that the therapy applied was efficient, but also that the series of skeletal and dental changes observed did not cause a temporary impact, but an impact that is compatible with the conditions of stability in the long term. However, further studies are necessary to longitudinally assess the post-treatment phase. Finally, it is important to emphasize the undesirable effect that the use of the Herbst appliance can cause to individuals with increased buccal inclination of the lower incisors at treatment onset.

CONCLUSIONS

Based on the results of treatment of adolescents with Class II malocclusion and mandibular retrognathism performed in two phases (Herbst and pre-adjusted orthodontic appliance) it is reasonable to conclude that both skeletal and dental changes, when performed together, allowed the correction of the malocclusion. The mandible grew significantly more than the maxilla, which favored sagittal maxillomandibular adjustment. The dental changes (distalization of upper molars) that overcorrected the malocclusion in phase I partially relapsed in phase II, without compromising the correction of the malocclusion. The facial type was preserved.

REFERENCES

1. Pancherz H. Treatment of Class II malocclusions by jumping the bite with the Herbst appliance. A cephalometric investigation. Am J Orthod.1979;76(4):423-42.
2. Pancherz H, Hansen K. Occlusal changes during and after Herbst treatment: a cephalometric investigation. Eur J Orthod. 1986;8(4):215-28.
3. Pancherz H, Fackel U. The skeletofacial growth pattern pre and post-dentofacial orthopaedics. A long-term study of Class II malocclusions treated with the Herbst appliance. Eur J Orthod. 1990;12(2):209-18.
4. Pancherz H, Ruf S. The Herbst appliance. Research based clinical management. Quintessence; 2008. cap. 6, p. 43-6.
5. Hägg U, Pancherz H. Dentofacial orthopaedics in relation to chronological age, growth period and skeletal development. An analysis of 72 male patients with Class II division 1 malocclusion treated with Herbst appliance. Eur J Orthod. 1988;10(3):169-76.
6. McNamara JA Jr, Howe RP, Dischinger TG. A comparison of the Herbst and Fränkel appliances in the treatment of Class II malocclusion. Am J Orthod Dentofacial Orthop. 1990;98(2):134-44.
7. Schiavoni R, Grenga V, Macri V. Treatment of Class II high angle malocclusions with the Herbst appliance: a cephalometric investigation. Am J Orthod Dentofacial Orthop. 1992;102(5):393-409.

8. Windmiller EC. The acrylic-splint Herbst appliance: a cephalometric evaluation. Am J Orthod Dentofacial Orthop. 1993;104(1):73-84.

9. Lai M, McNamara JA Jr. An evaluation of two-phase treatment with the Herbst appliance and preadjusted edgewise therapy. Semin Orthod. 1998;4(1):46-58.

10. Franchi L, Baccetti T, McNamara JA Jr. Treatment and posttreatment effects of acrylic splint Herbst appliance therapy. Am J Orthod Dentofacial Orthop. 1999;115(4):429-38.

11. Manfredi C, Cimino R, Trani A, Pancherz H. Skeletal changes of Herbst appliance therapy investigated with more conventional cephalometrics and European norms. Angle Orthod. 2001;71(3):170-6.

12. Schütz TCB, Vigorito JW, Rodrigues CRMD, Domínguez-Rodríguez GC. Avaliação cefalométrico-radiográfica das modificações dentoalveolares decorrentes do tratamento com o aparelho Herbst em adolescentes com maloclusão de Classe II, divisão 1ª de Angle – Parte I. Ortodontia. 2002;35(4):22-34.

13. Schütz TCB, Vigorito JW, Domínguez-Rodríguez GC. Avaliação cefalométrico-radiográfica das modificações esqueléticas e do perfil facial decorrentes do tratamento com o aparelho Herbst em adolescentes com maloclusão de Classe II, divisão 1ª de Angle – Parte II. Ortodontia. 2003;36(1):44-61.

14. Ruf S. Short and long-term effects of the Herbst appliance on temporomandibular joint function. Semin Orthod. 2003;9(1):74-86.

15. Schaefer AT, McNamara JA Jr, Franchi L, Baccetti T. A cephalometric comparison of treatment with the Twin-block and stainless steel crown Herbst appliances followed by fixed appliance therapy. Am J Orthod Dentofacial Orthop. 2004;126(1):7-15.

16. VanLaecken R, Martin CA, Dischinger T, Razmus T, Ngan P. Treatment effects of the edgewise Herbst appliance: a cephalometric and tomographic investigation. Am J Orthod Dentofacial Orthop. 2006;130(5):582-93.

17. Ruf S, Pancherz H. Herbst/multibracket appliance treatment of Class II division 1 malocclusions in early and late adulthood. A prospective cephalometric study of consecutively treated subjects. Eur J Orthod. 2006;76(2):352-60.

18. Bock N, Pancherz H. Herbst treatment of Class II division 1 malocclusions in retrognathic and prognathic facial types. Angle Orthod. 2006;76(6):930-41.

19. Aidar LA, Dominguez GC, Abrahão M, Yamashita HK, Vigorito JW. Effects of Herbst appliance treatment on temporomandibular joint disc position and morphology: a prospective magnetic resonance imaging study. Am J Orthod Dentofacial Orthop. 2009;136(3):412-24.

20. Aidar LA, Dominguez GC, Yamashita HK, Abrahão M.Changes in temporomandibular joint disc position and form following Herbst and fixed orthodontic treatment. Angle Orthod. 2010;80(5):843-52.

21. Siara-Olds NJ, Pangrazio-Kulbersh V, Berger J, Bayirli B. Long-term dentoskeletal changes with the Bionator, Herbst, Twin Block, and MARA Functional Appliances. Angle Orthod. 2010;80(1):18-29.

22. Schütz TC, Dominguez GC, Hallinan MP, Cunha TC, Tufik S. Class II correction improves nocturnal breathing in adolescents. Angle Orthod. 2011;81(2):222-8.

23. Vigorito FA, Domínguez GC. Comparação dos efeitos dento-esqueléticos decorrentes do tratamento realizado em duas fases (com aparelho de Herbst e aparelho fixo pré-ajustado) em adolescentes com retrognatismo mandibular. Ortodontia. 2007;40(4):263-70.

24. Howe RP, McNamara JA Jr. Clinical management of the bonded Herbst appliance. J Clin Orthod. 1983;17(7):456-63.

25. Tollero I, Baccetti T, Franchi L, Tanasescu CD. Role of the posterior transverse interarch discrepancy in Class II, division 1 malocclusion during the mixed dentition phase. Am J Orthod Dentofacial Orthop. 1996;110(4):417-22.

26. Houston WJB. The analysis of errors in orthodontic measurements. Am J Orthod. 1983;83(5):383-90.

27. Flores-Mir C, Ayeh, Goswani A, Charkhandeh S. Skeletal and dental changes in class II division 1 malocclusions treated with Splint-Type Herbst appliances: a systematic review. Angle Orthod. 2007;77(2):376-81.

28. Franchi L, Baccetti T, McNamara JA. Mandibular growth as related to cervical vertebral maturation and body height. Am J Orthod Dentofacial Orthop. 2000;118(3):335-40.

29. Pancherz H, Ruf S, Kohlhas P. Effective condylar growth and chin position changes in Herbst treatment: a cephalometric roentgenographic long-term study. Am J Orthod Dentofacial Orthop. 1998;114(4):437-46.

30. Ruf S, Pancherz H. The effect of Herbst appliance on the mandibular plane: a cephalometric roentgenographic study. Am J Orthod Dentofacial Orthop. 1996;110(2):225-9.

20

Assessment of upper airways measurements in patients with mandibular skeletal Class II malocclusion

Nayanna Nadja e Silva[1], Rosa Helena Wanderley Lacerda[2], Alexandre Wellos Cunha Silva[3], Tania Braga Ramos[4]

Objective: Mandibular Class II malocclusions seem to interfere in upper airways measurements. The aim of this study was to assess the upper airways measurements of patients with skeletal Class II malocclusion in order to investigate the association between these measurements and the position and length of the mandible as well as mandibular growth trend, comparing the Class II group with a Class I one. **Methods:** A total of 80 lateral cephalograms from 80 individuals aged between 10 and 17 years old were assessed. Forty radiographs of Class I malocclusion individuals were matched by age with forty radiographs of individuals with mandibular Class II malocclusion. McNamara Jr., Ricketts, Downs and Jarabak's measurements were used for cephalometric evaluation. Data were submitted to descriptive and inferential statistical analysis by means of SPSS 20.0 statistical package. Student's t-test, Pearson correlation and intraclass correlation coefficient were used. A 95% confidence interval and 5% significance level were adopted to interpret the results. **Results:** There were differences between groups. Oropharynx and nasopharynx sizes as well as mandibular position and length were found to be reduced in Class II individuals. There was a statistically significant positive correlation between the size of the oropharynx and Xi-Pm, Co-Gn and SNB measurements. In addition, the size of the nasopharynx was found to be correlated with Xi-Pm, Co-Gn, facial depth, SNB, facial axis and FMA. **Conclusion:** Individuals with mandibular Class II malocclusion were shown to have upper airways measurements diminished. There was a correlation between mandibular length and position and the size of oropharynx and nasopharynx.

Keywords: Angle Class II malocclusion. Oropharynx. Nasopharynx. Airway obstruction.

[1] Specialist in Orthodontics, Associação Brasileira de Odontologia (ABO-PB), João Pessoa, Paraíba, Brazil.

[2] Coordinator, Postgraduate Program in Orthodontics, Associação Brasileira de Odontologia (ABO-PB), João Pessoa, Paraíba, Brazil.

[3] Professor, Postgraduate Program in Orthodontics, Associação Brasileira de Odontologia (ABO-PB), João Pessoa, Paraíba, Brazil.

[4] Professor of Orthognathic Surgery, Postgraduate Program in Orthodontics, Associação Brasileira de Odontologia (ABO-PB), João Pessoa, Paraíba, Brazil.

» The authors report no commercial, proprietary or financial interest in the products or companies described in this article.

Rosa Helena Wanderley Lacerda
Associação Brasileira de Ortodontia
Rui Barbosa 38 , João Pessoa, Paraíba - CEP: 58.020-040 - Brazil
E-mail: rhelenawanderley@msn.com

INTRODUCTION

Skeletal Class II malocclusion is a dentofacial deformity caused by a growth disorder of the bones frequently associated with mandibular retrusion relative to upper facial structures.[1] This deformity is also associated with functional disorders, mainly affecting upper airways and the temporomandibular joint.[2,3]

Patients with skeletal Class II malocclusion who have this deformity due to deficiency in mandibular growth present with a retrognathic mandible either because of growth vector or by deficient mandibular length.

According to Muto et al,[4] craniofacial abnormalities, including mandibular retrognathism, short mandibular body length and backward/downward rotation, can lead to decreased pharyngeal airway. These findings indicate that nasopharyngeal obstruction may be related to changes in mandibular morphology.[5]

The study of upper airways and their relationship with mandibular position and size is extremely important in orthodontic diagnosis because of their association with obstructive respiratory disorders, especially sleep apnea. This knowledge is definitive to the indication of mandibular advancement, whether orthopedic or surgical, for treatment of these disorders.

Several studies have been carried out with a view to measuring the pharyngeal airway; however, comparison with Class I individuals and the correlation between the variables involved in Class II malocclusion and airways measurements are still scarce, which encouraged the present study.

MATERIAL AND METHODS

This study was submitted to and approved by the Ethics Committee on Human Research through Plataforma Brasil, following the norms of the law 466/2012, under approval protocol #835.928.

The sample comprised 80 digital lateral cephalograms belonging to 80 patients of both sexes, without associated abnormalities, aged between 10-17 years, with a mean age of 12.3 years, treated by postgraduate orthodontic students (ABO/PB, Brazil). Of the 80 images, 40 were from patients with mandibular Class II malocclusion, whose diagnosis was confirmed by Xi-Pm, Co-Gn, Go-Me, facial depth and SNB measurements (at least three of these measures should be reduced so that the image would not be withdrawn from the sample). The other 40 radiographs belonged to Class I individuals. Groups were matched by age.

Anatomical tracings of all radiographic images were made on acetate paper, in a dark room, by an examiner using graphite pencil (point 0.3). Each film was traced by one investigator and checked by a second one, so as to verify the accuracy of anatomical outline determination and landmark placement. Measurements of mandibular length and spatial position, as well as size of nasopharyngeal and oropharyngeal airways, were taken using the cephalograms (Fig 1, Table 1).

Measurements were taken twice, with a 10-day interval in between, with the aid of a millimeter ruler and a 180° protractor. The first assessment was carried out with the entire sample while the second one was carried out with 30% of the sample.

Procedures of statistical inference were performed based on parametric statistics. Correlation coefficient and intraclass correlation coefficient (ICC) were used to assess intraexaminer agreement. The choice for statistical test was based on normal distribution of data, according to Komogorov-Smirnov normality test ($p > 0.05$). Intergroup comparison was performed by Student's t-test and Pearson r correlation coefficient. For descriptive procedures, absolute and relative data and measurements of central tendency and variability were presented. A 95% confidence interval and 5% significance level ($p < 0.05$) were adopted to interpret the results. Data were submitted to SPSS 20.0 statistical package for Windows and analyzed by means of descriptive and inferential statistics.

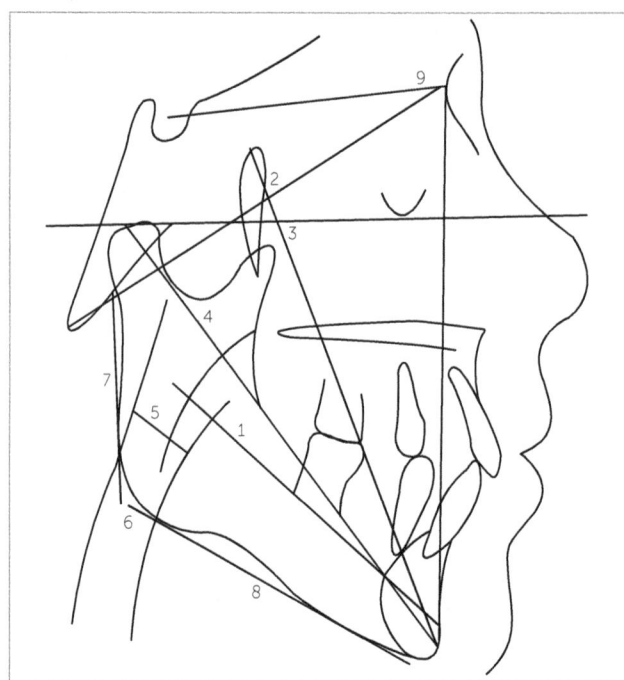

Figure 1 - Cephalogram and cephalometric measurements used.

Table 1 - Cephalometric measurements used.

Measure	Clinical standard	Appropriate age	Description
1. Xi-Pm	65 ± 3 mm	9 years (1.6/year)	Axis of the mandibular body – a line extending from point Xi to the mental protuberance.
2. Facial axis (Ba.NA x Frankfurt)	90 ± 3°	Does not change upon growth	Provides the direction of growth of the chin and the ratio between facial height and depth.
3. Facial depth (NA-Pog x Frankfurt)	87 ± 3°	9 years (0.33/ year)	Indicates the anteroposterior position of the mandible.
4. Co-Gn (Effective mandibular length)			Consists in the geometric relationship between the maxillomandibular length, directly linked either to patient's age or sex.
5. Oropharynx	10 to 12 mm		Measured by the width of the pharynx at the point where the posterior border of the tongue (in the radiograph) crosses the lower border of the mandible up to the posterior pharyngeal wall.
6. Nasopharynx	Mixed dentition: 12 mm Permanent dentition: 17.4 mm		It is measured linearly from a midpoint on the posterior wall of the soft palate to the posterior pharyngeal wall where there is the greatest closure of the airway.
7. Ar-Go	44 mm	11 years (male: 1.01 – 7.2) (female: 0.71 – 4.2)	Height of the mandibular ramus.
8. Go-Me	71 mm	11 years (male: 1.11 -7.11) (female: 0.73 – 3.12)	Length of the mandibular body.
9. SNB	80°		Anteroposterior position of the mandible in relation to the base of the cranium.

RESULTS

In order to assess the reliability of measurements of oropharynx and nasopharynx, mandibular length, mandibular position and direction of mandibular growth, the examiner conducted two assessments which were followed by determination of intraexaminer agreement. This calculation was done using intraclass correlation coefficient (ICC). Results were statistically significant and indicated intraclass coefficients ranging from 0.97 (facial depth) and 1.00 (oropharynx), thereby denoting strong intraexaminer agreement (Table 2).

As for upper airways measurements, statistically significant differences were found between both groups ($p < 0.001$). That is, the size of nasopharynx and oropharynx is reduced in Class II individuals (Fig 2).

The same results were observed for mandibular length, with significant differences between groups. The following measurements were found to be greater in Class I individuals: Xi-Pm, Co-Gn and Go-Me (Table 3, Fig 3).

As shown in Table 3, measurements of mandibular position also indicated significant differences between groups, with facial depth and SNB being greater among Class I individuals (Table 3). These results are graphically shown in Figure 4.

Measurements related to the direction of mandibular growth also differed significantly between groups. Facial axis and Ar-Go were greater in Class I individuals, while FMA was found to be greater in Class II individuals (Table 3, Fig 5).

In order to assess the correlation between oropharynx/nasopharynx size and mandibular length, position as well as growth, Pearson r correlation coefficient was performed.

Significant positive correlations were observed between the oropharynx and Xi-Pm, Co-Gn and SNB. Moreover, there were also correlations between the nasopharynx and Xi-Pm, Co-Gn, facial depth, SNB, facial axis and Ar-Go. Given that such correlations were positive, it is concluded that the greater the measurements of upper airways, the greater the variables, as reported herein. Correlation coefficients ranged from 0.24 to 0.37; thus, indicating weak to moderate correlations between variables (Table 4).

Table 2 - Assessment of intraexaminer agreement.

Measures	ICC	p	Interpretation
Xi-Pm	0.99	< 0.001	Strong intra-examiner agreement
Co-Gn	0.99	< 0.001	Strong intra-examiner agreement
Go-Me	0.99	< 0.001	Strong intra-examiner agreement
Facial depth	0.97	< 0.001	Strong intra-examiner agreement
SNB	0.99	< 0.001	Strong intra-examiner agreement
Facial axis	0.99	< 0.001	Strong intra-examiner agreement
Ar-Go	0.99	< 0.001	Strong intra-examiner agreement
FMA	0.99	< 0.001	Strong intra-examiner agreement
Oropharynx	1.00	-	Perfect agreement
Nasopharynx	0.99	< 0.001	Strong intra-examiner agreement

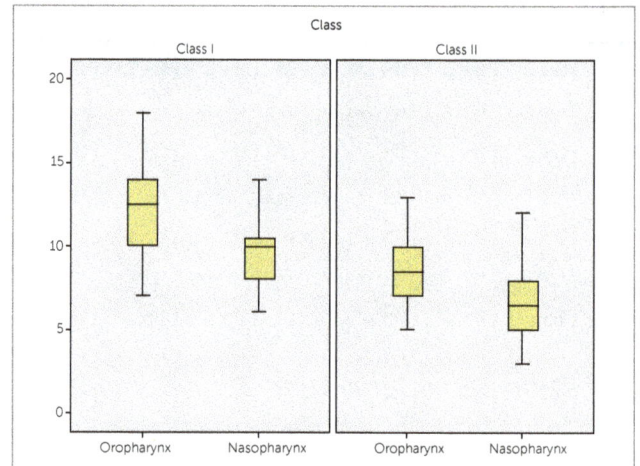

Figure 2 - Assessment of upper airway measurements of Class I and Class II groups.

Table 3 - Assessment of upper airways measurements, mandibular length, mandibular position and direction of mandibular growth of each group.

General measures	Specific measures	Class I Mean ± SD	Class I Min-Max	Class II Mean ± SD	Class II Min-Max	t (p)
Upper airways	Oropharynx	12.2±2.5	7 – 18	8.6±1.7	5 – 13	7.4 (< 0.001)
	Nasopharynx	9.4±1.9	6 – 14	6.7±1.9	3 – 12	6.2 (< 0.001)
Mandibular length	Xi-Pm	77.5±5.4	67 – 94	72.4±4.8	61 – 83	4.4 (< 0.001)
	Co-Gn	115.6±6.7	100 – 134	109.7±7.5	94 – 128	3.6 (< 0.001)
	Go-Me	73.5±11.2	13 – 90	69.4±4.9	57 – 80	2.0 (0.04)
Mandibular position	Facial depth	89.4±2.4	84 – 94	86.1±2.5	79 – 91	5.8 (< 0.001)
	SNB	79.7±2.9	74 – 88	74.5±2.9	68 – 84	7.8 (< 0.001)
Direction of the mandibular growth	Facial axis	90.5±3.7	80 – 100	87.4±3.6	78 – 93	3.8 (< 0.001)
	Ar-Go	43.9±4.1	37 – 51	40.5±4.8	31 – 50	3.3 (0.001)
	FMA	24.9±3.8	14 – 31	27.0±4.9	14 - 36	2.0 (0.04)

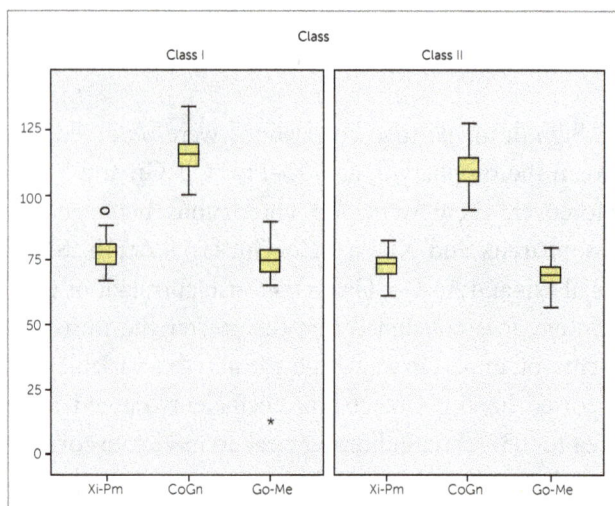

Figure 3 - Assessment of mandibular length of Class I and Class II groups.

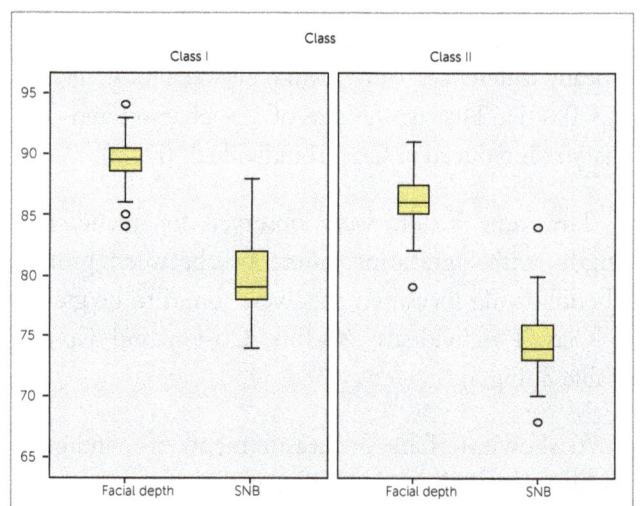

Figure 4 - Assessment of mandibular position of Class I and Class II groups.

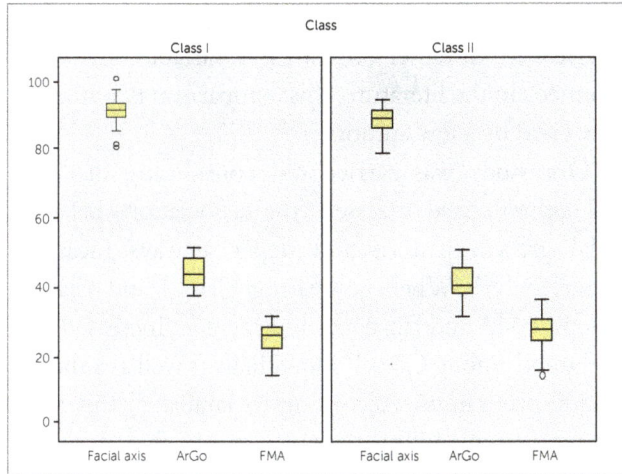

Figure 5 - Assessment of mandibular growth of Class I and Class II groups.

Table 4 - Correlation between upper airways measurements and mandibular length, position as well as direction of mandibular growth in both groups.

Measures	r	P	%	Interpretation
			Oropharynx	
Xi-Pm	0.31	0.004	9.6%	Significant, positive and moderate correlation
Co-Gn	0.24	0.02	5.7%	Significant, positive and weak correlation
Go-Me	0.13	0.23	1.6%	There was no correlation between variables
Facial depth	0.21	0.06	4.4%	There was no correlation between variables
SNB	0.37	0.001	13.6%	Significant, positive and moderate correlation
Facial axis	0.12	0.26	1.4%	There was no correlation between variables
Ar-Go	0.12	0.28	1.4%	There was no correlation between variables
FMA	-0.07	0.52	0.4%	There was no correlation between variables
			Nasopharynx	
Xi-Pm	0.37	0.001	13.6%	Significant, positive and moderate correlation
Co-Gn	0.32	0.003	10.2%	Significant, positive and moderate correlation
Go-Me	0.18	0.11	3.2%	There was no correlation between variables
Facial depth	0.29	0.009	8.4%	Significant, positive and weak correlation
SNB	0.34	0.002	11.5%	Significant, positive and moderate correlation
Facial axis	0.28	0.01	7.8%	Significant, positive and weak correlation
Ar-Go	0.29	0.007	8.4%	Significant, positive and weak correlation
FMA	-0.13	0.24	1.6%	There was no correlation between variables

DISCUSSION

Although some recent studies have reported a need for tridimensional evaluation by magnetic resonance,[6,7,8] its high cost and lack of standardization of patient's head position still hamper the use of this method for research. According to Muto et al,[9] a change of 10° in craniofacial tilt may affect measurement taking in the area of upper airways in approximately 4 mm. Lateral cephalograms have been used in this type of assessment as part of patients' basic orthodontic records, with the advantage of having low costs and low radiation dose, being of easy access, and providing standardization of measures with high reproducibility for diagnosis.[6,10,11] These advantages render this method common in research,[7,9,12,13,14] which validates the methodology adopted in the present study and allows comparison of results. The reproducibility of the method was confirmed statistically, with strong intraexaminer agreement.

The studied sample comprised patients aged between 10 and 17 years old, with a mean age of 12.3 years, similarly to other studies,[5,12,15,16]. Because there are minor changes in the nasopharynx as a result of growth,[17] the sample was matched by age; thus, avoiding potential bias as regards data interpretation. In terms of sex, groups were similar, although we found three more males than females in the Class II group.

Regarding airways measurements, there were significant differences between groups, with Class I patients having oropharynx and nasopharynx greater in size (Table 3, Fig 2). These findings corroborate the majority of studies found in the literature.[14,18,19,20] The studies by Freitas et al[12] as well as Memon, Fida and Shaikh[21] found no interference of malocclusion in oropharynx and nasopharynx width when they compared Class I to Class II patients. Differences in our results may be related to the methods employed, since those studies included a Class II sample based on dental occlusion and may have included subjects with Class II resulting from maxillary prognathism, whereas in our study, mandibular Class II was confirmed cephalometrically.

In order to have a better understanding of which factors inherent to malocclusion could be related to changes in upper airways, we initially diagnosed differences in skeletal features between groups, as follows: mandibular length (Xi-Pm, Co-Gn and Go-Me), mandibular position (facial depth and SNB), and direction of growth (facial axis, Ar-Go and FMA).

As regards mandibular length, measurements found in the Class I group were greater than those found in the Class II group (Table 3, Fig 3), thereby confirming mandibular Class II diagnosis. These data validate the assumption that mandibular length can be related to the size of upper airways, which is in agreement with Muto et al[4] who pointed out that craniofacial abnormalities, including mandibular retrognathism, short mandibular body and downward rotation, may cause a decrease in the size of airways, as reported by other studies.[9,13,19,22,23] The same behavior was observed in the variables related to spatial position of the mandible. As expected, the mandible in the Class II group was found retropositioned in relation to the cranial base when compared to the Class I group. This information allows us to conclude that both position and length of the mandible, i.e., the effective length of the mandible, must be considered in the diagnosis of patients with

Class II malocclusion. Nevertheless, a greater or less interference of either one of these variables cannot be assumed. In the literature, this comparison is scarce and only cited by a few authors.[1,23,24]

Our study was carried out considering that several others have assessed the association between facial growth pattern and upper airways measurements.[5,12,15,16,19] When comparing Class I and Class II groups, FMA and facial axis indicated an increased vertical trend among Class II individuals as well as a shorter mandibular ramus. According to Jarabak,[25] this finding refers to mandibular morphology with a clockwise growth pattern. This same feature was reported in the study by Joseph et al[15] who used a sample of individuals with Class II malocclusion. This information does not allow us to claim that all mandibular Class II individuals will have a vertical growth trend, although such feature was found in the sample. However, there seem to be an association between vertical pattern and reduced airways measurements, which has already been reported by several studies.[5,12,14,19]

The correlation between oropharynx and nasopharynx was studied separately from other variables, as shown in Table 4. There was a positive correlation between the size of the oropharynx and mandibular length, represented by Xi-Pm and Co-Gn, and the position of the mandible, represented by SNB. In agreement with our findings, studies carried out in the last five years[7,20,23,24] have concluded that mandibular length and position influence airways measurements.

Although Class II malocclusion patients have mostly presented with a vertical growth pattern in relation to Class I individuals, our results could not support a correlation between vertical pattern and a shorter oropharynx. We did not observe a positive correlation between growth pattern measurements (FMA, Ar-Go and facial axis) and the size of the oropharynx, even though there was an association. This is in agreement with the reports by Castro and Vasconcelos.[16] On the other hand, Freitas et al,[12] Zhong et al[19] as well as Ucar and Uysal[5] found a correlation between growth pattern and the size of the oropharynx.

When assessing airways measurements and growth pattern, Joseph et al[15] showed a correspondence between dolichocephalic individuals and shorter airways, particularly the nasopharynx. This is in agreement with our findings, as seen in Table 5 which shows a significant positive correlation between Ar-Go values and the size of the nasopharynx. In addition, they showed a positive correlation between Xi-Pm, Co-Gn, facial depth, SNB and facial axis; thus, concluding that mandibular length and position are related to the size of the nasopharynx.

Mandibular retrusion is one of the factors that may cause obstructive sleep apnea syndrome (OSA), characterized by a collapse site hindering the passage of air located in the pharynx. A reduction in this region can be the etiology of this syndrome both in children and adults. Characterized by respiratory disorders and nocturnal snoring, OSA may cause psychological and social impairment for the individual.[11,22,23]

As the results of our study suggest that mandibular length and position as well as the direction of growth can influence measurements of pharyngeal airways, we emphasize the importance of mandibular advancement in growing children through orthopedics by means of functional appliances; and in adults, with surgical advancement in order to promote enlargement of airways for functional and quality of life improvement, as well as decreased morbidity.[8,13,14,26,27]

CONCLUSION

» Individuals with mandibular Class II malocclusion were shown to have upper airways measurements reduced when compared to Class I individuals.

» Mandibular length is related to a decrease in upper airways measurements. Similarly, anteroposterior positioning of the mandible exerts influence on airways measurements.

» There was a tendency of facial growth pattern with a positive, but weak correlation with the sizes of the nasopharynx, but not with the oropharynx.

REFERENCES

1. McNamara Jr JA. Components of class II malocclusion in children 8-10 years of age. Angle Orthod. 1981;51(3):177-201.
2. Alcazar NMPV, Freitas MR, Janson G, Henriques JFC, Freitas KMS. Estudo cefalométrico comparativo dos espaços naso e bucofaríngeo nas más oclusões Classe I e Classe II, Divisão 1, sem tratamento ortodôntico, com diferentes padrões de crescimento. Rev Dental Press Ortod Ortop Facial. 2004;9(4):68-76.
3. Joseph AA, Elbowaa J, Cisneros GJ, Eisigsb A. Cephalometric comparative study of the soft tissue airway dimensions in persons with hyperdivergent and normodivergent facial pattern. J Oral Maxillofac surg. 1998;56:135-9.
4. Muto T, Yamazaki A, Takeda S. A cephalometric evaluation of the pharyngeal airway space in patients with mandibular retrognathia and prognathia, and normal subjects. Int J Oral Maxillofac Surg. 2008;37(3):228-31.
5. Ucar FI, Uysal T. Orofacial dimensions in subjects with Class I malocclusion and different growth patterns. Angle Orthod. 2011;81(3):460-8.
6. Pirilä-Parkkinen K, Löppönen H, Nieminen P, Tolonen U, Pääkkö E, Pirttiniemi P. Validity of upper airway assessment in children: a clinical, cephalometric, and MRI study. Angle Orthod. 2011;81(3):433-9.
7. Kim Y-J, Hong J-S, Hwang Y-I, Park Y-H. Three-dimensional analysis of pharyngeal airway in preadolescent children with different anteroposterior skeletal patterns. Am J Orthod Dentofacial Orthop. 2010;137(3):303-11.
8. Schutz TCB, Dominguez GC, Pradella-Hallinan M, Cunha TCA, Tufik S. Class II correction improves nocturnal breathing in adolescents. Angle Orthod. 2011;81(2):222-28.
9. Muto T, Yamazaki A, Takeda S, Kawakami J, Tsuji Y, Shibata T, Mizoguchi I. Relationship between the pharyngeal airway space and craniofacial morphology, taking into account head posture. Int J Oral Maxillofac Surg. 2006;35:132-6.
10. Major MP, Flores-Mir C, Major PW. Assessment of lateral cephalometric diagnosis of adenoid hypertrophy and posterior upper airway obstruction: a systematic review. Am J Orthod Dentofacial Orthop. 2006;130(6):700-8.
11. Bittencourt LRA, Haddad FLM. Diagnóstico e abordagem clínica do paciente com distúrbio respiratório do sono. In: Fabro CD, Chaves CM Jr, Tufik S. A odontologia na medicina do sono. Maringá: Dental Press; 2012. cap. 6, p. 144-58.
12. Freitas MR, Alcazar NM, Janson G, De Freitas KM, Henriques JFC. Upper and lower pharyngeal airways in subjects with Class I and Class II malocclusions and different growth patterns. Am J Orthod Dentofacial Orthop. 2006;130(6):742-45.
13. Susarla AM, Abramson ZR, Dodson TB, Kaban LB. Cephalometric measurement of upper airway length correlates with the presence and severity of obstructive sleep apnea. J Oral Maxillofac Surg. 2010;68:2846-55.
14. Restrepo C, Santamaria S, Pela EZ, Tapias A. Oropharyngeal airway dimensions after treatment with functional appliances in class II retrognathic children. J Oral Rehabil. 2011;38(8):588-94.
15. Joseph AA, Elbaum J, Cisneros GJ, Eisig SB. A cephalometric comparative study of the soft tissue airway dimensions in persons with hyperdivergent and normodivergent facial patterns. J Oral Maxillofac Surg.1998;56(2):135-9
16. Castro AMA, Vasconcelos MHF. Avaliação da influência do tipo facial nos tamanhos dos espaços aéreos nasofaríngeo e bucofaríngeo. Rev Dental Press Ortod Ortop Facial. 2008;13(6):43-50.
17. McNamara JA Jr. A method of cephalometric evaluation. Am J Orthod. 1984;86(6):449-69.
18. Mergen DC, Jacobs RM. The size of nasopharynx associated with normal occlusion and Class II malocclusion. Angle Orthod. 1970;40(4):342-6.
19. Zhong Z, Tang Z, Gao X, Zeng XL. A comparison study of upper airway among different skeletal craniofacial patterns in nonsnoring Chinese children. Angle Orthod. 2010;80(2):267-74.
20. El H, Palomo JM. Airway volume for different dentofacial skeletal patterns. Am J Orthod Dentofacial Orthop. 2011;139(6):511-21.
21. Memon S, Fida M, Shaikh A. Comparison of different craniofacial patterns with pharyngeal widths. J Coll Physicians Surg Pak. 2012;22(5):302-6.
22. Schwab RJ, Goldbert AN. Upper airway assessment: radiographic and other imagining techniques. Otolaryngol Clin North Am. 1998;31(6):931-68.
23. Guarim JA. Evaluation of the growth mandibular in a buccal respirator after the treatment with the use of the orthopedical prefabricated apparel. Rev Paul Odontol. 2009;32:15-23.
24. Kim JS, Kim JK, Hong SC, Cho JH. Changes in the upper airway after counterclockwise maxillomandibular advancement in young Korean women with class II malocclusion deformity. J Oral Maxillofac Surg. 2013;71:1603-5.
25. Jarabak JR, Fizzel JA. Technique and treatment with light wire edgewise appliances. 2nd ed. St. Louis: Mosby; 1972.
26. Lye KW. Effect of orthognathic surgery on the posterior airway space (PAS). Ann Acad Med Singapore. 2008;37(8):677-82.
27. Faria AC, Santos AC, Silva-Júnior SN, Xavier SN, Mello-Filho FV. Change in retrolingual airway space after maxillomandibular advancement surgery in OSA patients: evaluation with magnetic resonance imaging. Rev Bras Cir Craniomaxilofac. 2011;14 (3):145-8.

21

Base of the skull morphology and Class III malocclusion in patients with unilateral cleft lip and palate

Mariana Maciel Tinano[1], Milene Aparecida Torres Saar Martins[2], Cristiane Baccin Bendo[3], Ênio Mazzieiro[4]

Objective: The aim of the present study was to determine the morphological differences in the base of the skull of individuals with cleft lip and palate and Class III malocclusion in comparison to control groups with Class I and Class III malocclusion. **Methods:** A total of 89 individuals (males and females) aged between 5 and 27 years old (Class I, n = 32; Class III, n = 29; and Class III individuals with unilateral cleft lip and palate, n = 28) attending PUC-MG Dental Center and Cleft Lip/Palate Care Center of Baleia Hospital and PUC-MG (CENTRARE) were selected. Linear and angular measurements of the base of the skull, maxilla and mandible were performed and assessed by a single calibrated examiner by means of cephalometric radiographs. Statistical analysis involved ANCOVA and Bonferroni correction. **Results:** No significant differences with regard to the base of the skull were found between the control group (Class I) and individuals with cleft lip and palate (P > 0.017). The cleft lip/palate group differed from the Class III group only with regard to CI.Sp.Ba (P = 0.015). Individuals with cleft lip and palate had a significantly shorter maxillary length (Co-A) in comparison to the control group (P < 0.001). No significant differences were found in the mandible (Co-Gn) of the control group and individuals with cleft lip and palate (P = 1.000). **Conclusion:** The present findings suggest that there are no significant differences in the base of the skull of individuals Class I or Class III and individuals with cleft lip and palate and Class III malocclusion.

Keywords: Angle Class III malocclusion. Base of the skull. Cleft lip and palate.

[1] PhD resident in Child and Adolescent Health, School of Medicine — Federal University of Minas Gerais (UFMG).

[2] Postdoc resident in Pediatric Dentistry, Federal University of Minas Gerais (UFMG).

[3] Assistant professor, Department of Orthodontics and Pediatric Dentistry, Federal University of Minas Gerais (UFMG).

[4] PhD in Orthodontics, University of São Paulo (USP).

» The authors report no commercial, proprietary or financial interest in the products or companies described in this article.

Mariana Maciel Tinano
E-mail: maritinano@yahoo.com.br

INTRODUCTION

Correlations between the development of the base of the skull and maxillofacial components have been demonstrated in facial development studies.[1-4] The morphology of the base of the skull may be an important factor in the anteroposterior relationship of the maxilla and mandible as well as in determining Class III malocclusion.[5,6,7]

Class III malocclusion results from a combination of morphological abnormalities of the base of the skull, maxilla and mandible as well as in vertical facial dimensions.[5,8-11] Morphological variability in the craniofacial complex of individuals with Class III sagittal relationship suggests the influence of the base of the skull in the development of this type of malocclusion. Individuals with greater flexure of the base of the skull angle reveal a reduction in the horizontal dimension of the middle cranial fossa, with a consequent tendency toward nasomaxilllary retrognathism, a more forward positioning of the mandible and a prognathic craniofacial profile.[12] Moreover, a lower angle between the ramus of the mandible and the base of the skull, a smaller and more retrognathic maxilla and a larger and more prominent mandible can lead to Class III malocclusion associated with Class III facial pattern.[11,13]

The development of the craniofacial complex in patients with cleft lip and palate has been studied in an attempt to establish the mechanisms and determinant factors of facial development in such individuals. A number of studies state that the base of the skull is intrinsically different in shape and size in patients with cleft lip and palate.[14-18] This difference may affect the growth and positioning of facial structures, with an increased flexure of the base of the skull, thereby favoring the development of a Class III skeletal relationship. Nevertheless, other studies report that individuals with cleft lip and palate do not present significant differences in the base of the skull of which development is normal.[19,20,21] Abnormalities in intermaxillary and interalveolar sagittal relationships in such patients may stem primarily from a reduction in the depth of the maxilla, with no changes in the rotation or length of the ramus of the mandible.[22] Thus, the anteroposterior deformities often found in such individuals may actually result from surgical trauma, adaptive changes or a combination of both.

The literature does not reach a consensus regarding base of skull morphology in patients with unilateral cleft lip and palate. Additionally, there is considerable lack of current studies on this subject. For this reason, the aim of the present study was to compare the morphology of the base of the skull in individuals with unilateral cleft lip and palate and Class III malocclusion with control individuals with Class I and Class III malocclusion.

MATERIAL AND METHODS

This study was approved by the Catholic University of Minas Gerais Institutional Review Board (PUC-MG) under protocol CAAE - 0012.0.213.000-07.

Sample

The sample comprised 89 lateral cephalograms collected from the files of PUC-MG Dental Research Center and the Cleft Lip/Palate Care Center of Baleia Hospital and PUC-MG (CENTRARE). All cephalograms were taken from male and female patients at orthodontic treatment onset. Patients were aged between 5 and 27 years old (mean = 12.9; median = 12.0).

The sample was divided into three study groups: 1- Control group comprising 32 cephalograms of Class I individuals with no history of orthodontic treatment; 2- Group 2 comprising 29 cephalograms of Class III individuals with no history of orthodontic treatment; and 3- Group 3 comprising 28 cephalograms of nonsyndromic, unilateral cleft lip/palate Class III individuals having undergone correction for cleft lip/palate at an early age (lip surgery at a mean age of 6 months, and palate surgery at a mean age of 18 months).

Measurement methods

Cephalometric tracings were performed manually on acetate paper and based on patients' cephalograms. All tracings were performed by a single calibrated examiner. Intraexaminer agreement was assessed by paired Student's t-test. Linear and angular measurements were performed on two separate occasions with a 10-day interval in between. The p-value generated by the paired Student's t-test was 0.446 for linear measurements and 0.392 for angular measurements, thereby demonstrating no significant differences between measurements taken on the two different occasions.

The cephalometric landmarks used in the present study were as described by Jacobson:[23] sella (S), nasion (N), basion (Ba), A-point (A), condyle (Co), gnathion (Gn), posterior clinoid process (Cl) and sphenoid (Sp). Linear (S-N, S-Ba, Co-A, Co-Gn, Ba-Cl, Sp-Cl, Ba-Sp and Cl-I) and angular (Ba.S.N, Ba.Cl.Sp, Cl.Ba.Sp and Cl.Sp.Ba) measurements were taken as shown in Figure 1. The height of the base of the skull (Cl-I) was measured by the distance of a straight line from Cl and S landmarks and a point intercepting the greater wing of the sphenoid bone at a point established as point I (I) (Fig 1).

Data analysis

Statistical Package for Social Sciences (SPSS for Windows, version 19.0, SPSS Inc., Chicago, IL, USA) was used for data analysis. Initially, the three groups were analyzed with regard to age. As Shapiro-Wilk test determined that this variable was not normally distributed, Kruskal-Wallis test was used and revealed significant differences among the three groups with regard to age($P = 0.032$).

Conversely, Shapiro-Wilk test determined that linear and angular measurements were normally distributed, for this reason, analysis of covariance (ANCOVA) was used for statistical analysis of data. Analysis of covariance is justified by the potential interference of age in the mean linear and angular measurements. In cases of significant differences among groups, Bonferroni correction was used to identify in which groups the difference was found. To prevent errors arising from multiple comparisons, the significance level (0.05) was divided by the number of comparisons;[24] thus, p-values less than 0.017 were considered statistically significant (0.05 divided by 3).

RESULTS

Table 1 displays the angular measurements in the three groups. The cleft lip/palate group had intermediate measurements of the base of the skull that ranged between the control and Class III groups. No significant differences were found between the cleft lip/palate group and the control group (Class I). The cleft lip/palate group significantly differed from the Class III group only with regard to Cl.Sp.Ba ($P = 0.015$). Significant differences in Ba.S.N, Ba.Cl.Sp and Cl.Sp.Ba were found between the control (Class I) and Class III groups. The lowest Ba.S.N was found in the Class III group, thereby indicating greater flexure of the base of the skull angle in comparison to the other groups (Fig 2).

Table 2 displays the linear measurements in the three groups. Mean Co-A (maxilla) was greater in the control group (Class I) (90.8 mm) and lower in the cleft lip/palate group (85.1 mm). This difference was statistically significant ($P < 0.001$). Considering a p-value lower than 0.017 as statistically significant (as determined by Bonferroni correction), no significant difference was found between the Class III group and the cleft lip/palate group ($P = 0.032$). Mean length of the mandible (Co-Gn) was greater in the cleft lip/palate group (116.3 mm) in comparison to the other groups. However, this difference was not statistically significant. While no significant differences were found with regard to angular measurements, the linear measurements of the base of the skull were lower, except for S-N and Ba-Sp.

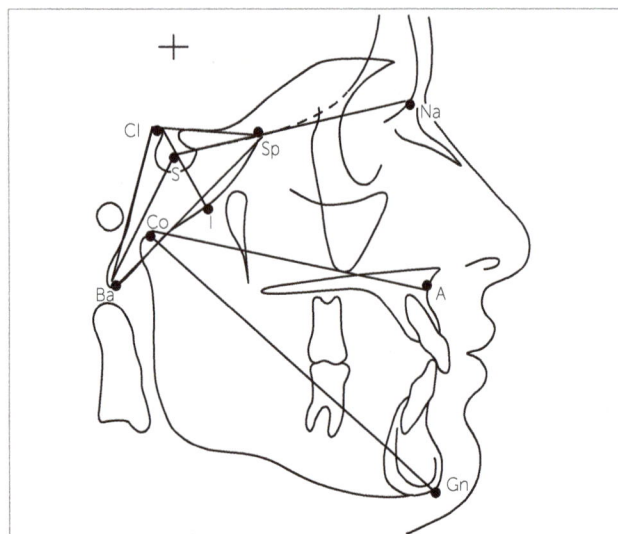

Figure 1 - Cephalometric landmarks, linear and angular measurements.

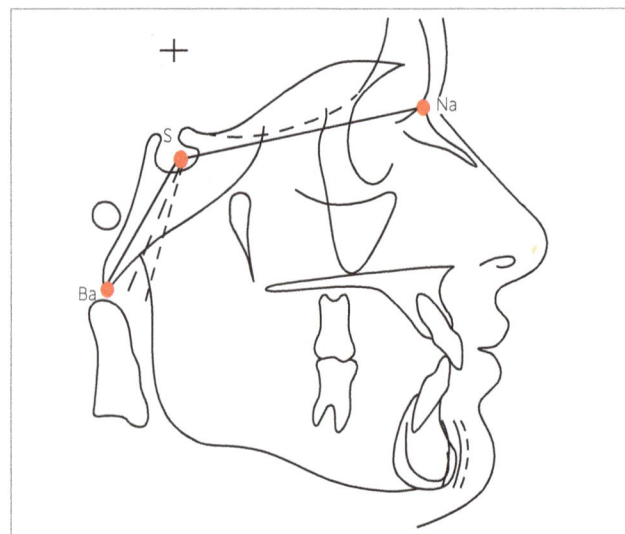

Figure 2 - Ba.S.N angular measurements demonstrating flexure of the base of the skull angle.

Table 1 - Mean angular measurements in different groups.

Variable	Groups			P-value*	Comparison between groups		
	Control (G1)	Class III (G2)	Cleft (G3)		G1 x G2	G1 x G3	G2 x G3
	Mean ± SD	Mean ± SD	Mean ± SD				
Ba.S.N	130.1 ± 5.0	125.6 ± 4.5	127.9 ± 5.0	0.002	**0.001**	0.275	0.192
Ba.Cl.Sp	114.7 ± 6.9	108.5 ± 6.9	113.2 ± 5.2	0.002	**0.002**	1.000	0.037
Cl.Ba.Sp	23.4 ± 2.6	25.2 ± 2.8	24.3 ± 2.7	0.080	-	-	-
Cl.Sp.Ba	42.1 ± 5.3	46.3 ± 5.5	42.5 ± 3.6	0.003	**0.004**	1.000	**0.015**

*Analysis of covariance adjusted for age. SD= standard deviation; G1= group 1; G2= group 2; G3= group 3.
Bonferroni correction= P < 0.017; p-values in bold significant at 0.017.

Table 2 - Mean linear measurements in different groups.

Variable	Groups			P-value*	Comparison among groups		
	Control (G1)	Class III (G2)	Cleft (G3)		G1 x G2	G1 x G3	G2 x G3
	Mean ± SD	Mean ± SD	Mean ± SD				
S-N	70.4 ± 5.1	68.5 ± 4.2	71.4 ± 4.9	0.591	–	–	–
S-Ba	46.5 ± 3.0	45.9 ± 3.0	45.3 ± 4.0	0.049	1.000	0.113	0.082
Co-A	90.8 ± 7.8	86.1 ± 6.0	85.1 ± 7.0	< 0.001	0.208	**< 0.001**	0.032
Co-Gn	114.7 ± 9.7	114.6 ± 10.9	116.3 ± 9.7	0.029	0.050	1.000	0.069
Ba-Cl	49.4 ± 3.6	49.2 ± 3.2	48.1 ± 4.5	0.051	-	-	-
Sp-Cl	29.3 ± 2.5	29.5 ± 2.7	29.1 ± 2.9	0.726	-	-	-
Ba-Sp	66.8 ± 3.5	64.3 ± 3.6	64.9 ± 5.5	0.072	-	-	-
Cl-I	25.1 ± 2.6	25.9 ± 2.4	24.6 ± 3.2	0.028	0.191	1.000	0.027

*Analysis of covariance adjusted for age. SD= standard deviation; G1= group 1; G2= group 2; G3= group 3.
Bonferroni correction = P < 0.017; p-value in bold significant at 0.017.

DISCUSSION

In the present study, no significant differences were found with regard to the linear measurements of the base of the skull (S-Ba, Ba-Cl, Sp-Cl, Ba-Sp and Cl-l) (P > 0.017), even though they were lower in the cleft lip/palate group in comparison to control (Class I). These results are in agreement with others studies[17,20,25] reporting that shorter measurements may be attributed to the small body children with cleft lip/palate normally have.

No significant differences were found for S-N among groups; however, mean S-N was greater in the cleft lip/palate group in comparison to the other groups. This is in disagreement with others studies[15,16,26,27,28] reporting lower S-N in children with cleft lip and palate, thereby suggesting a relative difference in the craniofacial morphology of such individuals. Nevertheless, the majority of the aforementioned studies included individuals with different types and degrees of cleft lip and palate, which may explain the divergent findings.

Significant difference was found in Co-A between the control (Class I) and the cleft lip/palate group (P < 0.001), as the former had the greatest whereas the latter had the shortest measurement among the three groups, thereby suggesting a deficiency in the effective length of the maxilla in this group. This result is in agreement with other studies[29-33] reporting the effect of surgical procedures on the anteroposterior growth and development of the maxilla in children with cleft lip and palate due to the formation of fibrous scar tissue at the surgery site. However, it is not yet clear whether maxillary retrognathism may also be related to intrinsic development deficiencies in such individuals. In some studies,[25,34,35] the maxilla of individuals with cleft lip and palate was reduced in size in both operated and non-operated groups, thus suggesting that maxillary retrognathism may not be related to surgical procedures only, but may also be due to intrinsic factors of the condition itself.

No statistically significant difference was found with regard to the linear measurement of mandibular length (Co-Gn) (P > 0.017), which is in agreement with other studies[21,25,26,36,37] reporting that the mandible of individuals with cleft lip and palate is equal in length to that of individuals without this condition. Likewise, no significant differences were found between the control and the Class III malocclusion group, which is in disagreement with other studies[9,10] concluding that mandibular length progressively increases with age of Class III individuals.

No significant difference was found in the base of the skull angle (Ba.S.N), particularly between control and cleft lip/palate group (P = 0.275). This is in agreement with previous studies[16,19,20,25,27] reporting that the malocclusion found in this group is much more the result of maxillary retrognathism caused by surgical trauma than the presence of a more flexed base of the skull, thereby determining the emergence of mandibular prognathism. However, significant differences were found between the control and the Class III malocclusion group, with a smaller angle in the latter group (125.6°). Other studies[8,10,38,39] also report that Class III individuals have morphological abnormalities in the craniofacial complex, with a reduction in the angle formed by the anterior and posterior segments of the base of the skull. The posterior base of the skull (S-Ba) exerts significant influence in the emergence of mandibular prognathism. This mandibular rotation caused by reduction in the angle may indicate an increase in the length of the linear measurement Cl-I due to the base of the skull being represented by a triangle in

this study. Thus, the greater height of the base of the skull in Class III individuals may be the consequence of greater flexure of this structure.

No significant differences were found between the control and the cleft lip/palate group regarding the angular measurements of the base of the skull (Ba. Cl.Sp, Cl.Ba.Sp and Cl.Sp.Ba), thereby confirming absence of morphological differences between the two groups. However, significant differences in Ba.Cl.Sp and Cl.Sp.Ba were found between the control and the Class III malocclusion group, thereby demonstrating morphological differences in the craniofacial complex of these two groups.

Based on the results of this study it is reasonable to assert that, the base of the skull in individuals with unilateral cleft lip and palate does not differ significantly from that of individuals with Class I malocclusion; its development is, therefore, normal. In contrast, craniofacial morphology in individuals with Class III malocclusion differs significantly from that of individuals with Class I malocclusion, thereby suggesting that structural alterations in this morphology may influence the emergence of Class III malocclusion.

CONCLUSION

No significant differences in the base of the skull of Class I or Class III individuals and cleft lip/palate individuals with Class III malocclusion were found. Results suggest that Class III malocclusion in cleft lip/palate patients might be associated with the length of the maxilla, only.

REFERENCES

1. Bjork, A. Base of the skull. Am J Orthod.1955;41:198-225.
2. Hopkins GB, Houston WJ, James GA. The base of the skull as an aetiological factor in malocclusion. Angle Orthod. 1968;38(3):250-5.
3. Enlow D, Kuroda T, Lewis A. The morphological and morphogenetic basis for craniofacial form and pattern. Angle Orthod.1971;41:161-88.
4. Enlow D, McNamara Jr JA. The neurocranial basis for facial form and pattern. Angle Orthod. 1973;43:256-70.
5. Sanborn RT. Differences between the facial skeletal patterns of class III malocclusion and normal occlusion. Angle Orthod. 1955;25(4):208-222.
6. Guyer EC, Ellis EE 3rd, McNamara JA Jr, Behrents RG. Components of class III malocclusion in juveniles and adolescents. Angle Orthod. 1986;56(1):7-30.
7. Chang HP, Liu PH, Tseng YC, Yang YH, Pan CY, Chou ST. Morphometric analysis of the base of the skull in Asians. Odontology. 2014;102(1):81-8.
8. Singh GD, McNamara Jr JA, Lozanoff S. Finite element analysis of base of the skull in subjects with class III malocclusion. Br J Orthod. 1997;24(2):103-12.
9. Miyajima K, McNamara JA Jr, Sana M, Murata S. An estimation of craniofacial growth in untreated class III female with anterior crossbite. Am J Orthod Dentofacial Orthop. 1997;112(4):425-34.

10. Mouakeh M. Cephalometric evaluation of craniofacial pattern of Syrian children with Class III malocclusion. Am J Orthod Dentofacial Orthop. 2001;119(6):640-9.
11. Chang HP, Hsieh SH, Tseng YC, Chou TM. Cranial-base morphology in children with class III malocclusion. Kaohsiung J Med Sci. 2005;21(4):159-65.
12. Lavelle CLB. A study of craniofacial form. Angle Orthod. 1979;49:65-72.
13. Battagel JM. The aetiological factors in Class III malocclusion. Eur J Orthod. 1993;15(5):347-70.
14. Moss ML. Malformations of skull base associated with cleft palate deformity. Plast Reconstr Surg (1946). 1956;17(3):226-34.
15. Dalh E. Craniofacial morphology in congenital clefts of lip and palate. Acta Odontol Scand.1970;28:83-100.
16. Hoswell BB, Gallup BV. Base of the skull morphology in cleft lip and palate: A cephalometric study from 7 to 18 years of age. J Oral Maxillofac Surg. 1992;50:681-5.
17. Harris EF. Size and form of base of the skull in isolated cleft lip and palate. Cleft Palate Craniofac J. 1993;30(2):170-4.

18. Cortés J, Granic X. Characteristic craniofacial features in a group of unilateral cleft lip and palate patients in Chile. Rev Stomatol Chir Maxillofac. 2006;107(5):347-53.

19. Brader AC. A cephalometric appraisal of morphological variations in base of the skull and associated pharyngeal structures. Angle Orthod. 1957;27:179-95.

20. Ross RB. Base of the skull in children with cleft lip and palate. Cleft Palate J. 1965;2:157-66.

21. Chierici G, Harvold E, Vargervik K. Morphogenetic experiments in cleft palate: mandibular response. Cleft Palate J. 1973;10:47-56.

22. Veleminská J. Analysis of intracranial relations in patients with unilateral cleft lip and palate using cluster and factor analysis. Acta Chir Plast. 2000;42(1):27-36.

23. Jacobson A. Radiographic Cephalometry. Chicago: Quintessence; 1995.

24. Nahler G. Dictionary of Pharmaceutical Medicine. New York: Springer-Verlag / Wien; 2009.

25. Bishara SE, Iversen WW. Cephalometric comparisons on the base of the skull and face in ndividuals with isolated clefts of the palate. Cleft Palate J. 1974;11:162-75.

26. Krogman WM, Mazaheri M, Harding RL, Ishiguro K, Bariana G, Meier J, et al. A longitudinal study of craniofacial growth pattern in children with clefts as compared to normal, birth to six years. Cleft Palate J. 1975;12(00):59-84.

27. Sandham A, Cheng L. Base of the skull and cleft lip and palate. Angle Orthod. 1988;58(2):163-8.

28. Trotman CA, Collett AR, McNamara JA Jr, Cohen SR. Analyses of craniofacial and dental morphology in monozygotic twins discordant for cleft lip and unilateral cleft lip and palate. Angle Orthod. 1993; 63:135-40.

29. Mestre JC, De Jesus J, Subtelny JD. Unoperated oral clefts at maturation. Angle Orthod. 1960;30:78-85.

30. Huang CS, Wang WI, Liou EJ, Chen YR, Chen PK, Noordhoff MS. Effects of cheiloplasty on maxillary dental arch development in infants with unilateral complete cleft lip and palate. Cleft Palate Craniofac J. 2002;39:513-6.

31. Singh GD, Rivera-Robles J, de Jesus-Vinas J. Longitudinal craniofacial growth patterns in patients with orofacial clefts: geometric morphometrics. Cleft Palate Craniofac J. 2004;41:136-43.

32. Liao YF, Mars M. Long-term effects of lip repair on dentofacial morphology in patients with unilateral cleft lip and palate. Cleft Palate Craniofac J. 2005;42:526-32.

33. Corbo M, Dujardin T, de Maertelaer V, Malevez C, Glineur R. Dentocraniofacial morphology of 21 patients with unilateral cleft lip and palate: a cephalometric study. Cleft Palate Craniofac J. 2005;42(6):618-24.

34. Hagerty RF, Hill MJ. Facial growth and dentition in the unoperated cleft palate. Fissurados. J Dent Res. 1963;42:412-21.

35. Blaine HL. Differential analysis of palate anomalies. J Dent Res. 1969;48(6):1042-8.

36. Capelozza Filho L, Normando AD, Silva Filho OG. Isolated influences of lip and palate surgery on facial growth: Comparison of operated and inoperated male adults with UCLP. Cleft Palate Craniofac J.1996;33:51-6.

37. Silva Filho OG, Calvano F, Assunção AG, Cavassan AO. Craniofacial morphology in children with complete unilateral cleft lip and palate: a comparison of two surgical protocols. Angle Orthod. 2001;71(4):274-84.

38. Tanabe Y, Taguchi Y, Noda T. Relationship between base of the skull structure and maxillofacial components in children aged 3-5 years. Eur J Orthod. 2002;24:175-81.

39. Andria LM, Leite LP, Prevatte TM, King LB. Correlation of the base of the skull angle and its components with others dental/skeletal variables and treatment time. Angle Orthod. 2004;74(3):361-6.

22

Bruxism in children and transverse plane of occlusion: Is there a relationship or not?

Ana Carla Raphaelli Nahás-Scocate[1], Fernando Vusberg Coelho[2], Viviane Chaves de Almeida[3]

Objective: To assess the occurrence of bruxism in deciduous dentition and a potential association between the habit and the presence or absence of posterior crossbite. **Methods:** A total of 940 patient files were assessed. They were gathered from the archives of University of São Paulo City - UNICID; however, 67 patient files were dismissed for not meeting the inclusion criteria. Therefore, 873 children, males and females, comprised the study sample. They were aged between 2-6 years old and came from six different public primary schools from the east of the city of São Paulo. Data were collected through questionnaires answered by parents/guardians and by clinical examinations carried out in the school environment in order to obtain the occlusal characteristics in the transverse direction. First, a descriptive statistical analysis of all variables was performed (age, sex, race, posterior crossbite, bruxism, headache and restless sleep); then, the samples were tested by means of chi-square test with significance level set at 0.05%. A logistic regression model was applied to identify the presence of bruxism. **Results:** The prevalence of this parafunctional habit was of 28.8%, with 84.5% of patients showing no posterior crossbite. Regarding the association of bruxism with crossbite, significant results were not found. Children with restless sleep have 2.1 times more chances of developing bruxism, whereas children with headache have 1.5 more chances. **Conclusion:** Transverse plane of occlusion was not associated with the habit of bruxism.

Keywords: Malocclusion. Bruxism. Epidemiology.

[1] Associate professor, Undergraduate and Postgraduate Program in Orthodontics, University of São Paulo City – UNICID.
[2] DDS, UNICID.
[3] MSc in Orthodontics, UNICID.

» The authors report no commercial, proprietary or financial interest in the products or companies described in this article.

Ana Carla Raphaelli Nahás-Scocate
Rua Cesário Galeno, 448/475 – Tatuapé – São Paulo/SP — Brazil
CEP: 03071-000 – E-mail: carlanahas@yahoo.com.br

INTRODUCTION

Bruxism is a parafunctional activity of the masticatory system characterized by clenching or grinding the teeth with rhythmic muscular contractions more frequent during sleep.[28] While this parafunctional activity is performed, nearly entirely in the subconscious level, neuromuscular protection mechanisms are absent,[19] thereby changing the masticatory system and causing temporomandibular disorders.[29]

Clinically, bruxism in children not only causes different levels of tooth surface wear, but also provides patients with muscle and joint discomfort. Furthermore, due to axial forces generated in patient's teeth, it can act as an adjuvant in the progression of destructive periodontal disease in children,[2] in addition to contributing to the development of false Class III, accelerated root resorption of deciduous teeth, changes in the chronology of permanent teeth irruption and promotion of dental crowding.[15] Thus, this habit should be diagnosed and managed as early as possible.[15]

There have been only a few published studies conducted to assess the prevalence of bruxism in children. This limitation prevents scientific parameters and association of bruxism with etiological factors to be established. The literature appears to be contradictory regarding the etiology of this parafunctional habit in childhood, thereby characterizing its origin as multifactorial, involving heredity, psychological and behavioral factors as well as occlusal interferences and certain pathologies.[4,14,17,18,20,21,28] Some authors report that occlusal factors such as overjet, overbite, molar and canine relationship, open bite and crossbite might play an important role in the development of this habit in children.[12,26,29]

Bruxism in children is also diagnosed with painful symptoms of Temporomandibular Disorders (TMD) of which it can be considered a possible causal factor.[26] Additionally, frequent headaches and restless sleep are associated with this habit.[3]

Thus, in this context, this study aimed at investigating the prevalence of bruxism in deciduous dentition, trying to relate it to occlusal factors, specifically the transverse plane of occlusion, so as to establish a causal factor alone, since several nuances are present in scientific research. In addition, the association of this parafunctional habit with restless sleep and headaches was also verified.

MATERIAL AND METHODS

Ethical aspects

This study was funded by the Brazilian National Council for Scientific and Technological Development - CNPq (Undergraduate Research) from 2008 to 2009. It is part of a project developed to assess the association between bruxism in children and posterior crossbite, conducted in accordance with the rules and principles adopted by Ethics and Research (13355774).

Sample selection

Clinical records of Brazilian children, males and females, aged between 2 years and 1 month old and 6 years and 11 months old, enrolled in 2005 in primary public schools located in the east of the city of São Paulo, were assessed. The initial sample comprised 940 children; however, 67 records were excluded for not meeting the inclusion criteria. Therefore, the final sample comprised 873 children of which 37.3% and 38.7% were 4 and 5 years old, respectively.

Inclusion criteria

The medical records of children included in this sample met the following inclusion criteria: Informed consent form signed by parents/guardians; questionnaire properly answered; children aged between 2 years and 1 month and 6 years and 11 months; complete deciduous dentition without erupted or erupting permanent teeth; absence of carious lesions or extensive loss of structure that compromised coronary occlusion; lack of early loss of deciduous teeth; absence of any kind of trauma; absence of visual and/or hearing and/or mental impairment; no previous orthodontic treatment and/or speech therapy.

Informed consent form and questionnaire

Parents/guardians were given detailed explanation about the objectives and design of data collection in the schools. Subsequently, an informed consent form was sent so as to notify them about the research, its importance and objectives. A questionnaire on parafunctional habits and other characteristics related to the overall health of children was also sent. The examiner did not interfere during questionnaire completion.

Examiner calibration

Three examiners were properly calibrated prior to clinical examination. The calibration process included the examination of occlusion in 24 children, performed twice with a 15-day interval in between. Data were subjected to Kappa statistics (K) for analysis of reproducibility. An index greater than 0.81 K and Pearson correlation coefficient (Rs > 0.90) were calculated. Results revealed excellent intra and inter-examiner reliability.

Clinical examination

All clinical examinations were performed in the school environment with the children sitting comfortably and facing abundant source of artificial light. First, they were asked to perform maximum mouth opening and then occlude in maximum intercuspation (MIH) for data collection.

To assess transverse posterior relationship between upper and lower dental arches, the following criteria were applied: Absent posterior crossbite (when the palatal cusps of upper posterior teeth occluded in the groove of mandibular posterior teeth), and presence of posterior crossbite (when the buccal cusps of upper posterior teeth occluded in the central sulcus of lower teeth, thereby establishing a transverse or inverted cross relationship on the back). Subsequently, both unilateral crossbites, whether with shift or true, as well as bilateral ones, were included.

Questionnaire

A questionnaire[13] comprising standardized questions about patient's history was answered by parents/guardians.[17] Based on the questionnaire, the presence of bruxism (yes or no), the period in which the child presented the parafunctional habit (daytime, night time or both), and the variables related to the presence of restless sleep (yes or no) as well as headaches (yes or no) were investigated. It is worth mentioning that the examiners did not interfere while the questionnaires were being filled out.

Data analysis

First, a descriptive statistical analysis of all variables (age, sex, race, posterior crossbite, bruxism, headache and restless sleep) was carried out. Subsequently, analyses of statistical significance were conducted by means of chi-square test in order to investigate possible associations between bruxism and other characteristics (sex, race, posterior crossbite, headache and restless sleep). The same test investigated a potential association between posterior crossbite, headache and restless sleep. At last, a logistic regression model was applied for the presence of bruxism, thus presenting the Odds Ratio (OR). The level of significance was set at 5%, i.e., test results were not statistically significant when P-value was less than or equal to 0.05.

RESULTS
Descriptive analysis of variables in the sample

Sample distribution according to age was predominantly composed of children between 4 and 5 years old (37.3% and 38.7%, respectively). Regarding patients' sex, the sample was very well divided and comprised 434 females (49.7%) and 439 males (50.3%). As for race, most children had brown skin (pardo) (58%), whereas only 0.4% had yellow skin.

The minority showed posterior crossbite, totaling 15.5% (n = 135) as distributed in Table 1. As for the prevalence of the parafunctional habit of bruxism, 26.5% of children had the habit at night, 2.2% during the day and 0.1% during the night and during the day, thereby representing a total of 28.8% of children with bruxism. Out of the total sample, 21.8% (n = 190) reported having headaches while 36.1% (n = 315) claimed to have restless sleep.

Association between bruxism and other variables

To assess a potential association between the presence of bruxism and other variables, the sample was divided as follows: "No" (when the child did not have bruxism) and "Yes" (when children showed signs of bruxism at night and/or day). The variable posterior crossbite was also treated in a similar way: "Absent" (when the child did not have posterior crossbite) and "Present" (when the child presented any type of posterior crossbite).

According to Table 2, the prevalence of bruxism was higher for males (30.5%) in comparison to females (27%). Likewise, black-skin children had higher prevalence (36.1%) when compared to other races. Among children with no posterior crossbite,

Bruxism in children and transverse plane of occlusion: Is there a relationship...

175

Table 1 - Sample distribution according to posterior crossbite (PCB)

PCB	Absent	Bilateral	Unil. shift R	Unil. shift L	Unil. true. R	Unil. true. L	Total
n	738	19	53	28	21	14	873
%	84.5	2.2	6.1	3.2	2.4	1.6	100

Table 2 - Sample distribution according to the presence of bruxism and variables of sex, posterior crossbite, headache, restless sleep and race.

Bruxism	Sex				Posterior crossbite				Headache				Restless sleep				Race							
	Female		Male		Absent		Present		No		Yes		No		Yes		Yellow		White		Black		Brown	
	n	%	n	%	n	%	n	%	n	%	n	%	n	%	n	%	n	%	n	%	n	%	n	%
No	317	73	305	69.5	510	69.1	112	83	505	73.9	117	61.6	432	77.4	190	60.3	4	100	225	74.5	39	63.9	354	70
Yes	117	27.0	134	30.5	228	30.9	23	17	178	26.1	73	38.4	126	22.6	125	39.7	0	0	77	25.5	22	36.1	152	30
Total	434	100	439	100	738	100	135	100	683	100	190	100	558	100	315	100	4	100	302	100	61	100	506	100

the percentage of bruxism (30.9%) was higher than children with posterior crossbite (17%). As for headaches, 38.4% reported headache and showed signs of bruxism, whereas 26.1% reported having no headache even though they showed signs of bruxism. Children with restless sleep presented a higher percentage of bruxism (39.7%) in comparison to those who did not report restless sleep (22.6%).

Table 3 presents the results of the chi-square test with significance level set at 5%. Results show a significant association between posterior crossbite (p = 0.0015), headache (p = 0.0012) and restless sleep (p < 0.0001).

Association between posterior crossbite, headache and restless sleep

Table 4 shows the result of sample distribution according to the presence of posterior crossbite, headache and restless sleep. Table 5 shows the result of sample distribution according to the presence of headache and restless sleep. A total of 31.7% of children who had restless sleep also had headaches. This represents nearly the double if compared to children who did not have restless sleep (16.1%). The chi-square test showed that there was only significant association between headache and restless sleep with p < 0.0001 (Table 6).

Logistic regression model for the presence of bruxism

A logistic regression model was applied for the presence or absence of bruxism (Table 7). Children without posterior crossbite were 2.2 times more

Table 3 - Chi-square test results.

Chi-square test	
Comparison with bruxism	P-value
Sex	0.2762
Race	0.1592
Posterior crossbite	0.0015*
Headache	0.0012*
Restless sleep	< 0.0001*

*Significant at 5%.

Table 4 - Sample distribution according to the presence of posterior crossbite associated with headache and restless sleep.

Posterior crossbite	Headache				Restless sleep			
	No		Yes		No		Yes	
	n	%	n	%	n	%	n	%
Absent	579	84.8	159	83.7	471	84.4	267	84.8
Present	104	15.2	31	16.3	87	15.6	48	15.2
Total	683	100	190	100	558	100	315	100

Table 5 - Sample distribution according to the presence of headache and restless sleep.

Headache	Restless sleep			
	Absent		Present	
	n	%	n	%
Absent	468	83.9	215	68.3
Present	90	16.1	100	31.7
Total	558	100	315	100

Table 6 - Chi-square test results.

Chi-square test	
Comparison	P-value
PCB X headache	0.7997
PCB X restless sleep	0.9671
Headache X restless sleep	< 0.0001*

*Significant at 5%.

Table 7 - Results of logistic regression model applied for the presence of bruxism.

| Characteristic | Chance ratio | 95% confidence interval | | P-value |
		Lower limit	Upper limit	
Posterior crossbite				
Present	1.0			
Absent	2.2	1.4	3.6	0.0011
Headache				
No	1.0			
Yes	1.5	1.1	2.2	0.0148
Restless sleep				
No	1.0			
Yes	2.1	1.6	2.9	<0.0001

likely to have bruxism in comparison to children with posterior crossbite. Children who complained of having headaches were 1.5 times more likely (50% more) to develop bruxism, in comparison to those who did not have headaches. Children with restless sleep have 2.1 more chances to develop bruxism, in comparison to children with peaceful sleep.

DISCUSSION

The prevalence of the parafunctional habit of bruxism in deciduous dentition has been the subject of some recent epidemiological studies. However, lack of uniformity and standardization of criteria to assess bruxism in children have resulted in a wide variation of its prevalence.[17,22,25,28]

The actual occurrence of bruxism in children cannot be easily registered because the presence of wear facets observed during clinical examination may indicate only a history of bruxism which may no longer be occurring at the time of evaluation. On the other hand, the beginning of the habit may not yet have caused the tooth to show signs of wear. Thus, although being subjective, the method of interviewing the children's parents is considered trustworthy to assess the prevalence of this habit, as it reflects the existence of dental noises produced by the child and which are actually perceived by parents. Therefore, even though prevalence was underestimated, the occurrence of false-positives is almost eliminated.[29]

The methods employed herein included a questionnaire answered by parents and/or guardians and followed a similar standard used in other studies.[5,13,14,17,30] The difficulty in diagnosing this parafunctional disturbance is widely known[29] even when diagnosis is based on polysomnography exams which were not performed in this sample. Such an exam becomes even more limited when dealing with children at the stage of primary dentition.

Results obtained herein showed a high prevalence of the parafunctional habit of bruxism, thus corroborating results of previous studies.[11,16,17,18,24,30] However, some studies[21,27] revealed even higher occurrences of around 45% whereas others revealed much lower occurrences as low as 6.4% in Turkey[1] and 11% in India.[5] It can be supposed that the origin of these differences (regarding the prevalence of bruxism in children) is possibly related to lack of uniformity in methodological research, cultural differences between countries, or even a variety of age groups.

Regarding patients' sex, some studies show that the parafunctional habit of bruxism in children has prevailed for males,[14,17,18] which was also found in this study. However, a study of Mexican children detected the presence of bruxism in 6% in female population compared to 1.5% in male population.[12] Other studies found no significant differences regarding sexual dimorphism.[5,7,9,28]

In the present study, the majority of children with bruxism did not present posterior crossbite when assessed statistically. However, the results support statistical analysis, thereby giving significance to factors of bruxism, headache and restless sleep. Bruxism is often associated with patient's emotional state and is more common among anxious children.[6,23]

When the chi-square test was applied, the only factors showing a statistically significant association were headache and restless sleep. Nevertheless, posterior crossbite was not significantly associated with headache and restless sleep. These data confirm what the literature already proves: There is a correlation between the presence of restless sleep in children with headache.[8,10]

The logistic regression model showed that children without posterior crossbite were 2.2 more likely to have bruxism, in comparison to children with posterior crossbite. Children who complained of headache were 1.5 times more likely to develop bruxism, in comparison to those who did not complain of headaches. Also, children with restless sleep were 2.1 more likely to have bruxism, in comparison to children with peaceful sleep.

Researchers believe bruxism is strongly correlated with children's emotional state[6,8,10,17,23] (anxiety, hyperactivity, restless sleep), which was also considered in this paper. Additionally, according to some studies,[4,14,18,20,21,28] children's general health, occurrence of malocclusion (absent, mild, moderate and severe) and the presence of other parafunctional oral habits can also be paired with bruxism. However, in contrast to these studies, the results of the present study showed no significant relationship between the presence of bruxism and posterior crossbite, i.e., the occlusal factor.

In this context, the combination of several etiologic factors present in a single individual greatly increases the likelihood of bruxism in children. Furthermore, its high prevalence is being considered an intrinsic problem of modern society. Thus, different treatment modalities available nowadays should be individualized for each patient.

Early diagnosis is important to reduce the consequences of this parafunctional activity. Clinician's treatment protocol should be directed towards reducing psychological stress and treating signs and symptoms, since bruxism cannot be permanently eliminated. One should opt for conservative therapy, with reversible and not invasive control as well as continuous follow-up. Due to its multifactorial etiology, bruxism treatment should involve professionals such as pediatricians, psychologists, pediatric dentists and otolaryngologists.

CONCLUSIONS

The parafunctional habit of bruxism was prevalent in 28.8% of the total sample studied. There was no significant relationship between this parafunctional habit and the transverse plane of occlusion. However, headache and restless sleep were significantly associated with bruxism in children.

REFERENCES

1. Agargun MY, Clli AS, Sener SS, Bilici M, Ozer OA, Selvi Y, Karacan E. The prevalence of parasomnias in preadolescent School-aged Children: a Turkish sample. Sleep. 2004;27(4):701-5.

2. Ahmad R. Bruxism in children. J Pedod. 1986;10(2):105-26.

3. Ángeles ET, Gáldos AC, Sanches LR, Martinez CS. Prevalência de bruxismo em pacientes de primeira vez en el Instituto Nacional de Pediatria. Acta Pediatr Méx. 2003;24(2):95-3.

4. Antonio AG, Pierro VSS, Maia LC. Bruxism in children: a warning sign for psychological problems. J Can Dent Assoc. 2006;72(2):155-60.

5. Bharti B, Malhi P, Kashyap S. Patterns and problems of sleep in school going children. Indian Pediatr. 2006;43(1):35-8.

6. Cariola TC. O desenho da figura humana de crianças com bruxismo. Bol Psicol. 2006;56(124);37-52.

7. Ferreira AM, Clemente V, Gozal D, Gomes A, Silva FC. Snoring in portuguese primary school children. Pediatrics. 2000;106(5):64.

8. Francesco DCR, Passerotii G, Paulucci B, Miniti A. Respiração oral na criança: repercussões diferentes de acordo com o diagnóstico. Rev Bras Otorrinolaringol. 2004;70(5):665-70.

9. Fukumizu M, Kaga M, Kohyama J, Hayes MJ. Sleep-related nighttime crying (yonaki) in Japan: a community-based study. Pediatrics. 2005;115(1):217-24.

10. Gorayeb MAM, Gorayeb R. Cefaléia associada a indicadores de transtornos de ansiedade em uma amostra de escolares de Ribeirão Preto, SP. Arq Neuropsiquiatr. 2002;60(3B):764-8.

11. Gregório PB, Athanazio RA, Bitencourt AGV, Neves FBCS, Hora F. Sintomas da síndrome de apnéia-hipopnéia obstrutiva do sono em crianças. J Bras Pneumol. 2008;34(6):356-61.

12. Jaime MEM. Frequencia de maloclusiones y su associación con hábitos perniciosos en una población de niños mexicanos de 6 a 12 años de edad. Rev ADM. 2004;61(6):209-14.

13. Junqueira TH, Nahás-Scocate AC, Valle-Corotti KM, Conti AC, Trevisan S. Association of infantile bruxism and the terminal relationships of the primary second molars. Braz Oral Res. 2013;27(1):42-7.

14. Liu X, Ma Y, Wang Y, Rao Y. Brief report: an epidemiologic survey of the prevalence of sleep disorders among children 2 to 12 years old in Beijing, China. Pediatrics. 2005;115(1):266-8.

15. Loos PJ, Aaron GA. Standards for management of the pediatric patient with acute pain in the temporomandibular joint or muscles of mastication. Pediatric Dent. 1989;11(4):331.

16. Mendes LR, Fernandes A, Garcia FT. Hábitos e perturbações do sono em idade escolar. Acta Pediatr Port. 2004;35:341-7.

17. Nahás-Scocate ACR, Trevisan S, Junqueira TH, Fuziy A. Associação entre o bruxismo infantil e as características oclusais, sono e dor de cabeça. Rev Assoc Paul Cir Dent. 2012;66(1):18-22.

18. Ng Dk, Kwok K, Cheung JM, Leung S, Chan CH. Prevalence of sleep problems in Hong Kong primary school children. Chest. 2005;128(3):1315-23.

19. Okeson JP. Temporomandibular disorders in children. Pediatric Dent. 1989;11(4):325-9.

20. Pavarina AC, Bussadori CMC, Alencar Jr FGP. Aspectos dos hábitos parafuncionais de interesse para o clínico geral. J Bras Clin Estet Odontol. 1999;3(13):86-90.

21. Petit D, Touchette E, Tremblay RE, Boivin M, Montplaisiur J. Dyssomnias and parasomnias in early childhood. Pediatrics. 2007;119(5):1016-25.

22. Pizzol KED C, Carvalho JCQ, Konishi F, Marcomini EMS, Giusti JSM. Bruxismo na infância: fatores etiológicos e possíveis tratamentos. Rev Odontol UNESP. 2006;35(2):157-63.

23. Porto FR, Machado LR, Leite ICG. Variáveis associadas ao desenvolvimento do bruxismo em crianças de 4 a 12 anos. J Bras Odontopediatr Odontol Bebê. 1999;2(10):447-53.

24. Reimão R, Lefevre A B, Diament AJ. Prevalência de distúrbios do sono na infância. Pediat. 1983;5:49-55.

25. Rodrigues KC, Ditterich RG, Shintcovsk RL, Tanaka O. Bruxismo: uma revisão da literatura. Publ UEPG Ci Biol Saúde. 2006;12(3):13-21.

26. Santos ECA, Bertoz FA, Pignatta LMB, Arantes FM. Avaliação clínica de sinais e sintomas da disfunção temporomandibular em crianças. Rev Dental Press Ortod Ortop Facial. 2006;11(2):29-34.

27. Serra-Negra JMC, Vilela LC, Rosa AR, Andrade ELSP, Paiva SM, Pordeus IA. Hábitos bucais deletérios: os filhos imitam as mães na adoção destes hábitos? Rev Odonto Ciênc. 2006;21(52):146-52.

28. Shinkai RSA, Santos LM, Silva FA, Santos MN. Contribuição ao estudo da prevalência de bruxismo excêntrico noturno em crianças de 2 a 11 anos de idade. Rev Odontol Univ São Paulo. 1998;12(1):29-37.

29. Vanderas AP, Manetas KJ. Relationship between malocclusion and bruxism in children and adolescents: a review. Pediatric Dent. 1995;17(1):7-12.

30. Villa MT, Torres AM, Soto BB, Gomar MR, Langa MJS, Sierra YAIU. Relación entre el trastorno por défict de atención e hiperactividad y los trastornos del sueño. Resultado de um estúdio epidemiológico em la población escolar de la ciudad de Gandía. An pediatr (barc). 2008;69(3):251-7.

23

Angle Class II correction with MARA appliance

Kelly Chiqueto[1], José Fernando Castanha Henriques[2], Sérgio Estelita Cavalcante Barros[3], Guilherme Janson[4]

Objective: To assess the effects produced by the MARA appliance in the treatment of Angle's Class II, division 1 malocclusion. **Methods:** The sample consisted of 44 young patients divided into two groups: The MARA Group, with initial mean age of 11.99 years, treated with the MARA appliance for an average period of 1.11 years, and the Control Group, with initial mean age of 11.63 years, monitored for a mean period of 1.18 years with no treatment. Lateral cephalograms were used to compare the groups using cephalometric variables in the initial and final phases. For these comparisons, Student's *t* test was employed. **Results:** MARA appliance produced the following effects: Maxillary growth restriction, no change in mandibular development, improvement in maxillomandibular relationship, increased lower anterior facial height and counterclockwise rotation of the functional occlusal plane. In the upper arch, the incisors moved lingually and retruded, while the molars moved distally and tipped distally. In the lower arch, the incisors proclined and protruded, whereas the molars mesialized and tipped mesially. Finally, there was a significant reduction in overbite and overjet, with an obvious improvement in molar relationship. **Conclusions:** It was concluded that the MARA appliance proved effective in correcting Angle's Class II, division 1 malocclusion while inducing skeletal changes and particularly dental changes.

Keywords: Angle's Class II malocclusion. Functional orthodontic appliances. Mandibular advancement.

[1] MSc and PhD in Orthodontics, FOB-USP. Coordinator of the Specialization Course in Orthodontics, ABCD-BA.
[2] Full Professor, Pediatric Dentistry, Orthodontics and Social Health Department, FOB-USP.
[3] Post-Doc in Orthodontics, FOB-USP. Adjunct Professor of Orthodontics, Federal University of Rio Grande do Sul, UFRGS.
[4] Full Professor and Head of the Pediatric Dentistry, Orthodontics and Social Health Department, FOB-USP.

» The author reports no commercial, proprietary or financial interest in the products or companies described in this article.

Kelly Chiqueto
Av. Bento Gonçalves, 1515 - apto 1904C, Santo Antônio – Porto Alegre/RS
CEP: 90.650-002 – E-mail: kellychiqueto@yahoo.com.br

INTRODUCTION AND LITERATURE REVIEW

Although functional appliances have been around for quite some time, their use, mode of action and effects are still shrouded in controversy. Deciding on the most effective technique to use in the treatment of growing patients with Class II malocclusion has been the subject of much debate in orthodontic literature. Advocates of functional appliances highlight their role in stimulating mandibular growth as a result of positioning the mandible anteriorly.[16] Histological studies in animals have consistently shown a significant increase in cell activity when the mandible is kept in an advanced position.[34,35] In this context, it is speculated that a similar effect can be seen in humans using functional appliances, thereby helping to correct Class II malocclusion.[16]

The fact that functional appliances are not successful is generally attributed to a lack of patient compliance in the use of the appliances and also to severity of the malocclusion.[8] Therefore, to be effective in treating Angle's Class II, division 1 malocclusion, an appliance should generate the skeletal and dental effects necessary to correct the discrepancy between the basal bones while reducing overjet, thus eliminating the need for patient compliance. Such appliance would also ideally allow the simultaneous (orthopedic and orthodontic) placement of a fixed orthodontic appliance in one single step, thereby speeding up treatment. Thus, Class II correction would be facili-

tated since it would perform aligning and leveling, while at the same time correcting the anteroposterior relationship. This advantage is not observed in non-extraction Class II treatment using a fixed orthodontic appliance combined with headgear or elastics, since patient compliance would still be an issue, as is the case with removable functional appliances.

Mandibular Anterior Repositioning Appliance (MARA) is a fixed functional appliance, which therefore works irrespective of patient cooperation. It comprises four steel crowns cemented on the permanent first molars (Fig 1). These crowns have loops that connect only when the patient occludes.[2,10] Given that the MARA does not feature any systems involving telescopic tubes or springs connecting the jaws permanently, it allows greater freedom of mandibular movement.[10] A lingual arch and transpalatal bar are incorporated to the appliance to stabilize the upper and lower molars, respectively.

Once installed, the appliance prevents the mandible from closing in a more retruded or in a Class II position, quickly teaching the patient to position the mandible anteriorly both during function and at rest. Mandibular advancement can be accomplished by inserting steel bands in the loop of the upper crown. There are four band sizes ranging from 1 to 4 mm in length. Thus, advancement can be gradual, while the patient is given the opportunity to adapt to the appliance.

The MARA allows concurrent use with a rapid maxillary expansion appliance and a total or partial fixed orthodontic appliance. To achieve orthopedic effects, a treatment time of 12 months is recommended.[25]

Some studies describe the skeletal and dental effects produced by the MARA.[10,11,13,26,28] However, only two systematic studies have been published on the dental and skeletal changes observed in the correction of Class II, division 1. In 2003, Pangrazio-Kulbersh et al[26] evaluated the cephalometric effects produced by the MARA in 30 patients (12 male and 18 female)

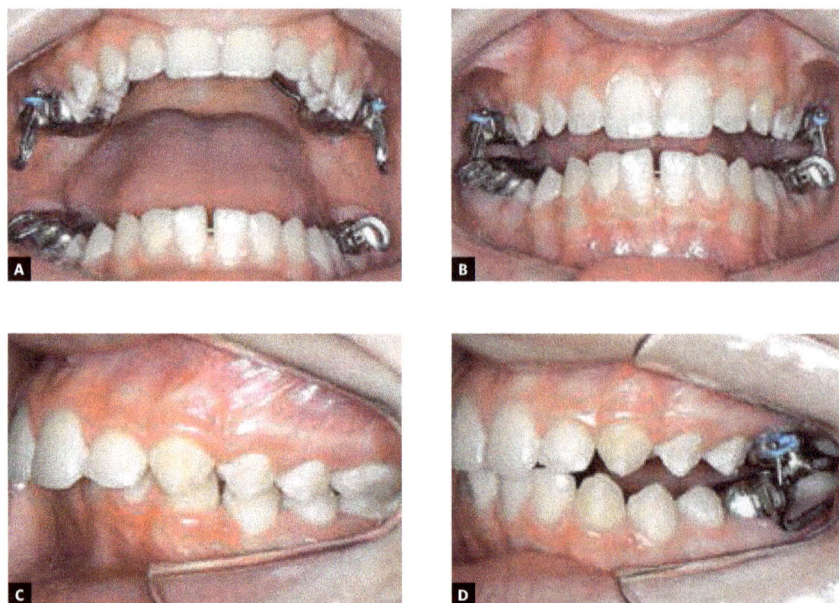

Figure 1 - A) MARA appliance in place with its components. B) The loops on the crowns create occlusal interference and hinder Class II occlusion. C, D) Photos taken before and after placement of the appliance.

with initial ages ranging from 9.5 to 15.8 years, after a mean treatment time of 10.7 months (8-17 months), and compared these with patients treated using the Herbst and Fränkel appliances and with patients with untreated Class II malocclusion. Results showed that the MARA appliance was effective in correcting Class II malocclusion by means of skeletal and dental changes. Proper molar relationship was obtained by means of 47% of skeletal changes and 53% of dental changes. Skeletal changes showed an increase in mandibular length and in anterior and posterior facial heights, but were ineffective in redirecting the maxilla. On the other hand, the dental effects included distalization of maxillary molars, mesialization of molars and incisors, and mild proclination of the lower incisors. In comparing the MARA with the Fränkel and Herbst appliances, the former showed greater dentoalveolar effects than Fränkel, and less maxillary redirecting and less inclination of maxillary incisors than the Herbst.

Another study[11] only assessed the effects of the MARA appliance on the lower incisors in children (10.6 years), adolescents (14.9 years) and adults (33.7 years). It was used concurrently with a fixed orthodontic appliance for a period of 1.7 years in children, 1.3 years in adolescents, and 1.5 years in adults. In children, it was observed that the incisors protruded by 0.4 mm and inclined labially by 1.7°. Adolescents showed a 1.0 mm protrusion and a 3.6° proclination, whereas in adults, there was a 1.7 mm protrusion and 4.5° proclination. They therefore concluded that the MARA appliance was effective in treating Class II patients in all groups, and the changes in the lower incisors were more substantial in adults than in adolescents and children. These changes were regarded as negligible compared to other fixed functional appliances, whereas the use of the MARA combined with a fixed orthodontic appliance allowed a good control of lower incisor inclination.

More conclusive studies about the major dental and skeletal changes that result from the use of the MARA appliance are warranted as evaluations to support the evidence of such changes are extremely important. The main reason being that MARA is a fixed oral appliance designed to correct Class II malocclusion irrespective of patient compliance. It is thus an extremely effective and rapid solution for this kind of malocclusion.[32] Therefore, this study aimed to evaluate through lateral cephalograms the skeletal and dental effects produced by the MARA appliance during correction of Angle's Class II, division 1 malocclusion.

MATERIAL AND METHODS

This research project was approved by the Ethics Committee of the School of Dentistry of Bauru (FOB-USP) and all patients signed an informed consent form before participating in the study.

Inclusion criteria were as follows: Bilateral Angle's Class II, division 1 malocclusion, mandibular retrusion, no agenesis or loss of permanent teeth, no supernumerary teeth, no crowding or only mild crowding in the upper and lower dental arches, moderate or severe overjet, no previous orthodontic treatment. Thus, the sample consisted of 44 young patients divided into two groups.

The MARA group comprised 22 patients, 15 male and 7 female, with initial mean age of 11.99 years ± 1.20 years (minimum = 10.30, maximum = 15 years) treated with the MARA orthopedic appliance for an average of 1.00 year (minimum = 0.77, maximum = 1.25 years).

Patients started orthopedic treatment with the MARA appliance and were treated by the same student of the Doctoral Course in Dentistry, area of concentration: Orthodontics, FOB-USP. Care was taken to insert the appliance within one month after the initial radiograph was taken. The MARA was installed with a transpalatal bar and a lingual arch in all patients. Only one patient presented initially with posterior crossbite involving only the first molars and was then subjected to rapid maxillary expansion with a Hyrax appliance. The patients in this group were not subjected in advance to tooth alignment and leveling, nor interproximal stripping. All were treated until 2 mm, on average, beyond Class I molar relationship was obtained. Malocclusion correction was deemed successful when an occlusion in centric relation was achieved, i.e., when the mandible was positioned in a centric relation (CR) that matched the position of maximum intercuspation (MI). After achieving this relationship, the appliance was kept in place for 6 months for retention purposes. The MARA appliance was thereafter removed and the patient's final radiograph taken.

» The Control Group comprised 22 patients, 15 male and 7 female, who did not undergo any type of orthodontic or orthopedic functional treatment during the observation period evaluated in this study.

The initial mean age was 11.63 years ± 1.03 years (minimum = 10.16, maximum = 13.88 years); they were then monitored for a mean period of 1.18 years (minimum = 0.80, maximum = 2.01 years).

The patients were selected from a sample provided by the Center for the Study of Growth, FOB-USP, where a group of children was X-rayed and checked annually by the Department of Orthodontics with the purpose of developing a longitudinal sample of occlusions in children spanning from primary to permanent dentition. Subsequently, all patients were referred for orthodontic treatment, but some either chose to postpone intervention to a later date, or showed no interest in the treatment, which allowed the authors to define a control group.

The 44 children in the study sample met the following criteria:

» Bilateral Angle's Class II, division 1 malocclusion.
» Mandibular retrusion.
» No agenesis or no permanent teeth missing.
» No supernumerary teeth.
» No crowding, or mild crowding in the upper and lower arches.
» Moderate or severe overjet.
» No previous orthodontic treatment.

Cephalometric method

The cephalometric tracing was performed on acetate tracing paper (Ultraphan) by the same researcher and then digitized (Numonics AccuGrid xnT, model A30TL.F - Numonics Corporation, Montgomeryville, Pa). Data were analyzed with Dentofacial Planner 7.2 software (Dentofacial Planner Software Inc., Toronto, Ontario, Canada); a 9.8% magnification factor was corrected in the radiographs of the MARA Group MARA and 6% in the radiographs of the Control Group, since they were taken by different X-ray machines.

The lines and reference planes used in the study are shown in Figure 2A, comprising:

A) Line SN.
B) Frankfort plane.
C) Palatal plane.
D) Functional occlusal plane.
E) Mandibular plane - GoGn.
F) Mandibular plane - GoMe.
G) Long axis of the upper incisor.

H) Long axis of lower incisor.
I) Long axis of the molar.
J) Long axis of the molar.
K) NA line.
L) NB line.
M) ANSperp line.
N) Pogperp line.

The skeletal cephalometric measures are shown in Figure 2B, the dental measures are shown in Figure 2C and the dental relations corresponding to overjet (OJ), overbite (OB) and molar ratio (MR) are shown in Figure 2D.

Superimposition of initial and final tracings in the MARA group.

Statistical analysis and method error

Statistical analysis was performed with Statistica for Windows 6.0 software (StatSoft Inc.). All results were considered statistically significant at $p < 0.05$.

To evaluate the method error, 20 randomly selected radiographs were once again traced and measured. Paired t test was applied in order to estimate systematic error. To evaluate random error, Dahlberg's test was used with the following formula: $Se^2 = \Sigma d^2/2n$, where Se stands for Dahlberg's error; d^2 is the sum of the squares of the differences between the first and second measurements, and 2n represents twice the number of cases in which the measurements were repeated.

Before starting the comparisons between groups, Kolmogorov-Smirnov test was applied and revealed that all variables had a normal distribution, thus allowing the application of parametric statistical tests.

Initial cephalometric compatibility and comparison of cephalometric changes were assessed using Student's t test.

RESULTS

Table 1 depicts the results of assessing initial cephalometric compatibility between the groups. It was observed that overjet was the only measure that showed statistically significant difference, with the MARA group reaching the highest overjet values.

To differentiate the effects produced by the functional appliance on the normal growth that occurred during the evaluation time, the changes found in cephalometric variables for MARA were compared with those of the Control Group (Table 2). As regards to skeletal changes, the results showed that in

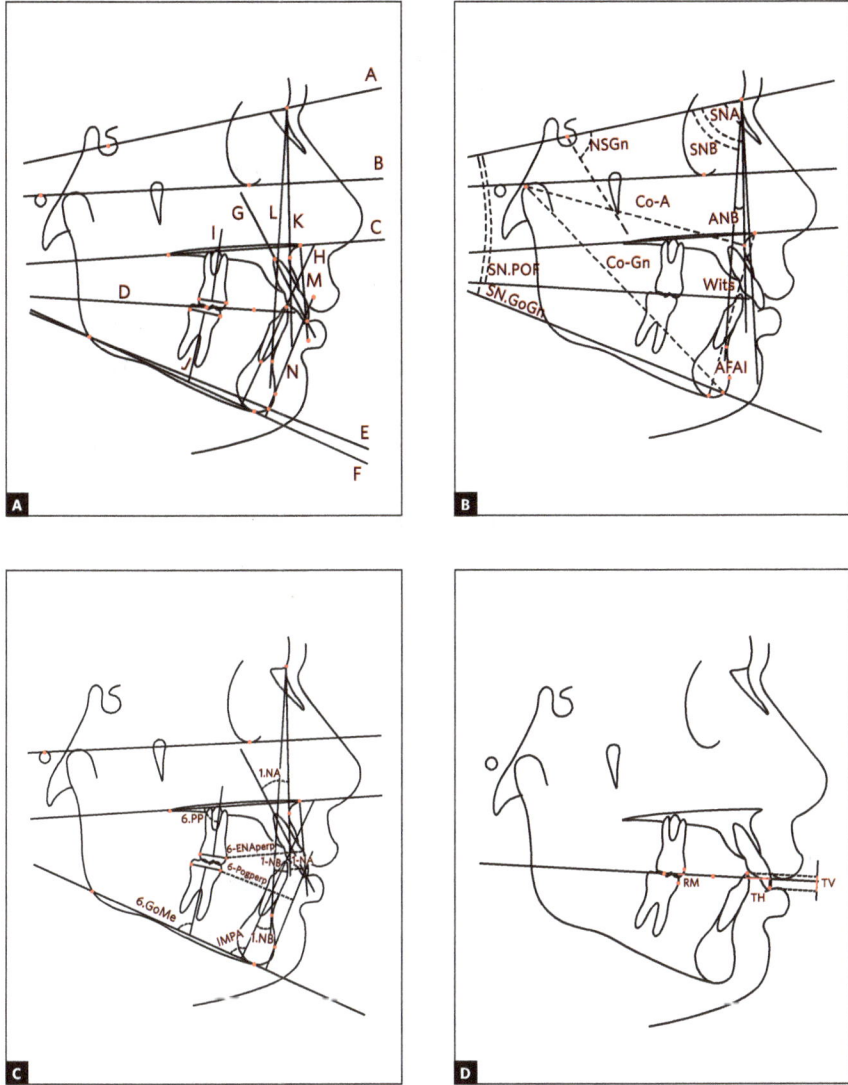

Figure 2 - Cephalometric tracings. **A)** Reference lines and planes. **B)** Skeletal cephalometric measures. **C)** Dental cephalometric measures. **D)** Dental relations: overjet (OJ), overbite (OB) and molar relationship (MR).

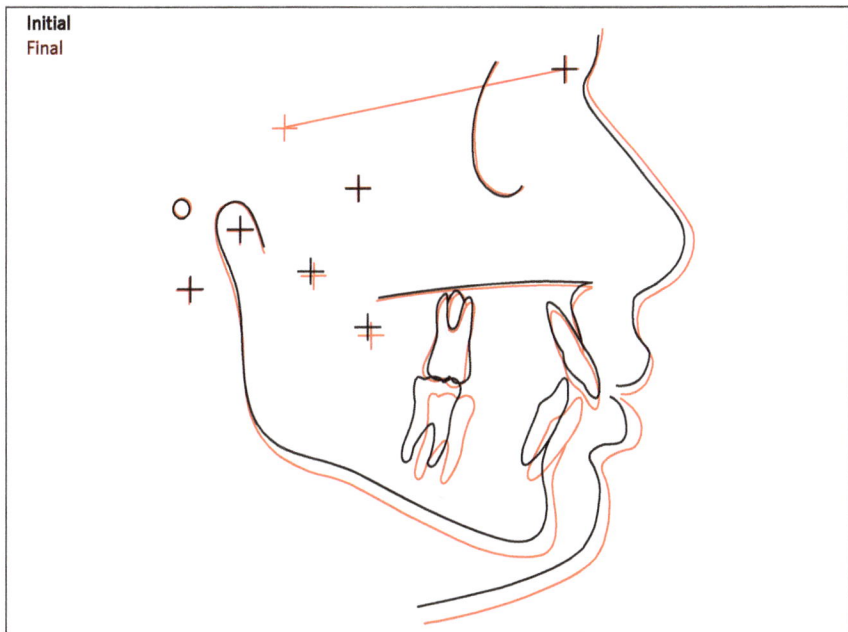

Figure 3 - Superimposition of initial and final tracings in the MARA group.

the MARA group, the maxilla showed a slight retrusion and less growth. The mandible showed no significant differences in length and position, the maxillomandibular relationship improved significantly, the growth pattern was not affected, the lower anterior facial height increased and the occlusal plane experienced a counterclockwise rotation. The dentoalveolar changes found in the MARA Group were: Greater lingual inclination and retrusion of upper incisors, crown distalization and distal tipping of the long axis of the upper molars, considerable buccal inclination and protrusion of the lower incisors, and mesialization and mesial tipping of mandibular molars. A reduction in overjet and overbite was noted in the dental relations as well as a significant improvement in the molar relationship in the MARA Group.

DISCUSSION

The initial degree of compatibility between study groups directly influences the reliability of the results of any cephalometric study. In this study, the groups were compatible in terms of initial age, observation time, gender distribution, initial severity and all cephalometric variables, except overjet, which appeared greater in the MARA Group. A difference between groups can be ascribed to the need for a greater overjet that enabled mandibular advancement until the total correction of anteroposterior discrepancy between the arches was reached. Since the Control Group did not follow this protocol, some anterosuperior crowding was to be expected, which may have contributed to a smaller overjet.

Considering the skeletal changes produced by the MARA appliance, there was a restriction in maxillary

Table 1 - Results of *t* test to assess initial cephalometric compatibility between groups.

Variables	MARA (n=22)	Control (n=22)	p
SNA (degrees)	81.12 ± 3.03	80.64 ± 3.74	0.645
Co-A (mm)	85.12 ± 3.89	83.33 ± 5.23	0.203
SNB (degrees)	75.89 ± 2.83	75.95 ± 3.93	0.954
Co-Gn (mm)	105.54 ± 5.36	104.10 ± 6.33	0.366
ANB (degrees)	5.23 ± 1.20	4.69 ± 1.88	0.264
Wits (mm)	4.06 ± 2.09	3.06 ± 1.46	0.072
SN.GoGn (degrees)	31.30 ± 4.53	31.39 ± 5.34	0.949
NSGn (degrees)	68.39 ± 2.82	67.73 ± 4.25	0.544
LAFH (mm)	61.08 ± 3.82	60.83 ± 3.50	0.822
SN.FH (degrees)	20.51 ± 4.33	21.54 ± 5.48	0.495
1.NA (degrees)	25.82 ± 5.03	24.79 ± 6.03	0.542
1-NA (mm)	5.71 ± 2.19	4.90 ± 2.16	0.222
6-ENAperp (mm)	-29.18 ± 2.14	-29.99 ± 2.40	0.244
6.PP (degrees)	74.45 ± 4.94	73.41 ± 3.72	0.434
IMPA (degrees)	94.91 ± 3.84	93.95 ± 6.27	0.539
1.NB (degrees)	24.63 ± 3.44	24.14 ± 5.45	0.722
1-NB (mm)	4.90 ± 1.68	4.49 ± 1.82	0.437
6-Pogperp (mm)	-29.67 ± 1.48	-30.55 ± 2.56	0.173
6.GoMe (degrees)	81.57 ± 3.99	80.58 ± 3.55	0.388
Overjet (mm)	9.12 ± 1.78	7.99 ± 1.81	0.042
Overbite (mm)	5.02 ± 2.12	4.09 ± 2.41	0.180
Molar relationship (mm)	-1.21 ± 1.22	-0.55 ± 1.21	0.079

Table 2 - Results of comparing changes in cephalometric variables of the MARA and Control groups.

Variables	MARA group (n=22)	Control group (n=22)	p
SNA (degrees)	-0.64 ± 0.89	0.15 ± 0.72	0.002
Co-A (mm)	0.82 ± 1.51	2.41 ± 1.33	0.000
SNB (degrees)	0.81 ± 0.85	0.43 ± 0.82	0.131
Co-Gn (mm)	4.23 ± 1.80	3.77 ± 1.81	0.699
ANB (degrees)	-1.47 ± 0.91	-0.29 ± 0.82	0.000
Wits (mm)	-3.15 ± 1.46	0.08 ± 1.21	0.000
SN.GoGn (degrees)	0.45 ± 1.16	-0.19 ± 1.07	0.062
NSGn (degrees)	0.32 ± 0.68	0.05 ± 0.79	0.216
LAFH (mm)	2.56 ± 1.41	1.54 ± 1.21	0.013
SN.FH (degrees)	-4.52 ± 3.85	-0.80 ± 2.12	0.000
1.NA (degrees)	-3.32 ± 3.66	0.05 ± 2.88	0.001
1-NA (mm)	-0.90 ± 1.33	0.34 ± 1.30	0.004
6-ENAperp (mm)	-1.79 ± 0.96	0.05 ± 1.17	0.000
6.PP (degrees)	-5.58 ± 4.14	2.18 ± 2.45	0.000
IMPA (degrees)	5.39 ± 3.81	0.43 ± 2.84	0.000
1.NB (degrees)	6.60 ± 4.07	0.62 ± 2.59	0.000
1-NB (mm)	1.83 ± 0.81	0.10 ± 0.66	0.000
6-Pogperp (mm)	1.04 ± 0.76	-0.42 ± 1.12	0.038
6.GoMe (degrees)	1.00 ± 2.62	-0.42 ± 1.95	0.047
Overjet (mm)	-5.46 ± 2.01	0.07 ± 1.17	0.000
Overbite (mm)	-2.87 ± 1.76	0.30 ± 1.11	0.000
Molar relationship (mm)	5.41 ± 1.38	0.22 ± 0.66	0.000

growth due to a decrease in the SNA angle (0.6°) and much lessened growth in Co-A (0.8 mm) compared to the control group (2.4 mm). It should be remembered that functional appliances exert upward and backward forces on the maxilla. This "headgear effect" is caused by tension in the facial muscles in an attempt to reposition the mandible back to its uppermost and posterior-most position.[5,7,14,22] Given that the appliance contacts the upper arch, forces arising from the muscles and soft tissues are delivered by the appliance to the teeth and maxilla.

On the other hand, Pangrazio-Kulbersh et al[26] evaluated the effects of the MARA and although the SNA and A-Nperp values indicated maxillary retrusion, this change did not prove statistically significant compared to controls, despite a decrease of 0.4° and 0.2 mm in annualized SNA and A-Nperp values. Almeida et al[4] also found no significant change in the sagittal position of the jaw after treatment with the Herbst appliance, despite a greater decrease observed in the SNA angle (-0.9°) in the Herbst group compared with controls (-0.5°).

No statistically significant difference was found between groups regarding changes in the mandible. Although a greater protrusion of the mandible was expected with the orthopedic treatment due to its permanent anterior position, changes in the Control Group were found to be similar.

The effect of functional orthopedic treatment during mandibular growth currently poses fierce controversy and disagreement among authors. Pangrazio-Kulbersh et al[26] found a statistically significant increase in length and some protrusion after treatment with the MARA and with Herbst in terms of control.

Some studies also report a significant protrusion after treatment with other types of fixed functional appliances such as Jasper Jumper[12] and Herbst,[4,14,18] whereas other studies found no significant changes in growth or sagittal position of the mandible.[6,15,20]

It is noteworthy that most scientific publications[7,17,24,31] report an increase in the length of the mandible immediately following removal of the appliance, i.e., an increase in sagittal growth. Ruf and Pancherz[30] concluded that the anterior-most position of the mandible after treatment appears to result from remodeling of the condylar joint and mandibular fossa. Popowich, Nebbe and Major[27] conducted a review of the skeletal effects of the Herbst appliance and concluded that most studies using Magnetic Resonance Imaging (MRI) or Computed Tomography (CT) are not conclusive.

Functional appliances induce a rapid, if temporary, anterior mandibular displacement during the first phase of treatment. This anterior repositioning of the mandible extends the retrodiscal tissues which, in turn, deliver forces to the condyle and articular fossa, thereby stimulating the process of bone remodeling in this region.[34] Once the stimulus is removed, the process gradually loses intensity until it reaches baseline levels.[33]

DeVincenzo[9] reported in their study that a major relapse of mandibular length increase occurs as a result of functional orthopedic treatment during the early phase of orthodontic treatment.

It is speculated that treatment with the MARA appliance may have generated this greater stimulus towards growth in the first six months or until a centric occlusion relationship was attained (CR=MI). Thereafter, while keeping the appliance for retention, growth may have declined, and eventually the total sum was equivalent to the total mandibular growth found in the Control Group. No values were found above those genetically programmed.

There was a significant improvement in the relationship between basal bones. These changes can result from a combination of several effects on the dento-skeletal structures associated with normal craniofacial growth. In this study, the improvement observed in the relationship between basal bones may have occurred as a result of maxillary retrusion combined with normal growth and anterior displacement of the mandible.

A statistically significant increase in lower anterior facial height was observed. Pancherz[21] demonstrated that the Herbst appliance caused a temporary increase in lower anterior facial height. McNamara Jr, Howe and Dischinger[17] reported an increase in anterior and posterior facial height, which did not negatively influence the mandibular plane angle. Nahás[19] also found that the craniofacial growth pattern was not affected by treatment with the Herbst, as observed in this study.

There was a counterclockwise rotation in the functional occlusal plane (FOP) due to extrusion of the premolars, which were used as reference in constructing the FOP. The MARA appliance allowed this extrusion due to a posterior open bite (Fig 1D), thus helping to correct the curve of Spee, and helping to determine a new FOP position.

The differences between groups are more evident and significant for the dentoalveolar variables, as noted by Almeida et al,[3] Neves[20] and Lima.[15]

Regarding changes in inclination and anteroposterior positioning of the upper incisors, these teeth exhibited lingual inclination and retrusion. The upper molars showed crown distalization and distal tipping. Distalization of first molars is advocated by some authors.[7,17,19,24] Valant and Sinclair[31] found that the effects of the Herbst appliance on the maxilla (restricted displacement) and on the upper teeth (molar distalization) were similar to those of a headgear.

The lower incisors tipped labially significantly in patients treated orthopedically. The MARA appliance is used as a lingual arch to stabilize mandibular molars. Since the resultant force is applied anteriorly, the effects of molar mesialization are reflected mostly in the incisors. Proclination therefore occurs in these teeth. Gönner et al[11] observed a 3.6° labial inclination in adolescents, and 4.5° in adults treated with the MARA appliance.

Neves[20] and Lima[15] found a 2.6° incisor proclination at the end of treatment with the Jasper Jumper. However, as noted by the authors, increased proclination must have occurred in the lower incisors during the period when the Jasper Jumper was in place. Later, after the Jasper Jumper was removed and during the finishing phase, there may have been some lingual inclination (retroclination) of these teeth, resulting from both natural tendency to relapse and lingual torque placed in the antero-inferior region of the rectangular archwire. In assessing the effects of the Herbst appliance on the mixed dentition, Almeida et al[4] found a significant proclination of the incisors, reflected in a 5° increase in IMPA. Pancherz and Hansen[23] compared five types of lower anchorage provided by the Herbst appliance and concluded that none was effective in controlling lower incisor proclination. However, Ruf, Hansen and Pancherz[29] reported that despite a considerable lower incisor proclination, no gingival recession was observed at the end of treatment, corroborating other authors who argue that such increased inclination has not been shown to be harmful.[1]

Lower molars in the MARA Group experienced mesialization and mesial tipping statistically higher than in the Control Group. In correcting Angle's Class II malocclusion it is desirable to move the molars mesially. This molar mesialization effect has been reported in several studies.[17,21,31]

Regarding dental relationships, overbite and overjet were significantly reduced by the MARA appliance. Furthermore, molar relationship showed significant improvement. The pronounced proclination noted in the lower incisors probably resulted from an evident correction of the molar relationship, and also contributed to a greater reduction in overbite.

CONCLUSIONS

MARA appliance was effective in correcting Angle's Class II, division 1 malocclusion, producing more dentoalveolar than skeletal effects, with skeletal changes occurring predominantly in the maxilla — where maxillary growth was restrained —, and no significant effects on the mandible. In addition, the MARA appliance increased the vertical dimension of the face. Regarding dental changes, the upper incisors were inclined lingually and retruded. The upper molars showed distalization and distal tipping. The lower incisors inclined labially and protruded. The lower molars showed mesialization and mesial tipping. The MARA caused some significant improvement in dental relations (overbite and overjet, and molar relationship).

REFERENCES

1. Allais D, Melsen B. Does labial movement of lower incisors influence the level of the gingival margin? A case-control study of adult orthodontic patients. Eur J Orthod. 2003;25(4):343-52.
2. Allen-Noble PS. Clinical management of the MARA: A manual for orthodontists and staff. Sturtevant: Ormco Corporation; 2002.
3. Almeida MR, Henriques JF, Almeida RR, Almeida-Pedrin RR, Ursi W. Treatment effects produced by the Bionator appliance. Comparison with an untreated Class II sample. Eur J Orthod. 2004;26(1):65-72.
4. Ameida MRA, Henriques JFC, Almeida RR, Ursi W, Almeida-Pedrin RR, McNamara JA Jr. Efeitos dentoesqueléticos produzidos pelo aparelho de Herbst na dentadura mista. Rev Dental Press Ortod Ortop Facial. 2006;11(5):21-34.
5. Angelieri F. Comparação dos efeitos cefalométricos promovidos pelos aparelhos extrabucal cervical e pendulum [tese]. Bauru (SP): Universidade de São Paulo; 2005.
6. Covell DA Jr, Trammell DW, Boero RP, West R. A cephalometric study of Class II division 1 malocclusions treated with the Jasper Jumper appliance. Angle Orthod. 1999;69(4):311-20.
7. Croft RS, Buschang PH, English JD, Meyer R. A cephalometric and tomographic evaluation of Herbst treatment in the mixed dentition. Am J Orthod Dentofacial Orthop. 1999;116(4):435-43.
8. Cureton SL, Regennitter F, Orbell MG An accurate, inexpensive headgear timer. J Clin Orthod. 1991;25(12):749-54.
9. DeVincenzo JP. Changes in mandibular length before, during, and after successful orthopedic correction of Class II malocclusions, using a functional appliance. Am J Orthod Dentofacial Orthop. 1991;99(3):241-57.
10. Eckhart JE, White LW. Class II therapy with the Mandibular Anterior Repositioning Appliance. World J Orthod. 2003;4(2):135-44.
11. Gönner U, Ozkan V, Jahn E, Toll DE. Effect of the MARA appliance on the position of the lower anteriors in children, adolescents and adults with Class II malocclusion. J Orofac Orthop. 2007;68(5):397-412.
12. Karacay S, Akin E, Olmez H, Gurton AU, Sagdic D. Forsus Nitinol Flat Spring and Jasper Jumper corrections of Class II division 1 malocclusions. Angle Orthod. 2006;76(4):666-72.
13. Kinzinger G, Ostheimer J, Förster F, Kwandt PB, Reul H, Diedrich P. Development of a new fixed functional appliance for treatment of skeletal Class II malocclusion first report. J Orofac Orthop. 2002;63(5):384-99.
14. Küçükkeleş N, Ilhan I, Orgun IA. Treatment efficiency in skeletal Class II patients treated with the jasper jumper. Angle Orthod. 2007;77(3):449-56.
15. Lima KJS. Comparação das alterações dentoesqueléticas promovidas pelos aparelhos Jasper Jumper e Ativador combinado à ancoragem extrabucal seguido de aparelho fixo, no tratamento da má oclusão de Classe II, 1ª divisão [tese]. Bauru (SP): Universidade de São Paulo; 2007.
16. McNamara JA Jr, Bookstein FL, Shaughnessy TG. Skeletal and dental changes following functional regulator therapy on Class II patients. Am J Orthod. 1985;88(2):91-110.
17. McNamara JA Jr, Howe RP, Dischinger TG. A comparison of the Herbst and Frankel appliances in the treatment of Class II malocclusion. Am J Orthod Dentofacial Orthop. 1990;98(2):134-44.
18. Moro A, Janson G, de Freitas MR, Henriques JF, Petrelli NE, Lauris JP. Class II Correction with the Cantilever Bite Jumper. A variant of the Herbst. Angle Orthod. 2009;79(2):221-9.
19. Nahás ACR. Estudo cefalométrico das alterações dento-esqueléticas da má oclusão de Classe I, divisão 1 tratada com o aparelho de Herbst e o aparelho extrabucal de tração occipital [tese]. Bauru (SP): Faculdade de Odontologia de Bauru, Universidade de São Paulo; 2004.
20. Neves LS. Estudo comparativo dos efeitos do tratamento da má oclusão de Classe II, 1ª divisão com os aparelhos Jasper Jumper e Bionator, associados ao aparelho fixo [tese]. Bauru (SP): Faculdade de Odontologia de Bauru, Universidade de São Paulo; 2007.
21. Pancherz H. The Herbst appliance--its biologic effects and clinical use. Am J Orthod. 1985;87(1):1-20.
22. Pancherz H, Anehus-Pancherz M. The headgear effect of the Herbst appliance: a cephalometric long-term study. Am J Orthod Dentofacial Orthop. 1993;103(6):510-20.
23. Pancherz H, Hansen K. Occlusal changes during and after Herbst treatment: a cephalometric investigation. Eur J Orthod. 1986;8(4):215-28.
24. Pancherz H, Zieber K, Hoyer B. Cephalometric characteristics of Class II division 1 and Class II division 2 malocclusions: a comparative study in children. Angle Orthod. 1997;67(2):111-20.
25. Pangrazio-Kulbersh V. Entrevista. Rev Dental Press Ortod Ortop Facial. 2008;13(2):29-33.
26. Pangrazio-Kulbersh V, Berger JL, Chermak DS, Kaczynski R, Simon ES, Haerian A. Treatment effects of the mandibular anterior repositioning appliance on patients with Class II malocclusion. Am J Orthod Dentofacial Orthop. 2003;123(3):286-95.
27. Popowich K, Nebbe B, Major PW. Effect of Herbst treatment on temporomandibular joint morphology: a systematic literature review. Am J Orthod Dentofacial Orthop. 2003;123(4):388-94.
28. Rondeau B. MARA appliance. Funct Orthod. 2002;19(2):4-12, 14-6.
29. Ruf S, Hansen K, Pancherz H. Does orthodontic proclination of lower incisors in children and adolescents cause gingival recession? Am J Orthod Dentofacial Orthop. 1998;114(1):100-6.
30. Ruf S, Pancherz H. Does bite-jumping damage the TMJ? A prospective longitudinal clinical and MRI study of Herbst patients. Angle Orthod. 2000;70(3):183-99.
31. Valant JR, Sinclair PM. Treatment effects of the Herbst appliance. Am J Orthod Dentofacial Orthop. 1989;95(2):138-47.

32. Von Bremen J, Pancherz H. Efficiency of early and late Class II Division 1 treatment. Am J Orthod Dentofacial Orthop. 2002;121(1):31-7.

33. Voudouris JC, Kuftinec MM. Improved clinical use of Twin-block and Herbst as a result of radiating viscoelastic tissue forces on the condyle and fossa in treatment and long-term retention: growth relativity. Am J Orthod Dentofacial Orthop. 2000;117(3):247-66.

34. Voudouris JC, Woodside DG, Altuna G, Angelopoulos G, Bourque PJ, Lacouture CY, Kuftinec MM. Condyle-fossa modifications and muscle interactions during Herbst treatment, Part 2. Results and conclusions. Am J Orthod Dentofacial Orthop. 2003;124(1):13-29.

35. Voudouris JC, Woodside DG, Altuna G, Kuftinec MM, Angelopoulos G, Bourque PJ. Condyle-fossa modifications and muscle interactions during Herbst treatment, Part 1. New technological methods. Am J Orthod Dentofacial Orthop. 2003;123(6):604-13.

24

Self-esteem in adolescents with Angle Class I, II and III malocclusion in a Peruvian sample

Karla Florián-Vargas[1], Marcos J. Carruitero Honores[2], Eduardo Bernabé[3], Carlos Flores-Mir[4]

Objective: To compare self-esteem scores in 12 to 16-year-old adolescents with different Angle malocclusion types in a Peruvian sample. **Material and Methods:** A cross-sectional study was conducted in a sample of 276 adolescents (159, 52 and 65 with Angle Class I, II and III malocclusions, respectively) from Trujillo, Peru. Participants were asked to complete the Rosenberg Self-Esteem Scale (RSES) and were also clinically examined, so as to have Angle malocclusion classification determined. Analysis of covariance (ANCOVA) was used to compare RSES scores among adolescents with Class I, II and III malocclusions, with participants' demographic factors being controlled. **Results:** Mean RSES scores for adolescents with Class I, II and III malocclusions were 20.47 ± 3.96, 21.96 ± 3.27 and 21.26 ± 4.81, respectively. The ANCOVA test showed that adolescents with Class II malocclusion had a significantly higher RSES score than those with Class I malocclusion, but there were no differences between other malocclusion groups. Supplemental analysis suggested that only those with Class II, Division 2 malocclusion might have greater self-esteem when compared to adolescents with Class I malocclusion. **Conclusion:** This study shows that, in general, self-esteem did not vary according to adolescents' malocclusion in the sample studied. Surprisingly, only adolescents with Class II malocclusion, particularly Class II, Division 2, reported better self-esteem than those with Class I malocclusion. A more detailed analysis assessing the impact of anterior occlusal features should be conducted.

Keywords: Self-esteem. Malocclusion classification. Adolescents.

[1] Dentist, Private Practice, Trujillo, Peru.
[2] Assistant professor, Universidad Privada Antenor Orrego, Trujillo, Peru.
[3] Senior lecturer, King's College London Dental Institute, Division of Population and Patient Health, London, United Kingdom.
[4] Associate professor and Head of the Division of Orthodontics, University of Alberta, Edmonton, Canada.

Marcos J. Carruitero Honores
E-mail: mcarruiteroh@upao.edu.pe

» The authors report no commercial, proprietary or financial interest in the products or companies described in this article.

INTRODUCTION

The physical, social and psychological consequences of a malocclusion have been topics of research for a long time. However, the related evidence is still conflicting. Although studies generally report an association between malocclusion and quality of life scores, the strength of evidence is relatively low. There is a need for standardized methods to enhance comparability between studies.[1,2,3] In addition, other subjective domains, such as well-being, happiness and self-esteem, have remained largely unexplored in relation to malocclusion.

Self-esteem can be defined as the perception of one's own ability to effectively master or deal with the surrounding environment, and it is affected by the reactions of others towards an individual.[4,5,6] It was initially claimed that facial features, especially those related to oral aesthetics, may have a high potential to influence self-esteem, especially during life stages when there is intense social and affective interaction.[7] However, the scarce literature on the subject provides conflicting evidence, with some authors arguing that malocclusion affects patients' self-esteem;[8,9] while others report weak to nonsignificant effects of malocclusion[10] or orthodontic treatment.[11,12,13] Reasons are probably related to the multifactorial nature of self-esteem and how individuals may weight individual factors differently. Further research is needed to shed some light onto this research area. There have been no studies reported in Peruvian people, in spite of differences that would need additional investigation, specifically to this population.

The aim of this study was to compare self-esteem scores in 12 to 16-year-old adolescents with different types of Angle malocclusions in a Peruvian sample. It was hypothesized that adolescents with Class II and III malocclusions would report lower levels of self-esteem than those with Class I malocclusion.

MATERIAL AND METHODS
Study sample

A cross-sectional study was conducted with a sample of 276 adolescents aged between 12 to 16 years old, recruited from a typical public school in the Porvenir District, Trujillo, Peru. The sample was selected from a population of 1083 students (550 males and 533 females), with the aid of a stratified random sampling method proportional to each level of study (332, 220

199, 193 and 139 students, from first to fifth grade, respectively). The study included adolescents with permanent dentition; and excluded those who had craniofacial syndromes or congenital malformations, any missing tooth (except for third molars) and had received or were undergoing orthodontic treatment.

A minimum sample size of 156 adolescents (52 comprising each one of the three Angle malocclusion groups) was required to estimate a mean difference in the Rosenberg Self-Esteem Score equal to or greater than 0.55 units between two of those groups, with an 80% statistical power, 95% confidence level and a common standard deviation of 1 unit.

The study protocol was approved by the Stomatology Permanent Research Committee of *Universidad Privada Antenor Orrego* (Trujillo, Peru). A written informed consent form from the participants' parents and an informed assent form from the adolescents were obtained before participation.

Data collection

Data were collected with the aid of a self-administered questionnaire and clinical examinations. The ten-item Rosenberg Self-Esteem Scale (RSES) was used to assess participants' global self-esteem.[5,14] Responses to the ten items were scored using a four-point scale ranging from 0 (strongly disagree) to 3 (strongly agree) with items 2, 5, 6, 8, and 9 reverse scored. Higher scores indicate higher self-esteem (possible scores range from 0 to 30). The Spanish version of the RSES was used for this study and showed good psychometric properties (validity and reliability) in a similar adolescent population.[15] Cronbach's alpha of the RSES was 0.70 in this sample.

Participants' type of malocclusion was classified according to Angle's classification which is mainly based on the anteroposterior position of the mandibular first permanent molar in relation to the maxillary first permanent molar, and complementarily on the anteroposterior position of anterior teeth. During clinical examination, participants were classified as having Class I (both molars are in good anteroposterior relationship), Class II (mandibular molar is posteriorly positioned) or Class III malocclusion (mandibular molar is anteriorly positioned).[16] One trained examiner carried out all clinical examinations in a separate room within the school facilities, under natural light and using a tongue depressor.

Ten individuals were re-examined after a week for reliability. Kappa values for intra- and inter-reliability were 1.00 and 0.85, respectively.

Statistical analysis

RSES total score showed a negatively skewed distribution, suggesting the use of nonparametric tests. However, we used analysis of covariance (ANCOVA) to compare the total score, as ANCOVA has several advantages over nonparametric tests.[17] It allows compensating for multiple comparisons by using an omnibus test, controlling for categorical and continuous confounders (adolescents' sex and age in years, respectively) and testing for interactions among explanatory variables.[17,18] Post-hoc comparisons between pairs of malocclusion groups were conducted by Scheffé's test and only if the omnibus test was statistically significant. A logistic regression analysis was used to evaluate the influence of malocclusion on low self-esteem.

RESULTS

A total of 276 12 to 16-year-old adolescents (141 girls and 135 boys) participated in the present study. Their mean age was 14.2 ± 1.3 years, with a quarter of the sample being 14 years old. According to Angle's classification, 57.6% of the sample had Class I malocclusion, 18.9% had Class II malocclusion and 23.5% Class III malocclusion (Table 1).

Table 2 shows the mean scores for RSES individual items and the total score. The mean RSES total score was 20.93 ± 4.09; range = 0 - 30. There was no

floor effect (minimum possible score), but four individuals had the maximum possible score (ceiling effect). Mean scores for RSES individual items ranged between 1.07 for the item "I wish I could have more respect for myself," and 2.53 for the item "I am able to do things as well as other people."

There were significant differences in the total self-esteem score between the three Angle's malocclusion groups (ANCOVA test, $p = 0.048$). Post-hoc comparisons showed that adolescents with Class II malocclusion had a significantly higher total self-esteem score than those with Class I malocclusion (21.96 *versus* 20.47 units). There were no significant differences between other malocclusion groups. Finally, the two-way interaction terms between malocclusion group and sex, and malocclusion group and age, were not significant ($p > 0.05$ in both cases).

In further exploratory analysis, due to limited numbers of participants with Class II, Divisions 1 and 2 malocclusion (30 and 22 individuals, respectively), there was significant difference in the RSES score between Class II, Division 2 (Mean = 22.59, SD = 2.50) and Class I malocclusion groups (independent group t-test, $p = 0.001$), but not between Class II, Division 1 (Mean = 21.50, SD = 3.70) and Class I malocclusion groups (independent group t-test, $p = 0.172$).

A logistic regression analysis was used to evaluate the influence of malocclusion on low self-esteem. According to this analysis, there was no influence of any type of malocclusion on low self-esteem ($R^2 = 0.01$, $p > 0.05$).

Table 1 - Description of the sample of adolescents (n = 276).

Characteristic		n	%
Sex	Girls	141	51.1
	Boys	135	49.9
Age	12 years	29	10.5
	13 years	58	21.0
	14 years	70	25.4
	15 years	62	22.5
	16 years	57	20.6
Angle's classification	Class I	159	57.6
	Class II	52	18.9
	Class III	65	23.5

Table 2 - Item and total scores for Rosenberg Self-Esteem Scale in the sample (n = 276).

Item	Mean	SD	Range
On the whole, I am satisfied with myself	2.42	0.60	0-3
At times, I think I am no good at all	2.38	0.58	0-3
I feel that I have a number of good qualities	2.25	0.65	0-3
I am able to do things as well as most other people	2.53	0.61	0-3
I feel I do not have much to be proud of	2.47	0.62	0-3
I certainly feel useless at times	1.75	0.90	0-3
I feel that I am a person of worth, at least on an equal plane with others	2.24	0.87	0-3
I wish I could have more respect for myself	1.07	0.95	0-3
All in all, I am inclined to feel that I am a failure	2.05	0.92	0-3
I take a positive attitude toward myself	1.77	1.01	0-3
Self-esteem total score	20.93	4.09	0-30

Table 3 - Comparison of self-esteem scores by malocclusion type (n = 276).

Malocclusion	n	Mean	SD	(95% CI)
Class I	159	20.47[a]	3.96	(19.85 – 21.09)
Class II	52	21.96[a]	3.27	(21.05 – 22.87)
Class III	65	21.26	4.81	(20.07 – 22.45)
p value		0.048		

ANCOVA was used for comparison, controlling for adolescents' sex and age (continuous form).
Superscripts indicate which groups were significantly different (Scheffé's post-hoc test was used).

DISCUSSION

Our findings showed that self-esteem scores, as measured by RSES, vary by certain Angle's malocclusion groups. Contrary to our hypothesis, only adolescents with Class II malocclusion reported higher self-esteem when compared to those with Class I malocclusion. No other groups were found to differ in terms of self-esteem scores. Our findings disagree with previous studies in which adolescents with Class II malocclusion had poorer self-esteem, which was measured by the child self-esteem scale, than those with Class I and III malocclusions.[9] In further supplemental, but exploratory analysis, we also found that it may be those with Class II, Division 2 malocclusion who have greater self-esteem compared to adolescents with Class I malocclusion.

We could speculate on possible explanations for the present findings. First, Class II, Division 2 malocclusion individuals tend to have a very prominent chin, straight or concave facial profile and strong facial muscular definition.[19] These features could very well be associated with a more aesthetic facial definition. The problem with this explanation is that prominent chins and strong

facial musculature are characteristics that are associated with male facial features and not female ones.

A second explanation relates to how adolescents' malocclusion was assessed in this study. Angle's classification remains the most commonly used classification of malocclusions and its universal acceptance by the dental profession is evidence of its practicability.[20] We chose this classification for the relationship it has with the facial profile of the patient,[21] which impacts on oneself and lay person's perception.[22] However, Angle's classification system was mainly based on the antero-posterior position of first molars,[16] and not all anterior dentoalveolar features that are likely to impact lay person's aesthetic preferences. Puzzling in Class II, Division 2, the usual dentoalveolar characteristics are proclined upper laterals, retroclined centrals, deep bite and excessive upper incisor display at smiling. These are not features that are normally aesthetically pleasant.[23,24] Evaluation of more specific features, such as overjet, overbite, dentoalveolar discrepancy, gingival exposure, labial competence and position, among others, may allow for a more precise discrimination and identification of which particular occlusal traits are linked to poor and high self-esteem, respectively. There is some preliminary evidence that crowding of anterior teeth may affect adolescents' self-esteem, particularly among girls.[8]

A final explanation is that malocclusion considered as an anteroposterior classification has no actual impact on adolescents' self-esteem. This is reflected by the fact that the differences found between Class II and Class I malocclusions may be statistically significant, but not clinically important. RSES ranges from 0 to 30 units, with values between 15 and 25 considered normal. Values below 15 and above 25 are indicative of low and high self-esteem, respectively.[5,14,25] All malocclusion groups had, on average, values within the normal range, suggesting that differences between groups may not be of clinical importance. Prior research has shown that malocclusion and orthodontic treatment have no impact on self-esteem.[10-13] Nevertheless, low self-esteem has been associated with the aesthetic impact of malocclusion, and that it significantly affects the quality of life of schoolchildren.[26] In addition, an anteroposterior classification of malocclusion does not consider the severity of malocclusion. This aspect could have affected the results, clinical significance and implications on the priority need for treatment, specifically when considering public health policies and resource allocation.

Some limitations of this study need to be discussed. First, all adolescents included in this study had some type of malocclusion, and, therefore, had some degree of need for orthodontic treatment. Having an alternative comparison group with no malocclusion might have produced different results. The absence of a control group could provide possible implications

on the outcomes found, mainly the possibility to compare the results with a normal occlusion. Furthermore, self-esteem could be influenced by several factors; a person may have high self-esteem in his or hers working life and low self-esteem in his or hers personal life. Also self-esteem could have hereditary characteristics, and genetics could play a role on it too. It is difficult to identify the pure contribution of malocclusion on the self-esteem of individuals. It would be necessary to consider these aspects in further investigations.

Second, we used RSES to measure adolescents' self-esteem and it is possible that results may be different if a different scale was used. However, RSES is one of the most widely used measures of global self-esteem in social sciences.[25] The popularity of RSES is due in part to its good psychometric properties, simplicity and brevity (only 10 questions that can be completed within 1-3 minutes). More importantly, it has been adapted to several languages, including Spanish,[16] and has been used in different populations and settings.[25,27] Overall, further research should evaluate self-esteem by means of multiple instruments and considering anterior teeth features, with and without malocclusion also classified in transversal and vertical ways.

CONCLUSION

This study shows that self-esteem may vary according to adolescents' malocclusion in the sample studied. Adolescents with Class II malocclusion (and more specifically, Class II, Division 2) report better self-esteem than those with Class I malocclusion. No differences were found between other malocclusion groups.

REFERENCES

1. Zhang M, McGrath C, Hagg U. The impact of malocclusion and its treatment on quality of life: a literature review. Int J Paediatr Dent. 2006 Nov;16(6):381-7.
2. Kiyak HA. Does orthodontic treatment affect patients' quality of life? J Dent Educ. 2008 Aug;72(8):886-94.
3. Liu Z, McGrath C, Hagg U. The impact of malocclusion/orthodontic treatment need on the quality of life. A systematic review. Angle Orthod. 2009 May;79(3):585-91.
4. Gecas V. The self-concept. Annu Rev Sociol. 1982;8(1):1-33.
5. Rosenberg M, Schooler C, Schoenbach C, Rosenberg F. Global self-esteem and specific self-esteem: Different concepts, different outcomes. Am Soc Rev 1995;60(1):141-56.
6. Haney P, Durlak JA. Changing self-esteem in children and adolescents: a meta-analytic review. J Clin Child Psychol. 1998 Dec;27(4):423-33.
7. Burden DJ. Oral health-related benefits of orthodontic treatment. Semin Orthod. 2007;13(2):76-80.

8. Jung MH. Evaluation of the effects of malocclusion and orthodontic treatment on self-esteem in an adolescent population. Am J Orthod Dentofacial Orthop. 2010 Aug;138(2):160-6.
9. Sun Y, Jiang C. [The impact of malocclusion on self-esteem of adolescents]. Zhonghua Kou Qiang Yi Xue Za Zhi. 2004 Jan;39(1):67-9.
10. Badran SA. The effect of malocclusion and self-perceived aesthetics on the self-esteem of a sample of Jordanian adolescents. Eur J Orthod. 2010 Dec;32(6):638-44.
11. Kenealy PM, Kingdon A, Richmond S, Shaw WC. The Cardiff dental study: a 20-year critical evaluation of the psychological health gain from orthodontic treatment. Br J Health Psychol. 2007 Feb;12(Pt 1):17-49.
12. Birkeland K, Bøe OE, Wisth PJ. Relationship between occlusion and satisfaction with dental appearance in orthodontically treated and untreated groups. A longitudinal study. Eur J Orthod. 2000 Oct;22(5):509-18.

13. Varela M, Garcia-Camba JE. Impact of orthodontics on the psychologic profile of adult patients: a prospective study. Am J Orthod Dentofacial Orthop. 1995 Aug;108(2):142-8.

14. Rosenberg M. Society and the adolescent self-image. Revised edition. New Jersey: Princeton University Press; 1965.

15. Martin-Albo J, Nuniez JL, Navarro JG, Grijalvo F. The Rosenberg Self-Esteem Scale: translation and validation in university students. Span J Psychol. 2007;10:458-67.

16. Angle EH. Classification of malocclusion. Dent Cosmos. 1899;41:248-64.

17. Hair JF Jr, Black WC, Babin BJ, Anderson RE. Multivariate data analysis. Upper Saddle River: Prentice Hall; 2009.

18. Huberty CJ, Olejnik S. Applied MANOVA and discriminant analysis. New Jersey: Wiley Interscience; 2006.

19. Moyers RE, Riolo ML, Guire KE, Wainright RL, Bookstein FL. Differential diagnosis of class II malocclusions. Part 1. Facial types associated with Class II malocclusions. Am J Orthod. 1980 Nov;78(5):477-94.

20. Peck S. The contributions of Edward H. Angle to dental public health. Community Dent Health. 2009 Sept;26(3):130-1.

21. Siriwat PP, Jarabak JR. Malocclusion and facial morphology, is there a relationship? An epidemiologic study. Angle Orthod. 1985 Apr;55(2):127-38.

22. Johnston C, Hunt O, Burden D, Stevenson M, Hepper P. Self-perception of dentofacial attractiveness among patients requiring orthognathic surgery. Angle Orthod. 2010 Mar;80(2):361-6.

23. Witt M, Flores-Mir C. Laypeople's preferences regarding frontal dentofacial esthetics: periodontal factors. J Am Dent Assoc. 2011 Aug;142(8):925-37.

24. Witt M Flores-Mir C. Laypeople's preferences regarding frontal dentofacial esthetics: tooth-related factors. J Am Dent Assoc. 2011 Jun;142(6):635-45.

25. Sinclair SJ, Blais MA, Gansler DA, Sandberg E, Bistis K, LoCicero A. Psychometric properties of the Rosenberg Self-Esteem Scale: overall and across demographic groups living within the United States. Eval Health Prof. 2010 Mar;33(1):56-80.

26. Marques LS, Ramos-Jorge ML, Paiva SM, Pordeus IA. Malocclusion: esthetic impact and quality of life among Brazilian schoolchildren. Am J Orthod Dentofacial Orthop. 2006 Mar;129(3):424-7.

27. Twenge JM, Campbell WK. Age and birth cohort differences in self-esteem: a cross-temporal meta-analysis. Pers Soc Psychol Rev. 2001 Nov;5(4):321-44.

Permissions

List of Contributors

Marisana Piano Seben and Aristeu Correa Bittencourt Neto
MSc in Orthodontics, Inga Dental School, Maringá/PR, Brazil

Fabricio Pinelli Valarelli
Assistant Professor, MSc Program at Inga Dental School, Maringá/PR, Brazil

Karina Maria Salvatore de Freitas and Rodrigo Hermont Cançado
Post-doc in Orthodontics, University of Toronto. Assistant Professor, Inga Dental School, Maringá/PR, Brazil

Kelly Chiqueto
MSc and PhD in Orthodontics, FOB-USP. Coordinator of the Specialization Course in Orthodontics, ABCD-BA

José Fernando Castanha Henriques
Full Professor, Pediatric Dentistry, Orthodontics and Social Health Department, FOB-USP

Sérgio Estelita Cavalcante Barros
Post-Doc in Orthodontics, FOB-USP. Adjunct Professor of Orthodontics, Federal University of Rio Grande do Sul, UFRGS

Guilherme Janson
Full Professor and Head of the Pediatric Dentistry, Orthodontics and Social Health Department, FOB-USP

Ana Carla Raphaelli Nahás-Scocate
Associate professor, Undergraduate and Postgraduate Program in Orthodontics, University of São Paulo City – UNICID

Fernando Vusberg Coelho
DDS, UNICID

Viviane Chaves de Almeida
MSc in Orthodontics, UNICID

Mariana Maciel Tinano
PhD resident in Child and Adolescent Health, School of Medicine — Federal University of Minas Gerais (UFMG)

Milene Aparecida Torres Saar Martins
Postdoc resident in Pediatric Dentistry, Federal University of Minas Gerais (UFMG)

Cristiane Baccin Bendo
Assistant professor, Department of Orthodontics and Pediatric Dentistry, Federal University of Minas Gerais (UFMG)

Ênio Mazzieiro
PhD in Orthodontics, University of São Paulo (USP)

Nayanna Nadja e Silva
Specialist in Orthodontics, Associação Brasileira de Odontologia (ABO-PB), João Pessoa, Paraíba, Brazil

Rosa Helena Wanderley Lacerda
Coordinator, Postgraduate Program in Orthodontics, Associação Brasileira de Odontologia (ABO-PB), João Pessoa, Paraíba, Brazil

Alexandre Wellos Cunha Silva
Professor, Postgraduate Program in Orthodontics, Associação Brasileira de Odontologia (ABO-PB), João Pessoa, Paraíba, Brazil

Tania Braga Ramos
Professor of Orthognathic Surgery, Postgraduate Program in Orthodontics, Associação Brasileira de Odontologia (ABO-PB), João Pessoa, Paraíba, Brazil

Fabio de Abreu Vigorito
PhD in Orthodontics, School of Dentistry, University of São Paulo (USP)

Gladys Cristina Dominguez
Full professor, Department of Orthodontics, University of São Paulo (USP)

Luís Antônio de Arruda Aidar
Full professor, Department of Orthodontics, University of Santa Cecília (UNISANTA)

Aniruddh Yashwant V.
Senior lecturer, Department of Orthodontics and Dentofacial Orthopedics, Indira Gandhi Institute of Dental Sciences, MGMCRI campus, SBV University, Pillayarkuppam, Pondicherry, India

Ravi K.
Professor and Head of Department, Department of Orthodontics and Dentofacial Orthopedics, SRM Dental College, Ramapuram, Chennai, India

Edeinton Arumugam
Associate professor, Department of Orthodontics and Dentofacial Orthopedics, SRM Dental College, Ramapuram, Chennai, India

Milton Meri Benitez Farret
Professor of Orthodontics, Undergraduate Program, Universidade Federal de Santa Maria, Santa Maria, Rio Grande do Sul, Brazil

Eduardo Martinelli de Lima
Adjunct professor of Orthodontics, Pontifícia Universidade Católica do Rio Grande do Sul (PUC/RS), Porto Alegre, Rio Grande do Sul, Brazil

Marcel M. Farret
PhD in Orthodontics, Pontifícia Universidade Católica do Rio Grande do Sul (PUCRS), Porto Alegre, Rio Grande do Sul, Brazil

Laura Lutz de Araújo
MSc in Orthodontics, Pontifícia Universidade Católica do Rio Grande do Sul (PUC/RS), Porto Alegre, Rio Grande do Sul, Brazil

Julia Garcia Costa and Thaís Magalhães Galindo
Orthodontics department, Universidade Federal Fluminense, Niterói, Brazil

Claudia Trindade Mattos and Adriana de Alcantara Cury-Saramago
Professor of Orthodontics, Dental Clinic department, Universidade Federal Fluminense, Niterói, Brazil

Natália Valli de Almeida and Giordani Santos Silveira
Masters student of Orthodontics, Fluminense Federal University (UFF)

Daniele Masterson Tavares Pereira
Specialist in Library science, Integrated Colleges of Jacarepaguá (FIJ)

Claudia Trindade Mattos
Adjunct professor, Department of Orthodontics, UFF

José Nelson Mucha
Full professor, Department of Orthodontics, UFF

Luciano Zilio Saikoski
MSc in Orthodontics, Ingá College (UNINGÁ)

Rodrigo Hermont Cançado and Karina Maria Salvatore de Freitas
Adjunct professor, Department of Orthodontics, postgraduate program, (UNINGÁ)

Fabrício Pinelli Valarelli
Adjunct professor, Department of Orthodontics, Ingá College (UNINGÁ)

Cristina Batista Miamoto, Lucas Guimarães Abreu and Saul Martins Paiva
Universidade Federal de Minas Gerais, Departamento de Odontopediatria e Ortodontia (Belo Horizonte/MG, Brazil)

Leandro Silva Marques
Universidade Federal dos Vales do Jequitinhonha e Mucuri, Departamento de Odontopediatria e Ortodontia (Diamantina/MG, Brazil)

Thiene Silva Normando
Master's student in Dentistry, Federal University of Pará (UFPA)

Regina Fátima Feio Barroso
Associate professor, UFPA

David Normando
Adjunct professor, UFPA

Mayara Paim Patel
PhD in Orthodontics, School of Dentistry — University of São Paulo/Bauru

José Fernando Castanha Henriques
Full professor, University of São Paulo, USP

Karina Maria Salvatore de Freitas
Adjunct professor, Masters program in Orthodontics, Ingá College, UNINGÁ

Roberto Henrique da Costa Grec
PhD resident in Orthodontics, School of Dentistry — University of São Paulo/ Bauru

Fundagul Bilgic
Assistant Professor, Mustafa Kemal University, Faculty of Dentistry, Department of Orthodontics, Hatay, Turkey

Ibrahim Erhan Gelgor
Professor, Kirikkale University, Faculty of Dentistry, Department of Orthodontics, Kirikkale, Turkey

Ahmet Arif Celebi
Lecturer, Ishik University, Faculty of Dentistry, Department of Orthodontics, Erbil, Iraq

Carolina Baratieri
Professor, Department of Orthodontics, Federal University of de Santa Catarina, UFSC

Matheus Alves Jr
PhD resident inOrthodontics, Federal University of Rio de Janeiro

Ana Maria Bolognese
Full professor, Department of Orthodontics, Federal University of Rio de Janeiro

Matilde C. G. Nojima and Lincoln I. Nojima
Professor, Department of Orthodontics, Federal University of Rio de Janeiro, UFRJ

Sônia Rodrigues Dutra
Private practice (Belo Horizonte/MG, Brazil)

Henrique Pretti, Cristiane Baccin Bendo and Miriam Pimenta Vale
Universidade Federal de Minas Gerais, Faculdade de Odontologia, Departamento de Odontopediatria e Ortodontia (Belo Horizonte/MG, Brazil)

Milene Torres Martins
Universidade Estadual de Montes Claros, Curso de Odontologia (Montes Claros/MG, Brazil)

Mayara Paim Patel
PhD in Orthodontics, College of Dentistry – Bauru/ University of São Paulo (USP)

José Fernando Castanha Henriques, Guilherme Janson and Marcos Roberto de Freitas
Full professor, Department of Pediatric Dentistry, Orthodontics and Collective Health, College of Dentistry – Bauru/ University of São Paulo (USP)

Renato Rodrigues de Almeida
Full professor, Department of Orthodontics, College of Dentistry – Bauru/ University of São Paulo (USP) and UNOPAR

Arnaldo Pinzan
Full professor, Department of Pediatric Dentistry, Orthodontics and Collective Health, College of Dentistry – Bauru/ University of São Paulo (USP)

Helder B. Jacob
PhD in Orthodontics, Araraquara Dental School/ São Paulo State University- UNESP, Araraquara, SP, Brazil. Post-doc in Orthodontics,Texas A&M Health Science Center

Peter H. Buschang
Professor, Baylor College of Dentistry, Texas A&M Health Science Center

Ary dos Santos-Pinto
Professor, Department of Orthodontics, Araraquara Dental School, São Paulo State University-UNESP, Araraquara, SP, Brazil

Darwin Vaz de Lima
Professor, Specialization Course in Orthodontic UNORP

Karina Maria Salvatore de Freitas
Post-Doctor in Orthodontics, University of Toront Head Professor of the Master Course in Orthodontic UNINGÁ

Marcos Roberto de Freitas, Guilherme Janson an José Fernando Castanha Henriques
Professor of Orthodontics, FOB-USP

Arnaldo Pinzan
Associate Professor of Orthodontics, FOB-USP

Paulo Roberto dos Santos-Pinto
Professor, Barretos University - UNIFEB

Lídia Parsekian Martins
PhD in Orthodontics. Assistant Professor, Children' Clinic Department, School of Dentistry of Araraqua - UNESP

Ary dos Santos-Pinto, Luiz Gonzaga Gandini Júnio and Dirceu Barnabé Raveli
Full Professor, Children's Clinic Department, Schoo of Dentistry of Araraquara - UNESP

Cristiane Celli Matheus dos Santos-Pinto
MSc in Orthodontics, FOB-USP. Professor, Ribeirão Preto University - UNAERP

Maged Sultan Alhammadi
Jazan University, College of Dentistry, Department of Preventive Sciences, Division of Orthodontics and Dentofacial Orthopedics (Jazan, Saudi Arabia)
Ibb University, Faculty of Oral and Dental Medicine, Department of Orthodontics and Dentofacial Orthopedics (Ibb, Republic of Yemen)

Esam Halboub
Jazan University, College of Dentistry, Department of Maxillofacial Surgery and Diagnostic Sciences (Jazan, Saudi Arabia)

Amr Labib
Cairo University, Faculty of Oral and Dental Medicine, Department of Orthodontics and Dentofacial Orthopedics (Cairo, Egypt)

Mona Salah Fayed
Cairo University, Faculty of Oral and Dental Medicine, Department of Orthodontics and Dentofacial Orthopedics (Cairo, Egypt)
University of Malaya, Faculty of Dentistry, Department of Pediatric Dentistry and Orthodontics (Kuala Lumpur, Malaysia)

restina El-Saaidi
oto University, Graduate School of Medicine, partment of Global Health and Socio-epidemiology yoto, Japan)

ulo Estevão Scanavini
Sc in Orthodontics, UMESP. Professor, Specialization urse in Orthodontics, APCD

enata Pilli Jóias
hD Student, Oral Biopathology, UNESP

Iaria Helena Ferreira Vasconcelos
hD in Orthodontics, FOB/USP. Professor, UMESP

Iarco Antonio Scanavini
hD in Orthodontics, USP. Professor, UMESP

Luiz Renato Paranhos
Post-Doc in Dentistry, UNICAMP. Adjunct Professor, Federal University of Sergipe

Karla Florián-Vargas
Dentist, Private Practice, Trujillo, Peru

Marcos J. Carruitero Honores
Assistant professor, Universidad Privada Antenor Orrego, Trujillo, Peru

Eduardo Bernabé
Senior lecturer, King's College London Dental Institute, Division of Population and Patient Health, London, United Kingdom

Carlos Flores-Mir
Associate professor and Head of the Division of Orthodontics, University of Alberta, Edmonton, Canada

Index

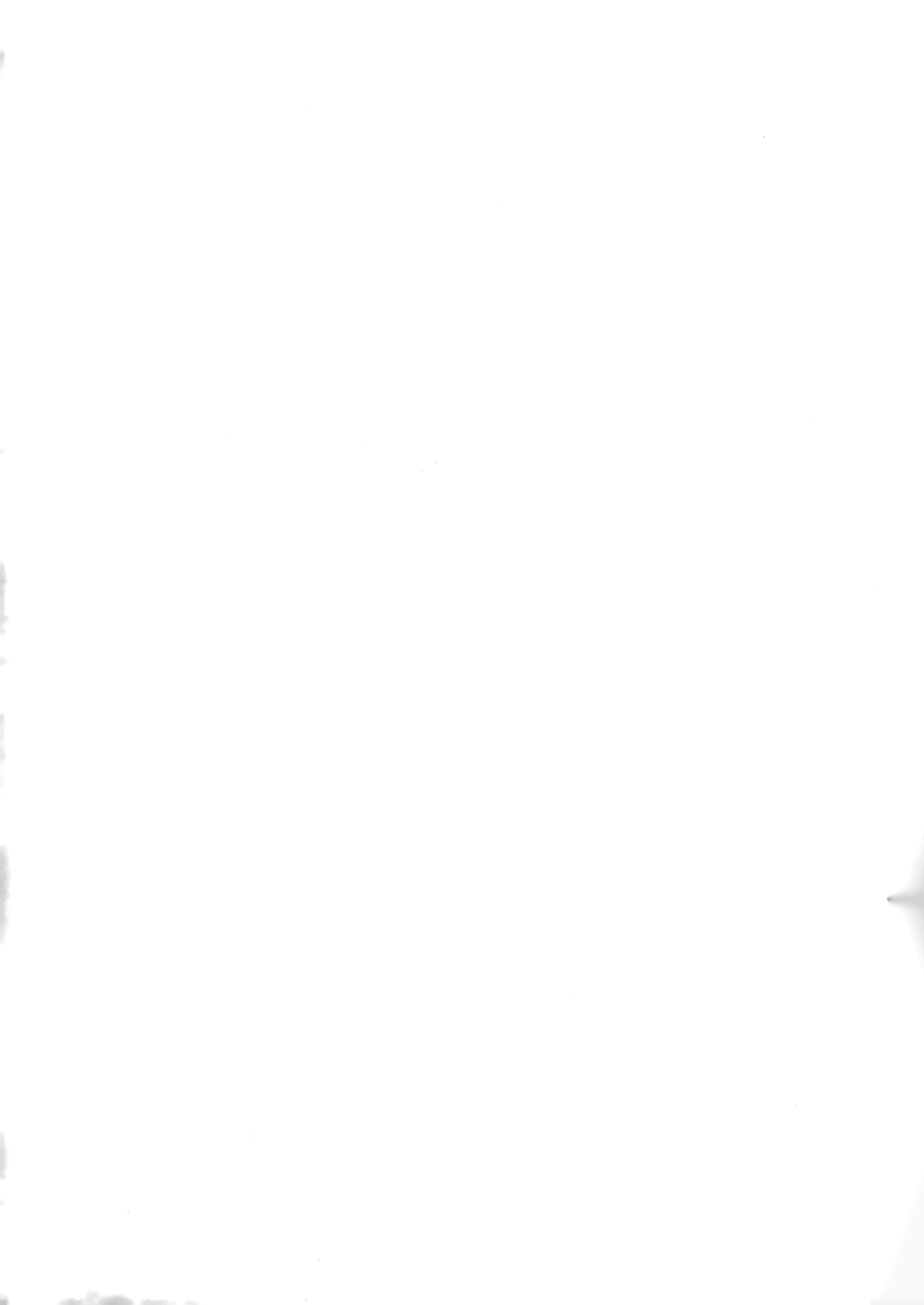